FRENZY IN EARLY MODERN ENGLAND

Today, frenzy is the stuff of newspaper headlines. Five hundred years ago, it described a disease which could kill its sufferers within days. This book offers the first full-length study of frenzy, providing a fresh perspective on early modern understandings of mental illness, mind–body relations, and personhood. Frenzy was frightening not just because it killed its sufferers, but because it changed them beyond recognition. It gave the impression that what was then the most precious part of the person – the soul – was as easy to damage as the body. *Frenzy in Early Modern England* deepens and complicates our sense of what madness meant in this period, both to those who assigned the label, and to those who lived with it. This is an important intervention in the often-fragmented historiography of early modern madness, combining intellectual, social, and cultural history with the history of medicine.

PHILIPPA CARTER is a historian of early modern Britain and Europe, with interests in medicine, natural knowledge, belief, and the body. She is a fellow of Sidney Sussex College, Cambridge, and assistant professor at the Department of History and Philosophy of Science, University of Cambridge.

CAMBRIDGE STUDIES IN EARLY MODERN BRITISH HISTORY

SERIES EDITORS

This is a series of monographs and studies covering many aspects of the history of the British Isles between the late fifteenth century and the early eighteenth century. It includes the work of established scholars and pioneering work by a new generation of scholars. It includes both reviews and revisions of major topics and books which open up new historical terrain or which reveal startling new perspectives on familiar subjects. All the volumes set detailed research within broader perspectives, and the books are intended for the use of students as well as of their teachers.

For a list of titles in the series go to
www.cambridge.org/earlymodernbritishhistory

FRENZY IN EARLY MODERN ENGLAND

Madness, Brain Disease and the Soul

PHILIPPA CARTER

University of Cambridge

CAMBRIDGE
UNIVERSITY PRESS

CAMBRIDGE
UNIVERSITY PRESS

Shaftesbury Road, Cambridge CB2 8EA, United Kingdom

One Liberty Plaza, 20th Floor, New York, NY 10006, USA

477 Williamstown Road, Port Melbourne, VIC 3207, Australia

314–321, 3rd Floor, Plot 3, Splendor Forum, Jasola District Centre, New Delhi – 110025, India

Cambridge University Press is part of Cambridge University Press & Assessment, a department of the University of Cambridge.

We share the University's mission to contribute to society through the pursuit of education, learning and research at the highest international levels of excellence.

www.cambridge.org
Information on this title: www.cambridge.org/9781009703710

DOI: 10.1017/9781009703697

When citing this work, please include a reference to the DOI 10.1017/9781009703697

First published 2026

Cover image: Rembrandt, Philosopher in Meditation, 1632
© GrandPalaisRmn (Musée du Louvre) / Tony Querrec

A catalogue record for this publication is available from the British Library

Library of Congress Cataloging-in-Publication Data
NAMES: Carter, Philippa author
TITLE: Frenzy in early modern England : madness, brain disease and the soul / Philippa Carter, University of Cambridge.
DESCRIPTION: Cambridge, United Kingdom ; New York, NY : Cambridge University Press, 2026. | Series: Cambridge studies in early modern British history | Includes bibliographical references and index.
IDENTIFIERS: LCCN 2026001782 (print) | LCCN 2026001783 (ebook) | ISBN 9781009703710 hardback | ISBN 9781009703673 paperback | ISBN 9781009703697 epub
SUBJECTS: LCSH: Mental illness–Great Britain–History–16th century | Mental illness–Great Britain–History–17th century | Mental illness–Great Britain–History–18th century | Mental illness–Great Britain–Religious aspects
CLASSIFICATION: LCC RC450.G7 C37 2026 (print) | LCC RC450.G7 (ebook)
LC record available at https://lccn.loc.gov/2026001782
LC ebook record available at https://lccn.loc.gov/2026001783

ISBN 978-1-009-70371-0 Hardback
ISBN 978-1-009-70367-3 Paperback

For my parents

Contents

Acknowledgements

I am grateful to Rosanna Barraclough, Liz Friend-Smith, and Lucy Rhymer at Cambridge University Press; to the Series Editors; and to the three anonymous readers who read the manuscript with generosity and care.

For reading and commenting on drafts of the manuscript, I owe thanks to Thomas Banbury, Beatrice Bottomley, Sara Caputo, Alison Carter, Maxime Guttin, Marie Van Haaster, Timo Houtekamer, Yijie Huang, Mika Hyman, Lauren Kassell, Sandra Liwanowska, Dániel Margóscy, Jakub Ochociński, Silvia De Renzi, Mónica Morado Vázquez, Sonia Wigh, and Ewa Zakrzewska. I am especially grateful to Maxime and Lauren for giving me the opportunity to workshop the book with the members of the European University Institute History of Science working group.

Alexandra Walsham, Lauren Kassell, and Mark Jenner have mentored me for almost a decade with no compensation other than my undying thanks. For kindness, wisdom, and encouragement, I am grateful to Cat Beck, Mary Brazelton, Lewis Bremner, Montserrat Cabré, Sara Caputo, Rosanna Dent, Róisín Donohoe, Mari Eyice, Mary Fissell, Marta Halina, Katharine Hodgkin, Peter Murray Jones, Sachiko Kusukawa, Elaine Leong, Sophie Mann, Charmian Mansell, Dániel Margóscy, Riikka Miettinen, Jonah Miller, Lea T. Olsan, Miri Rubin, Karin Sennefelt, Charu Singh, Grace Whorrall-Campbell, and Sonia Wigh. My friends and colleagues at Sidney Sussex College have been unfailingly supportive; special thanks to Eugenio Biagini, Tania Demetriou, Bernhard Fulda, Gary Gerstle, Emma Gilby, Brett Gray, Ruth Jackson-Ravenscroft, Tom Lambert, Rosamond McKitterick, Deirdre Serjeantson, Edward Wilson-Lee, and Clive Wilson (in memoriam).

For taking an interest in this project in its very early days, I would like to thank Peter Biller, Boyd Brogan, Leif Dixon, Ian Forrest, Adam Fox, Steven Gunn, Mark Jenner, Maaike van der Lugt, Richard Oosterhoff,

Richard Sowerby, Chiara Thumiger, Michael Walkden, and Tom Webster. I am indebted to Steven Gunn for generously sharing some of the preliminary data from his project 'Everyday Life and Fatal Hazard in Sixteenth-Century England' (co-led by Tomasz Gromelski).

I am grateful to all the librarians and archivists who have shared their expertise with me, and especially to Chris Barker, Sean Cunningham, Paul Dryburgh, James Freeman, Felix Lancashire, Patricia McGuire, Euan Rogers, Nicholas Rogers, and Sue Sampson. I could not have asked for better palaeography tutors than Gary Brannan, Linne Mooney, Marigold Norbye, Chris Stamatakis, and Andrew Zurcher. For teaching me to read Richard Napier's awful handwriting, thanks to Joanne Edge, Lauren Kassell, Robert Ralley, and John Young (in memoriam).

Special thanks to Kirstine Lines and Erin Norwood-Grundy.

Introduction

A Disease of the Person

On 7 November 1681, the English preacher Oliver Heywood was called to the house of a young man named Joshua Bates, who had fallen into 'a kind of a phrenzy'. After a fortnight, the disease 'grew to a perfect distraction', so that

> 4 men had much adoe to hold him, he was bound, raved, raged, in a formidable manner, made rimes, yea (which was sad) Satan used his tongue to swear many dreadful oaths, which he never did in all his life: he was much prayd for . . . that evening he grew quieter, had a quiet night – in the morning I went to see him, he was a sad object, put him into the hands of god by prayer, that evening at 10 o'clock he dyed, buryed Dec 24 81.[1]

At this point Heywood had been a minister for thirty-one years; he had buried many friends and neighbours in that time. But when he came to write up his spiritual observations on this episode, he faltered. This 'precious young man was profiting beyond his fellows in religion, many sober Christians did much admire the grace of god in him', he lamented.[2] To see a 'godly young man' cut off in his prime was always a cause for sorrow. Yet what seems to have pained Heywood the most was not the memory of Joshua's death, but of his last days alive.[3] 'Oh my Lord', he begged, 'what shall I say to these things? . . . Doth our Lord give them grace and then deprive them of the use of Reason? doth god sanctify their hearts and then leave them to the black humours of their bodys? . . . what glory can god have from frantick persons that have not the use of reason?'[4]

These questions belong to a specific person, time, place, and faith community – namely, to one late seventeenth-century English Protestant

[1] Oliver Heywood, 'Objects and Observations', in Joseph Horsfall Turner (ed.), *The Rev. Oliver Heywood, B.A., 1630–1702: His Autobiography, Diaries, Anecdote and Event Books*, 4 vols. (Bingley: T. Harrison, 1882), vol. 4, p. 31.

[2] Ibid., p. 34. [3] Ibid., p. 31. [4] Ibid., p. 33.

non-conformist minister. Yet they also speak to a more perennial human experience: the experience of losing a person – or of losing parts of a person which once seemed inalienable. In a 2021 tribute to his former mentor Jonathan Steinberg (1934–2021), the historian Christopher Clark wrote

> In the very last years of his life, Jonathan was engulfed by Alzheimer's disease. It was like watching someone shrink and get lost inside himself. He was still pondering enigmas: 'Something has happened to me. But I can't work out what it is. But something fundamental has changed'. I spent a day with him last September and we watched together a video of a wonderful lecture he had given about Bismarck at the University of Pennsylvania some years before. He was gripped by it. And when it was finished, he said: 'That man, Jonathan Steinberg, doesn't exist any more'.[5]

It is safe to say that early modern people saw fewer cases of age-related dementia than are seen worldwide today. What they *are* likely to have witnessed – and far more often – were the dramatic changes to demeanour, speech, and behaviour which accompanied the late stages of febrile illness. Frenzy – by its early modern definition both an 'inflammation of the brain' and a 'continual madness' – was one such illness. It gave the impression that what, for many, were the most precious and integral parts of the person – the 'reason', the 'understanding', and the 'will' – were as easy to destroy as the body. Frenzy troubled early modern people because it forced them to confront the seeming fragility of personhood. Offering a case study of a now-obsolete brain disease, this book explores what was at stake for those who were faced with the diagnosis. Its aim is to deepen and complicate our sense of what 'madness' meant in this period, both to the diagnosticians – the doctors, divines, polemicists, and jurors – and to all those who lived with the label.

Madness and Personhood

In recent years, it is historians of ancient medicine who have led the way in the study of diseases of mind. Chiara Thumiger and Peter Singer, among others, have tracked the shifting categorizations of mental illness in the writings of ancient and late antique medical theorists, ranging from the earliest Hippocratic authors (fifth century BCE) to the Byzantine

[5] Christopher Clark, 'Professor Jonathan Steinberg 1934–2021, in Memoriam'. Cambridge Faculty of History website (8 March 2021), www.hist.cam.ac.uk/news/professor-jonathan-steinberg-1934-2021-memoriam.

encyclopaedists (sixth century CE).[6] Most recently, Thumiger has turned her attention to the centuries-long history of *phrenitis*, the ancient disease category which gave rise to early modern frenzy.[7] Prior to this masterly overview, it was possible to count the scholarly works on *phrenitis* on one hand: a short but illuminating essay by Akio Sakai (1991), followed in 1992 by Danielle Jacquart's study of the disease's afterlife in the 'golden age' of Arabo-Islamic medicine, and in 2013 by Glenda McDonald's article on its treatment in the writings of the imperial physician Galen of Pergamon (129–216 CE).[8] This book builds on the work of these historians of medicine, showing the extent to which the early modern diagnosis at its centre was built on the foundations of ancient and medieval *phrenitis*. But the medical history of frenzy is only a part of the story told by this book, and even this part is not a simple picture of continuity. Many variants of the disease category came into currency in early modern England, a process which was accelerated by the quickening vernacularization of learned medicine. Some of these incarnations of frenzy resembled ancient *phrenitis* very closely; others did not.

In that respect, this book aligns more closely with the cultural history of madness than with the intellectual histories of medicine mentioned above. It would be misleading to set up a hard-and-fast dichotomy between these fields; few cultural historians of madness have underestimated the importance of the ancient medical tradition, and most historians of that tradition working today know better than to ignore its cultural context. What *is* fair to say is that the cultural historians of madness have tended to treat the diagnostic categories of learned medicine as one type of discursive construction among many. This approach characterizes many landmark works in the field – Michael MacDonald's *Mystical Bedlam: Madness, Anxiety and Healing in Seventeenth-Century England* (1981), William F. Bynum, Roy Porter, and Michael Shepherd's three-volume edited collection *The Anatomy of Madness* (1985–1988), Michael W. Dols's *Majnūn: The*

[6] Chiara Thumiger, *A History of the Mind and Mental Health in Classical Greek Medical Thought* (Cambridge: Cambridge University Press, 2017); Chiara Thumiger and Peter N. Singer (eds.), *Mental Illness in Ancient Medicine: From Celsus to Paul of Aegina* (Leiden: Brill, 2018).

[7] Chiara Thumiger, *Phrenitis and the Pathology of the Mind in Western Medical Thought, Fifth Century BCE to Twentieth Century CE* (Cambridge: Cambridge University Press, 2023).

[8] Akio Sakai, 'Phrenitis: Inflammation of the Mind and Body', *History of Psychiatry* 2(6) (1991), 193–205; Danielle Jacquart, 'Les Avatars de la phrénitis chez Avicenne et Rhazès', in Danielle Gourevitch (ed.), *Maladie et Maladies: Histoire et Conceptualisation. Mélanges en l'honneur de Mirko Grmek* (Geneva: Librairie Droz, 1992), pp. 181–192; Glenda C. McDonald, 'Galen on Mental Illness: A Physiological Approach to Phrenitis', *Bulletin of the Institute of Classical Studies. Supplement* 114 (2014), 135–151.

Madman in Medieval Islamic Society (1992), and H. C. Erik Midelfort's *A History of Madness in Sixteenth-Century Germany* (1999).[9] In seeking to give equal weight to medical, legal, religious and broader socio-cultural understandings of madness, I follow in these authors' footsteps.

What is striking about this potted bibliography are its dates of publication. It is a curious fact that, in the first two decades of the twenty-first century – a moment which has seen the zenith of the history of the self, the emotions, and the senses – interest in the history of madness has ebbed.[10] And perhaps this is not a coincidence. Early work in the history of emotions – eager to refute Norbert Elias's vision of a premodern society governed by the volatile explosions of the *id* – responded by stridently reasserting the rationality of premodern emotion. Emotional expression, these historians insisted, was necessarily orderly; it had to correspond with collectively intelligible 'codes' or 'scripts' in order to be read.[11] Pointing to the propositional content and social usefulness of emotion, they resisted not only the condescension of a purportedly 'rational' posterity, but also a long tradition of 'retrospective diagnosis', an approach which re-emerged in the 1970s as 'psychohistory'.[12] Although today this approach is generally condemned by academic historians, it lives on in the collective consciousness as an urge to armchair-psychologize famous historical figures. If the merest mention of 'mental illness' has been enough to send self-respecting early modernists running for the hills, it is easy to see why.

[9] Michael MacDonald, *Mystical Bedlam: Madness, Anxiety and Healing in Seventeenth-Century England* (Cambridge: Cambridge University Press, 1981); William F. Bynum, Roy Porter, and Michael Shepherd (eds.), *The Anatomy of Madness: Essays in the History of Psychiatry*, 3 vols. (London: Tavistock, 1985–1988); Michael W. Dols, *Majnūn: The Madman in Medieval Islamic Society* (Oxford: Oxford University Press, 1992); H. C. Erik Midelfort, *A History of Madness in Sixteenth-Century Germany* (Stanford, CA: Stanford University Press, 1999).

[10] There are notable exceptions: see, e.g., Katharine Hodgkin, *Madness in Seventeenth-Century Autobiography* (Basingstoke: Palgrave Macmillan, 2007); Elena Carrera, 'Madness and Melancholy in Sixteenth- and Seventeenth-Century Spain: New Evidence, New Approaches', *Bulletin of Spanish Studies* 87(8) (2010), 1–15; Elizabeth Mellyn, *Mad Tuscans and Their Families: A History of Mental Disorder in Early Modern Italy* (Philadelphia: University of Pennsylvania Press, 2014). In the last five years, a new generation of historians has begun to approach madness via disability studies; see, e.g., Catherine Beck, 'Patronage and Insanity: Tolerance, Reputation and Mental Disorder in the British Navy, 1740–1820', *Historical Research* 94(263) (2021), 73–95; Riikka Miettinen, 'Constructing "Mad" Religious Experiences in Early Modern Sweden', in Sari Katajala-Peltomaa and Raisa Maria Toivo (eds.), *Histories of Experience in the World of Lived Religion* (London: Palgrave Macmillan, 2022), pp. 163–194.

[11] Barbara Rosenwein (ed.), *Anger's Past: The Social Uses of an Emotion* (Ithaca, NY: Cornell University Press, 1998), pp. 2–3, 238–239.

[12] See Geoffrey Barraclough, 'Psychohistory Is Bunk', *The Guardian*, 3 March 1973; Philip Pomper, 'Problems of a Naturalistic Psychohistory', *History and Theory* 12(4) (1973), 367–388; Gerald Izenberg, 'Psychohistory and Intellectual History', *History and Theory* 14(2) (1975), 139–155.

But it is worth reflecting on the limits imposed by this determination to keep unreason at arm's length. The conceptual frameworks championed by historians of emotion – 'scripts', 'communities', 'practices' – have been enormously productive, but they prove less useful in helping us to understand instances where members of the same 'emotional community' responded to an individual's displays of affect with bafflement, incomprehension, concern, or outright fear – moments, in short, in which the act of communication seems to have gone badly wrong.[13] In their scrupulous refusal to pathologize emotional displays (even those read as 'madness' by contemporaries), historians have ended up limiting their analytic categories to 'disturbance' or 'distress'.[14] This approach certainly avoids pathologizing, but not necessarily reduction. For we cannot expect 'distress' to do justice to the full spectrum of experience described by those who were diagnosed as 'mad' in early modern England. Some of the 'frantic' individuals we will encounter in this book described feelings of rapturous delight, righteous anger, pride, ambition, or resignation. It seems safe to assume that the feelings of the 'mad' were as wide-ranging, complex, and fluctuating as those of the 'sane'. The difference was that their expressions of those feelings were read by observers as fundamentally inappropriate to the circumstances.

However we account for historians' wariness towards madness, the feeling has never been shared by literary scholars. This book engages with the vibrant body of scholarship on 'renaissance madness' which has sprung up over the last twenty years, including Carol T. Neely's *Distracted Subjects* (2004) and Helen Hackett's *The Elizabethan Mind* (2022).[15] Studies on melancholy have included Angus Gowland's *Worlds of Renaissance Melancholy* (2006), Jeremy Schmidt's *Melancholy and the Care of the Soul* (2007), and Mary Ann Lund's *Melancholy, Medicine and Religion in Early Modern England* (2010).[16] These are primarily studies of key works of

[13] Barbara Rosenwein, *Emotional Communities in the Early Middle Ages* (Ithaca, NY: Cornell University Press, 2007); Barbara Rosenwein et al., '*AHR* Conversation: The Historical Study of the Emotions', *American Historical Review* 117(5) (2012), 1516.

[14] Jonathan Willis, '"Strange Letters to the Queen": Mental and Emotional Distress in the Elizabethan State Papers', Tudor and Stuart History Seminar, London (29 April 2023); Jonathan Willis, '"Strange Enthusiastical Exhortations": Distress, Religious Identity, and the English Reformation', *Journal of Ecclesiastical History* 76(4) (2025), 760–789. I too have struggled to analyse these difficult texts.

[15] Carol T. Neely, *Distracted Subjects: Madness and Gender in Shakespeare and Early Modern Culture* (Ithaca, NY: Cornell University Press, 2004); Helen Hackett, *The Elizabethan Mind: Searching for the Self in an Age of Uncertainty* (New Haven, CT: Yale University Press, 2022).

[16] Angus Gowland, *The Worlds of Renaissance Melancholy: Robert Burton in Context* (Cambridge: Cambridge University Press, 2006); Jeremy Schmidt, *Melancholy and the Care of the Soul: Religion,*

English literature, and as such, certain figures tend to steal the limelight; chief among them, the Oxford divine and anatomist of melancholy Robert Burton (1577–1640) and the poet and playwright William Shakespeare (1564–1616). While acknowledging the enormous influence of these authors on perceptions of madness in early modern England, this book takes a different approach. While Burton and Shakespeare do make the occasional cameo (alongside other well-studied figures like Francis Bacon, Thomas Willis, and Henry More), most of the historical personalities who appear in this book left a much sparser paper trail. Among their number was the charwoman Alice Scot, who was struck by frenzy in the summer of 1597, and the housewife Margery Sagar, who in 1641 petitioned the Lancashire Quarter Sessions for help with her frantic husband. Setting glimpses of ordinary people's lives alongside works of medicine, natural philosophy, law, and theology, this book offers a history of frenzy in the round. It lends a fresh historical perspective to an ongoing interdisciplinary conversation about the meanings of early modern madness.

This book also speaks to related scholarly debates on early modern personhood (here loosely embracing 'selfhood', 'identity', 'subjectivity', and 'intersubjectivity').[17] I cannot hope to offer an adequate sketch of this vast and wide-ranging field here. Suffice to say that – over the course of the last century – scholars have done a very thorough job of shredding the birth certificate of Jakob Burckhardt's 'renaissance individual'.[18] In this book, I focus instead on a more recent claim about the historicity of selfhood. In *Being Brains: Making the Cerebral Subject* (2017), Fernando Vidal and Francisco Ortega argue that the identification of the self with the brain (or 'brainhood') is a modern phenomenon.[19] It was only in the post-Enlightenment West, Vidal and Ortega argue, that '*intellect*' came to stand

Moral Philosophy and Madness in Early Modern England (Aldershot: Ashgate, 2007); Mary Ann Lund, *Melancholy, Medicine and Religion in Early Modern England* (Cambridge: Cambridge University Press, 2010).

[17] For just a few recent contributions, see Nandini Dos (ed.), *Lives in Transit in Early Modern England: Identity and Belonging* (Amsterdam: Amsterdam University Press, 2022); James Simpson, 'Unwritten Virtues, Selves, and Texts: Early Modern Self-Erasure', *Journal of Medieval and Early Modern Studies* 52(3) (2022), 415–443; Neil Howard Keeble, '"Self-Confidence and Self-Conceit Render Men Fools": Seventeenth-Century "Self-" Compounds, Puritan Discourse and Early Modern Subjectivity', *Renaissance Studies* 37(3) (2023), 345–363.

[18] For an old but still useful overview, see John Martin, 'Inventing Sincerity, Refashioning Prudence: The Discovery of the Individual in Renaissance Europe', *American Historical Review* 102(5) (1997), 1309–1342.

[19] Fernando Vidal and Francisco Ortega, *Being Brains: Making the Cerebral Subject* (New York: Fordham University Press, 2017), p. 34.

> for a complex of psychological features, such as memory, consciousness, and self-awareness, whose possession defines both our individual personal identity and human personhood in general . . . But the *historical* point is that personhood was *not* always reduced to those psychological features and that therefore, as long as personhood was *not* thus redescribed, it could *not* be conceived of in terms of brainhood.[20]

The birth of this 'cerebral self' could be dated back to the late seventeenth century, and, even more precisely, to 1694 – the year of publication of the second edition of John Locke's *An Essay Concerning Humane Understanding.*[21] Thereafter, 'being an *I* or having a self was equated with memory, consciousness, and self-awareness. This is the "modern" self'.[22] Vidal and Ortega are not the only historians to tell this sort of story.[23] The aim of this book is not to play 'earlier than thou' with these scholars, or to insist that Locke's philosophy was less radical than it is sometimes made out to be. Instead, this is a history of understandings of personhood – encompassing 'mind', 'soul', 'brain', and 'body' – which neither began nor ended with Locke.[24]

Approaching Frenzy

Anyone who decides to study early modern madness is soon confronted by a problem which most historians will face sooner or later. The only methodologies which can justifiably be applied to the evidence at our disposal are discursive: we 'read' texts, images, and other material remains, and we try to recover their meanings. Any attempt to go 'beyond discourse' is necessarily speculative, and usually ends up resting on notions drawn, variously, from the natural, human, or social sciences, psychoanalysis, or the historian's gut.[25] The attempt to draw any firm conclusions about non- or pre-discursive elements of human societies from their discursive traces often looks – in retrospect – like a fool's errand. And the labelling of people who died hundreds of years ago with diagnoses found in the pages

20 Ibid., p. 25. 21 Ibid., pp. 25–26, 32–33. 22 Ibid., p. 25.

23 See, e.g., Roy Porter, *Flesh in the Age of Reason: How the Enlightenment Transformed the Way We See Our Bodies and Souls* (London: Penguin, 2003), ch. 6; Richard Sugg, *The Smoke of the Soul: Medicine, Physiology and Religion in Early Modern England* (London: Springer, 2013), ch. 9.

24 I have not seriously excluded Locke on point of principle; he just happened not to write about frenzy – or at least, not in his own name. In his days as a medical student, he probably authored or co-authored a few medical treatises which were later attributed to his mentor Thomas Sydenham. It is also thanks to Locke's diligent note-taking that we have transcripts of Thomas Willis's Oxford lectures.

25 Lyndal Roper, 'Beyond Discourse Theory', *Women's History Review* 19(2) (2010), 316–317.

of the American Psychiatric Association's *Diagnostic and Statistical Manual* (first ed. 1952) is a prime example.

Yet the social constructionist approach – in which madness is taken to lie in the eye of the historical beholder – also has its limits. While writing this book, I found that it offered little interpretive purchase on situations in which the onset of frenzy seems to have gone directly *against* the grain of all parties' attempts at meaning-making. In 1547, for example, when the English reformer John Bale received the news that his collaborator John Leland was 'in suche a frenesy at thys present, that lytle hope I haue of hys recouer[y]', he found himself at a loss.[26] Leland was supposed to have been the divinely appointed chronicler of the English Reformation. Two years later, Bale wrote dejectedly that 'Englande had yet neuer a greater losse. But what shall we saye? It hath pleased god that he shuld thus be depryued of hys wyttes, the lord knoweth best what he hath to do'.[27] Like Heywood, Bale did his best to work the plot twist into God's grand design, but it took time and effort. Frenzy *was* socially constructed – this is surely true of anything human beings have ever given a name. But sometimes its diagnosis was anything but strategic.

It is at this juncture that my approach departs somewhat from earlier cultural histories of madness.[28] Early on in this book's gestation, I tried to describe its subject matter to a woman who had spent most of her career working for various non-governmental organizations in the Global South. What interested me about frenzy, I explained, was that it was seen by early moderns *both* as a form of mental illness *and* as a brain disease, something akin to meningitis or encephalitis. Giving me a measured look, she replied that infections of the central nervous system were still common in the areas in which she had worked, and that she had seen their effects when untreated. Her comment has stayed with me. It was a reminder that, without rapid medical intervention, brain infection *did* – and *does* – produce frightening changes in speech, mood, and behaviour. It was a reminder that non-human agents – viruses, bacteria, parasites – can change human history of their own accord, quite heedless of the names they have been given. Acknowledging these facts does not lead me to embrace

[26] John Bale, *The laboryouse iourney [and] serche of Iohan Leylande, for Englandes antiquitees geuen of hym as a newe yeares gyfte to Kynge Henry the viij. in the. xxxvij. yeare of his reygne, with declaracyons enlarged* (London, 1549), sig. B3v.

[27] Ibid., sigs. B5r–v.

[28] See, e.g., Michael MacDonald, 'Insanity and the Realities of History in Early Modern England', *Psychological Medicine* 11(1) (1981), 11–25; Alexandra Walsham, '"Frantick Hacket": Prophecy, Sorcery, Insanity, and the Elizabethan Puritan Movement', *The Historical Journal* 41(1) (1998), 27–66.

retrospective diagnosis. I will never know how many of those once labelled as 'frantic' were suffering from brain infections; the central nervous systems in question are long gone. But there is no question that early modern England was hard-hit by infectious diseases – by deadly 'agues', 'sweats', and 'fevers'.[29] In the back of my mind, then, has been the notion that frenzy was *real*. That is, it took its shape not only from anecdotes and abstractions, but also from a specific constellation of signs observed in its sufferers: primarily, fever and mental alienation.

Likewise, where early modern authors describe the precise parts of the brain which were affected in cases of frenzy – usually the meninges – I have taken them at their word. Perhaps their descriptions were inaccurate by the standards of present-day biomedicine; this is not the point. After all, if pathogens were indeed at work, we cannot hope to know which ones, or the specific patterns of damage which they caused. What is clear is that a correlation was observed between the diseased appearance of the brain at post-mortem, on the one hand, and the patient's disturbed speech and behaviour before death, on the other. Although it does not have much palpable impact on the claims made in this book, I do not believe that these long-dead individuals' observations are explicable by recourse to discourse analysis alone.

Knowledge

Who were these observers? To claim 'understandings of frenzy' as the subject of this book begs the question: whose understandings? Thus far I have quoted John Bale (1495–1563) and Oliver Heywood (1630–1702), two well-read, university-educated men. But we should not assume that they held a monopoly on knowledge of this kind. On 21 May 1551, for example, the chief justice of Frankfurt, investigating whether or not a local housewife had died at the hands of her husband, asked a witness whether 'the fatal illness *phrenesie* first began on the seventh day after the beating' and 'whether the cranium and the *dura* and *pia mater* had been damaged by the bruising'. The witness was another housewife, Katharina Hansenn, and she replied with apparent confidence in her own assessment.[30]

[29] Mary Dobson, *Contours of Death and Disease in Early Modern England* (Cambridge: Cambridge University Press, 1997), pp. 287–367.

[30] Translation by J. Andrew Mendelsohn and Annemarie Kinzelbach, in 'Common Knowledge: Bodies, Evidence, and Expertise in Early Modern Germany', *Isis* 108(2) (2017), 261, 272.

J. Andrew Mendelsohn and Annemarie Kinzelbach have taken the proceedings from this trial as evidence that, in premodern Europe, the pool of 'common knowledge' was larger and more accessible than has often been supposed.[31] It is true that we should not underestimate the extent of oral and experiential knowledge among the illiterate. It does not seem implausible that Hansenn possessed the knowledge she claimed – if she had not seen many learned anatomical textbooks, she had probably seen more cracked skulls and calf brains than most of us today.

Unfortunately, I have found no equivalent Rosetta stone for early modern England. The words 'frenzy' and 'frantic' were in widespread circulation among the unlettered majority, but what their users meant by them is much harder to pin down. In 1985, Roy Porter called on historians of medicine to recapture 'the patient's view', filling in 'sufferers' characterizations and classifications of illnesses'. 'It is odd', he concluded, 'how deaf we have been to lay nosologies'.[32] Unfortunately, recovering 'lay nosologies' is easier said than done. It is much more common to find laypersons using the word 'frenzy' than spelling out exactly what they meant by it. This, of course, reflects the fact that most of them were not writing things down at all; this was predominantly a culture of oral knowledge. In the absence of evidence, common knowledge can be neither assumed nor ruled out.

The first half of this book focuses primarily on frenzy as it appears in learned, specialist traditions of knowledge: medicine, anatomy, and divinity. In the second half, however, I broaden my analytical scope, placing 'frenzy' alongside demotic equivalents like the 'wode ague'. Bracketing these terms together risks artificially superimposing specialist medical diagnoses onto non-specialist ones, but – to my mind – this is a better approach than remaining wilfully deaf to 'lay nosologies'. As will become clear, laypersons tended to take a pragmatic approach to identifying madness; it was not at all uncommon for them to hedge their bets by stating that the individual in question was suffering from a 'Lunacye or Frensye'.[33] This open-ended approach should not surprise us. The makers of these legal and administrative records were not concerned with producing accurate medical diagnoses; their goal was to make appropriate arrangements for the sick and the dead.

31 Ibid., pp. 259–261.

32 Roy Porter, 'The Patient's View: Doing Medical History from Below', *Theory and Society* 14 (1985), 175–198.

33 Kew, TNA, SP 12/194, f. 87r.

Limits

The local contexts in which these manuscripts were produced bring us to another set of remits defining this book: its focus on England from 1500 to 1700. *Phrenitis* was embedded in every early modern culture which had ever been influenced by the ancient Greek medical tradition. It was invoked by speakers and readers of Arabic, Latin, Greek, and the European vernaculars, as both a literal diagnosis and a trope. If I have decided to concentrate on one polity and one territory, my aim has been to keep focus and to avoid unwarranted generalization. Yet, while most of the authors studied here are English, their ideas were usually contributions to international conversations. I have tried to situate them in these contexts, and to pay attention to their far-flung interlocutors. The focus on England is intended to serve as a relatively stable vantage-point on frenzy, not as a containment zone.

For the sake of manageability, this book focuses not just on one period and one place, but also on one disease. There were three main categories of 'madness' in Europe's mainstream medical tradition: melancholy, mania, and frenzy. Of the three, melancholy has garnered by far the most attention as a subject of historical study. From Erwin Panofsky, Raymond Klibansky and Fritz Saxl's classic *Saturn and Melancholy* (1964) down to the work of Lund, Schmidt, and Gowland, melancholy seems to hold a singular attraction for scholars – related, perhaps, to its reputation as the quintessential scholar's disease.[34] Even in classic studies of early modern 'madness', such as those of Roy Porter and Michael MacDonald, mania and melancholy tend to be treated as a pair, while frenzy is set uneasily to one side.[35]

In fact, early modern authors also seem to have found melancholy both more interesting and more palatable a topic of discussion than its sibling diseases. Languishing in his Florentine palazzo, the self-diagnosed melancholic Marsilio Ficino (1433–1499) worked hard to glamorize his affliction. The result was a fusion of Plato's hymn to divine *mania* – a state of ecstatic inspiration reached only by poets and seers – with the

[34] Raymond Klibansky, Erwin Panofsky, and Fritz Saxl, *Saturn and Melancholy: Studies in the History of Natural Philosophy, Religion and Art* (London: Nelson, 1964); Gowland, *Renaissance Melancholy*; Schmidt, *Melancholy and the Care of the Soul*; Lund, *Melancholy, Medicine, and Religion*.

[35] Roy Porter, 'Madness and Its Institutions', in Andrew Wear (ed.), *Medicine in Society: Historical Essays* (Cambridge: Cambridge University Press, 1992), pp. 278–279; MacDonald, *Mystical Bedlam*, pp. 118–132, 146.

peripatetic view that 'all those men who have become extraordinary in philosophy, politics, poetry, or the arts are obviously melancholic'.[36] Both melancholy and mania were legible as signs of intellectual and spiritual distinction. Frenzy, on the other hand, was hot, sweaty, and often fatal. It was not the sort of thorn in the flesh which the tortured geniuses of Renaissance Europe were looking for. Nor does it map particularly well onto present-day understandings of mental illness. Yet it is precisely this awkwardness – for early moderns and for us – which makes the disease so illuminating. It merits a study in its own right.

On closer inspection, even the boundaries which early modern medical theorists drew between frenzy, mania, and melancholy prove surprisingly blurry. This will be discussed in more detail in Chapter 1, but it is worth briefly outlining the point here. According to Galen, black bile came in two kinds: natural and unnatural (in his terms, *preternatural*). This second kind of black bile was actually the burnt remains of another humour – usually yellow bile – and it produced extreme symptoms, ranging from violent attacks to prophetic visions.[37] Yet the disease which Galen was describing here was not melancholy, but *phrenitis*. Although Galen's medieval commentators developed sub-categories such as 'bestial melancholy' to preserve the distinctions between the classic triad of diseases, there was still plenty of occasion for confusion and conflation.[38] Where I have separated out frenzy from other forms of madness, I have sought to echo the analytic approach of the source at hand. Throughout the book, I have tried to be sensitive to conceptual fluidity as well as precision.

[36] Marsilio Ficino, *De vita libri tres* (Lyon, 1560); Aristotle (attrib.), 'Problem XXX.1', in Robert Mayhew and David C. Mirhady (trans.), *Problems, Volume II: Books 20–38*, LCL 317 (Cambridge, MA: Harvard University Press, 2011), quotation at pp. 276–277. See Winfried Schleiner, *Melancholy, Genius and Utopia in the Renaissance* (Wiesbaden: Harrassowitz, 1991); Noel Brann, *The Debate Over the Origin of Genius during the Italian Renaissance* (Leiden: Brill, 2002), pp. 82–83. I have usually found Plato's divine *mania* rendered as *furor* by early modern Latinists, and very rarely as *phrenitis*.

[37] Galen, 'De locis affectis', in Karl Gottlob Kühn (trans.), *Claudii Galeni Opera Omnia* (Leipzig: Cnobloch, 1821), vol. 8, lib. 3, pp. 177–178; 'De humoribus', in Karl Gottlob Kühn (trans.), *Claudii Galeni Opera Omnia* (Leipzig: Cnobloch, 1821), vol. 19, pp. 490–491. All further Latin translations are from Kühn's edition.

[38] Galen used the term *θηριώδης* (bestial, savage), which Latin translators rendered as *ferinus* (feral). Avicenna distinguished between the *phrenitis ferina* described by Galen (in Arabic *sibare*), 'bestial' mania, and a 'bestial' subspecies of *melancholia* (*lycanthropia*, in Arabic *cutubut*). See Avicenna [Ibn Sīnā], *al-Qānūn fī l-ṭibb*, book 3, part 1, sections 3:6 and 4:16–22, in Giovanni Costeo and Giovanni Paulo Mongio (eds.), *Avicennae Arabum medicorum principis...* [*Canon Medicinae*] (Venice, 1595), pp. 475, 487–488, 493–494. All translations are my own unless otherwise indicated.

Language

One unifying principle of my approach has been an attentiveness to rhetoric, in both the broad and narrow senses of the word. In the narrow sense, one thing which the learned authors who feature in this book had in common was that they had studied classical rhetoric as undergraduates.[39] They were well-versed in the art of persuasion. I have thus taken it as read that they used metaphors, similes, irony, and many other rhetorical techniques with purpose and skill. The invocation of frenzy was sometimes deadly serious; sometimes, it was the stuff of hyperbole. As such, I have sought to listen out for obvious shifts in register (although I have doubtless had my tone-deaf moments).

Attending to rhetoric in its broader sense, I have been influenced by the work of David Harley and Maria Devlin. Writing from a social constructionist perspective, Harley argued that the art of medicine is – and was – fundamentally rhetorical. The act of healing requires a 'plausible practitioner who can deploy a credible system in a successful negotiation that brings order to the patient's experience'.[40] More recently, Devlin has developed a similar approach in her readings of sermons, catechisms, morality plays, and dialogues composed in post-Reformation England. These are forms, she argues, of 'rhetorical theology'. While '[s]ystematic theology treats the logical relations between propositions without positing any particular speaker, audience, or occasion … [r]hetorical theology is always situated between teacher and believer and is governed by its purpose, often to persuade and to console'.[41]

Devlin's heuristic has helped me to keep my texts anchored to their social contexts. Most of the university-based philosophers who appear in this book, for example, were free from the pressing pastoral and didactic concerns of the Protestant ministers who quoted them. At points, I have distinguished between theorization and the strategic uses of theory. As with tonal register, however, I envision this difference on a sliding scale. None of the texts featuring in this book were written entirely without reference to 'speaker, audience, or occasion'. To borrow Harley's

[39] David Harley, 'Medical Metaphors in English Moral Theology, 1560–1660', *Journal of the History of Medicine and Allied Sciences* 48 (1993), 398–399.

[40] David Harley, 'Rhetoric and the Social Construction of Sickness and Healing', *Social History of Medicine* 12(3) (1999), 434.

[41] Maria Devlin, '"If It Were Made for Man, 'Twas Made for Me". Generic Damnation and Rhetorical Salvation in Reformation Preaching and Plays', in Jonathan Willis (ed.), *Sin and Salvation in Reformation England* (Farnham: Ashgate, 2015), p. 174.

formulation, 'knowledge is not merely representational; it is always praxis'.[42]

This is manifest in the fact that many early modern accounts of frenzy were stories, intended for reading or speaking aloud.[43] Physicians narrated the life course of the disease from beginning to end; coroners' juries narrated its terrible effects on the sufferer. In judgement books and martyrologies, God used frenzy to punish reprobates; in sermons, he used it to warn, chastise, and correct his own. Frenzy was a disease with a temporal trajectory of its own, but it was also a template for narratives about personhood: about ensoulment, rationality, identity, freedom, and what it meant to lose them.

Structure

This book consists of six chapters. Chapter 1 offers a case study of frenzy as a medical diagnosis. Beginning in 1500, it shows how the core elements of its profile – its definition, causes, signs, and prognosis – were adapted to fit the new medical philosophies which took hold in England over the course of the seventeenth century. Yet, despite their self-conscious renunciation of tradition, late seventeenth-century medical theorists continued to explain the disease in terms strikingly similar to those used by their predecessors: with reference to the diffusion of an animating principle – carried by a rarefied bodily medium known as 'animal spirit' – throughout the body. They sought to localize that impairment to a specific part of this system (the nerves) and to a specific organ (the brain). This chapter argues that it was the devastating effects of brain disease which galvanized medical theorists to seek to explain disorders of the mind as disruptions of the animal spirits.

Chapter 2 takes this story from the desk of the learned physician to the worktop of the experimental anatomist. Reading the work of the physician and anatomist Thomas Willis (1621–1675) alongside his various sixteenth- and seventeenth-century interlocutors, it situates his anatomical work within a longer tradition of brain cartography. The chapter argues that Willis's determination to map the functions of the brain onto its

42 Harley, 'Rhetoric', p. 414.

43 Here, like many before me, I am following in the footsteps of Natalie Zemon Davis. See Natalie Zemon Davis, *Fiction in the Archives: Pardon Tales and Their Tellers in Sixteenth-Century France* (Stanford, CA: Stanford University Press, 1987); Malcolm Gaskill, 'Reporting Murder: Fiction in the Archives in Early Modern England', *Social History* 23(1) (1998), 1–30; Mark Jackson, 'Fiction in the Archives? Sources for the Social History of Infanticide', *Archives* 27 (2002), 173–185.

structures was driven, in part, by his clinical experiences of frenzy. His explicit hope was that his anatomy would be the foundation stone on which a new, clinically useful 'Pathologie of the Brain and nervous stock, might be built'.[44] But not all of his hopes for the project were medical in nature, or even corporeal. At its commencement, he had been hoping to pinpoint the anatomical seat of the immortal, rational soul. Finding it would shore up two vital truths, both of which frenzy seemed to undermine: first, that there was a categorical difference between the human soul and that of all other living beings, and second, that the human soul alone would survive the death of the body.

Willis was not the only one who started off observing the effects of brain disease and ended up spearheading a campaign to underwrite the scriptural promise of human immortality. Chapter 3 turns from medicine to theology, in order to ask why frenzy tended to inflame this one particular theological sore spot. The default assumption of learned medical theory was that the functionality of the mind depended utterly on the health of the brain. This placed pressure on a Christian cosmology in which the soul had to be able to survive the death of the body. Frenzy forced contemporaries to ask how it was possible for the mind – a possession of that soul – to be impaired by organic disease. Reading a range of texts written by sixteenth- and seventeenth-century religious thinkers, this chapter examines their varied attempts to resolve this nagging problem.

The second part of the book turns to consider how the diagnosis of frenzy changed the lives of those who lived with it. Chapter 4 explores what the loss of the rational faculty known as the 'will' meant in practice. The English common law had its own framework for classifying madness, one which ran parallel to the medical nosologies explored in Chapter 1. This chapter looks at one of the specific legal settings in which these categories were applied: the coroner's inquest. Focusing on the crime of self-murder, it demonstrates the centrality of frenzy to what would later come to be termed the 'insanity defence'. Where suicide was suspected, it argues, a story about frenzy – told right – offered an escape route for suspects and their families.

Chapter 5 explores the ways in which the ideational link between 'reason' and 'rule' was used to justify real-life arrangements: if the 'ruling faculties' of the sufferer's mind were impaired, this merited the placement of that individual under the 'rule' of others. It looks at the tropes and

[44] Thomas Willis, 'The Anatomy of the Brain', in Samuel Pordage (trans.), *The remaining medical works of that famous and renowned physician Dr. Thomas Willis* (London, 1681), p. 53.

images which fuelled this thinking, from the 'great chain of being' to the biblical tale of Nebuchadnezzar. Looking at how householders, parishioners, physicians, mayors, and local magistrates thought about frenzy, it shows how these ideas transformed the spatial, material, and social circumstances of those who received the diagnosis. It considers some of the methods of 'cure' and 'correction' which were applied to sufferers, with the stated aim of restoring them to their right wits. Ultimately, this chapter argues, these promises of restoration rang hollow. Most of these methods had little to do with making sufferers 'rational', and everything to do with keeping them 'ruly'. If the high premium placed on the faculty of the 'reason' served to shore up the rigidly hierarchical order of social relations which obtained in early modern England (encompassing rank, age, gender, and species), frenzy threatened to expose the fragility of that same order.

The final chapter looks at the ways in which frenzy was weaponized during the religious and political upheavals of this era, beginning with the reign of Mary Tudor and ending with the Restoration of Charles II. As a trope, it was useful to polemicists, who knew that questioning their opponents' sanity was more effective than simply refuting their claims. As a literal diagnosis, it was useful to monarchs and statesmen, who had found that it was an excellent way to silence politically inconvenient people without making a show. This chapter shows how it was used to justify the indefinite incarceration of prophets, visionaries, and – eventually – kings. Yet the label had one serious drawback: it gave its recipients the gift of innocence. Frantic persons were incapable of crime, and could be neither convicted nor punished for their actions. If a recipient later became not just inconvenient but too dangerous to live, any previous diagnosis – no matter how spurious – had to be redacted from the record. This was a problem for religious polemicists too: the aim was to pathologize 'heretics', 'papists', 'puritans', and 'sectarians', not to excuse them from all wrongdoing. Eventually, the chapter argues, this flaw drove Anglican polemicists to abandon frenzy for a new diagnosis: 'melancholy enthusiasm'. This chapter thus draws together various thematic strands explored earlier in the book: the immobilizing effect of frenzy on an individual's powers of 'reason' and 'will'; the reversals of 'rule' which this predicament could justify; the exculpatory effect of a diagnosis, and the high cost paid by those who received one.

CHAPTER 1

Making the Diagnosis

Introduction

What *was* frenzy? Writing in the early sixteenth century, the English physician Andrew Boorde (1490–1549) had a fairly straightforward answer: it was an abscess (an 'Apostumacion') arising in the brain or its meninges, which caused an 'alienation of a mans minde and memorie'.[1] But the landscape of medical knowledge was changing in this period, and frenzy was changing with it. This chapter tracks frenzy's trajectory as a diagnosis between 1500 and 1700, drawing on a genre of medical text known as the *practica*. This was the medical student's time-honoured companion: a concise, user-friendly handbook which listed the diseases of the human body from head to toe. Like an encyclopaedia, the typical *practica* followed a predictable order: each disease was assigned its own chapter, and each chapter progressed from definitions to causes, signs, prognosis, and finally cures.[2] This was how early modern medical students would have learnt to diagnose frenzy, and – stepping into their shoes – we will follow the first four steps of their itinerary. We will return to consider cures in Chapter 5.

The text of the *practica* was relatively stable, but not all of its readers read it in the same way. To capture something of this diversity, this chapter

[1] Andrew Boorde, *The breuiarie of health* (London, 1587), f. 92v. What Galen had called 'swellings against nature' (παρὰ φύσιν ὄγκον), English medical writers called 'apostemes' (or sometimes 'tumours'). Here, I have glossed 'aposteme' as 'abscess', on the grounds that some Latinate medical translators treated them as synonyms. See, e.g., Bartholomew Traheron, 'Aposteme … In latyne it is called abscessus', in Traheron (trans.), Giovanni da Vigo, *The most excellent workes of chirurgerye* (London, 1543), sig. Zziir. Quotation from Galen from 'De tumoribus praeter naturam', in Karl Gottlob Kühn (trans.), *Claudii Galeni Opera Omnia*, vol. 7 (Leipzig: Cnobloch, 1821), p. 706.

[2] Faith Wallis (ed.), *Medieval Medicine: A Reader* (Toronto: University of Toronto Press, 2010), pp. 131–136; Ian Maclean, *Logic, Signs and Nature in the Renaissance: The Case of Learned Medicine* (Cambridge: Cambridge University Press, 2002), pp. 56–58, 68–69.

focuses on eight different medical practitioners. They can be grouped into two loose cohorts – the first coming of age in a time of relative stability in English medicine (1560–1640), and the second in a time of rapid change (1640–1700). The first cohort consists of the medical astrologers Simon Forman (1552–1611) and Richard Napier (1559–1634), the self-taught gentlewoman Lady Grace Mildmay (1552–1620), and the academic physician John Hall (c. 1574/75–1635). The second consists of the surgeon Richard Wiseman (1622–1703), the physicians Thomas Sydenham (1624–1689) and Thomas Willis (1621–1675), and the unlicensed practitioner William Salmon (1644–1713).

This is admittedly an eclectic line-up; of these eight practitioners, only four had any kind of medical qualification. But our focus here is on the diagnosis of frenzy, and university-trained physicians were far from being the only ones to make that diagnosis. Considering a wider range of medical practitioners reveals the gaps which could emerge between lay and learned understandings of frenzy. There was plenty of common ground; all eight of these individuals had read at least some of the same books, and most of them would have recognized the ancient Greek physician Hippocrates (460–370 BCE) as the 'father' of their art. Yet the type and extent of medical knowledge to which they had access varied widely, and it was determined – among other factors – by gender, location, wealth, education, and status. As we track change over two centuries, we also need to remain alert to this synchronic diversity. To this end, it is worth taking a moment to sketch out the circumstances in which each of these medical practitioners lived, worked, and wrote.

According to his autobiography, Simon Forman spent his early years starved of the learning he craved.[3] After his father's premature death, his mother took him out of school for several years to work. His local schoolmaster did not take his education seriously enough, and – soon after his admission to Oxford as a poor servitor – it became clear that his gentlemen patrons did not either. Forman left the university the following year, determined to take his learning into his own hands. And the syllabus he devised for himself was nothing if not wide-ranging: by the time he settled in London in 1591, he was styling himself as a magus, alchemist, astrologer, and physician.[4] In 1601, the London College of Physicians

[3] Simon Forman, 'The bocke of the life and generation of Simon', Oxford, Bodleian Library, MS Ashm. 208, ff. 136–142.

[4] Lauren Kassell, *Medicine and Magic in Elizabethan London, Simon Forman: Astrologer, Alchemist and Physician* (Oxford: Clarendon Press, 2005), pp. 19–30.

declared him 'an Intruder into the profession of Physick', among the worst of the 'unlearned and unlawful practitioners, lurking in many corners of the City'.[5] From 1596, Forman became the unlikely mentor of the shy, self-effacing Oxford graduate and Buckinghamshire rector Richard Napier. Napier soon found that he had a greater gift for healing than for preaching, and continued to practise Forman's methods from his rectory in Great Linford for two decades after his teacher's death.[6]

Born into the ranks of the Northamptonshire gentry, Lady Grace Mildmay's earliest training in medicine had been provided by her governess. This was part of her preparation for married life, during which she would be expected to manage the health of her whole household. In the event, Mildmay did not stop there: after marriage, she gradually expanded her practice to service her entire local parish. Her surviving papers indicate the bulk production and purchasing of medical supplies, self-education in Hippocratic-Galenic theory, and correspondence with a number of university-trained physicians.[7] Many of the latter – all of whom were male – disapproved of women practising medicine on point of principle. Yet one of them, the eye doctor Richard Banister, was willing to make an exception to the rule:

> in this generall reprehension [of female healers], I would not be accounted to cry out of all women without exception ... for I haue knowne some, whose worth and wisedome might be paraleled with principall men; whose cures were attended with due care, and ended with true charity: as the right religious and vertuous lady, the Lady Mildmay, of Apethorpe in the county of Northampton, who had her selfe good iudgment in many things; yet when the poore came home to her for help (for on such people did she plant her practice) in cases of Physicke, she would use the approbation of a Physician; in Chirurgerie, the aid of a Chirurgeon, and for the eyes, the assistance of my selfe.[8]

Mildmay's referral of patients with eye problems to Banister is not the only evidence we have of her good judgement; evidently, one key to her success was that she knew how to keep her better accredited colleagues sweet.

[5] London, Royal College of Physicians. *Annals*, MS 4143, f. 149r.

[6] MacDonald, *Mystical Bedlam*, pp. 13–26; Jonathan Andrews, 'Napier, Richard (1559–1634), Astrological Physician and Church of England Clergyman', *Oxford Dictionary of National Biography* (hereafter *ODNB*), 21 May 2009, https://doi.org/10.1093/ref:odnb/19763.

[7] Linda Pollock, 'Mildmay [née Sharington], Grace, Lady Mildmay (c. 1552–1620), Memoirist and Medical Practitioner', *ODNB*, 27 May 2010, https://doi.org/10.1093/ref:odnb/45817.

[8] Richard Banister, 'To the Reader', in *A treatise of one hundred and thirteene diseases of the eyes, and eye-liddes* (London, 1622), unnumbered page.

John Hall's trajectory was typical of the academic physician: eight years of study at Cambridge led to the award of an MA in 1597. The university's medical programme still lacked prestige at this time, and its graduates were encouraged to spend a few years shadowing their seniors and polishing their learning (ideally on the continent). This was probably the path taken by Hall, for it was not until around 1607 that he settled down and set up practice in the small town of Stratford-upon-Avon. Although he is best remembered today for marrying William Shakespeare's daughter, in his day Hall had no small reputation of his own – as a 'master of physick'.[9] He died in 1635, at the age of sixty. Like Forman, Napier, and Mildmay, Hall had spent most of his life as a subject of Elizabeth I and then James VI and I. Whether he knew it or not, that era – an era of glittering stagecraft and fragile domestic peace – was dying with him.

In 1642, the grievances which had festered between King Charles I and Parliament over the preceding two decades finally came to a head, and England slipped into the first of two devastating civil wars. At the time, the twenty-two-year-old surgeon-in-training Richard Wiseman was serving the final two years of his apprenticeship in London. The surgeon to whom he was apprenticed had been on the king's payroll prior to the war, and Wiseman seems to have remained stoutly loyal to his master's master; on qualifying, he immediately enlisted as a surgeon to the royalist army. He must have earned a reputation as a safe pair of hands: by 1646, he had been appointed the sole surgical attendant to the young Prince Charles. He accompanied the prince across the continent and back, before finally being taken prisoner at the battle of Worcester – the royalists' last stand – in September 1651. After two rounds of release and reimprisonment, Wiseman decided Cromwell's England was no place for him: he spent 1654–1657 in self-imposed exile, working as a ship surgeon to the Spanish navy. The wind finally changed in 1660, when the newly restored King Charles II reinstated him as his royal surgeon-in-ordinary. A decade later, having grown rich, respected, and increasingly frail in health, Wiseman's thoughts turned to writing. His magnum opus, *Severall Chirurgicall Treatises*, appeared in 1676. Wiseman did not live to see the book's success: the preface is dated to three months before his death.[10]

9 Greg Wells, *John Hall, Master of Physick: A Casebook from Shakespeare's Stratford* (Manchester: Manchester University Press, 2020), pp. 28–38.

10 John Kirkup, 'Wiseman, Richard (bap. 1620?, d. 1676), Surgeon', *ODNB*, 3 January 2008, https://doi.org/10.1093/ref:odnb/29792.

Among the wounded soldiers whom Wiseman may have seen lying on the battlefield at Worcester was a young man named Thomas Sydenham. His father belonged to the ranks of independent-minded, puritan-leaning, office-holding gentry who – from 1641 – would join the parliamentarian cause in their droves. The Sydenham boys had all enlisted to fight; by the time of his wounding in 1651, Thomas had lost his mother and two brothers to the conflict. Although he would later report that he had been left for dead at Worcester, help must have arrived in the end: he ended up spending several weeks in the care of his old Oxford college. Although Sydenham had begun his medical studies at Oxford at the end of the first war, and had been made a Bachelor of Medicine in 1648, it wasn't until the 1660s that he set up a full-time practice. The catalyst of this change was the same as it had been for Wiseman: the reinstatement of the Stuart monarch Charles II.[11]

What for Wiseman had been a new dawn was, for Sydenham, the start of a long night. In the late 1650s, he had still harboured hopes of making a career in politics; now those hopes were permanently dashed. Even his career prospects as a physician were seriously diminished by polite society's awareness of his parliamentarian past. Undeterred, and now styling himself 'Dr' (though he still had no qualification other than the honorary BM), Sydenham was examined and licensed by London's Royal College of Physicians. Unable to attract politically conservative elites, Sydenham found most of his patients among the middling and poorer sorts. It was in these years that he began to develop his idiosyncratic medical philosophy. A frustrated radical at heart, Sydenham was determined not merely to practise medicine, but to *reform* it. This meant conducting research which would not only break new ground, but whose outcomes would benefit the poor as well as the rich. Working in London's overcrowded hospitals, epidemic disease presented itself as an obvious topic. Influenced by Oxford's experimentalist natural philosophers, Sydenham decided that he would adopt their 'Baconian' method, trusting as 'fact' only what had been confirmed by his own observations. The one ancient medical author worth reading – in his view – was Hippocrates. Sydenham saw himself as the direct heir to the ancient Greek physician: it was he who had pioneered evidence-based medicine, and now at last someone was following in his footsteps. Sydenham would no doubt have been

11 Harold J. Cook, 'Sydenham, Thomas (bap. 1624, d. 1689), Physician', *ODNB*, 19 May 2011, https://doi.org/10.1093/ref:odnb/26864.

pleased – if not surprised – to learn that one day he would come to be known as 'the English Hippocrates'.[12]

He may have been less pleased to learn that one of the torchbearers of his legacy would be his younger contemporary William Salmon. Sydenham was an empiricist, but only his enemies would ever have called him an 'empiric'. Like 'quack' and 'mountebank', this was the kind of derogatory label used to paint irregular practitioners as snake-oil merchants. This was the brush with which Salmon was tarred, and not just by his enemies. Rumour had it that he had spent his boyhood apprenticed to a 'mountebank': he 'made speeches and wrote Panygyricks in praise of his master's Panaceas. He wrote Almanacks to direct the taking of his medicines, and made the stars vouch for their virtue'.[13] As far as we know, Salmon never gained any formal qualification. But this does not oblige us to accept the connotative baggage which comes with the label 'quack'. Salmon was a prolific writer and translator, publishing on medicine, anatomy, surgery, and pharmacology. He has been lambasted by posterity for his dilettantism, derivativeness, and energetic product-branding.[14] But these criticisms say more about modern notions of what a medical professional *should* be than about who Salmon was to his readers and clients. And although he published little original material, as a compiler, translator, and editor he was far from undiscriminating. Multilingual, enterprising, and creative – Sydenham might have said a little *too* creative – Salmon made his medical translations his own.

The great rupture in the life of Thomas Willis – as for Wiseman and Sydenham – was the outbreak of the first civil war. On its eve, Willis had been an undergraduate at Christ Church, Oxford, possibly on track for ordination. By its end, he had seen hard fighting, lost his father and stepmother to camp fever, and decided to become a physician. Returning to his old Oxford college, he began his medical studies in earnest, though like Sydenham his BM was awarded more in recognition of his wartime loyalty – in Willis's case, to the king – than of any academic achievement. By 1650, Willis had achieved modest success as a general

12 Andrew Cunningham, 'Thomas Sydenham: Epidemics, Experiment, and the "Good Old Cause"', in Roger French and Andrew Wear (eds.), *The Medical Revolution of the Seventeenth Century* (Cambridge: Cambridge University Press, 1989), pp. 164–190.

13 Philip K. Wilson, 'Salmon, William (1644–1713), Medical Empiric and Author', *ODNB*, 11 November 2021, https://doi.org/10.1093/ref:odnb/24559.

14 See ibid.; Charles J. S. Thompson, *The Quacks of Old London* (London: Brentano's, 1928), pp. 125–131; Craig Ashley Hanson, *The English Virtuoso: Art, Medicine, and Antiquarianism in the Age of Empiricism* (Chicago: University of Chicago Press, 2009), pp. 11, 18.

practitioner. Meanwhile, out of hours, he was joining his Oxford peers in a series of increasingly daring experiments in chemistry, physiology, and anatomy.[15] Appointed Oxford's Sedleian Professor in Natural Philosophy in 1660, Willis was free to devote himself to these studies. He assembled a like-minded research group, whose combined labours culminated in the publication of *Cerebri anatome* (1664).[16] This was the first dedicated anatomical study of the brain and nerves to be published in Europe, unparalleled in its detail and in the quality of its engravings. The book's English translator coined a new name for Willis's specialism – 'neurologie' – and medical historians have assigned him full rights of paternity ever since. Yet, despite his innovations, some of Willis's ideas about brain disease would have struck his predecessors as distinctly familiar.

Definitions

Resuming his medical studies in interwar Oxford, Willis had probably picked up at least one book with the word *practica* in the title. Of all the diseases he would have found listed there, frenzy had a particularly venerable (if complicated) pedigree. To gain a sense of why early modern readers sometimes struggled to define it, we will first need to take a brief tour through ancient Greece and Rome. The earliest mention of frenzy's Greek forebear – *phrenitis* – occurs in the Hippocratic Corpus, a multi-authored body of texts traditionally attributed to Hippocrates. In fact, the diagnosis probably predates the Corpus: one of these texts, the *Regimen in Acute Diseases* (c. 400 BCE), describes *phrenitis* as a disease classified as acute by 'the ancients'.[17] Throughout the Corpus, *phrenitis* is characterized by certain common signs, chief among them mental alienation, fever, sleeplessness, and restless plucking motions of the fingers.[18] In comparison to other ancient Greek diagnoses, *phrenitis* was already unusually well-defined. In fact, one recent study has described it as 'the only obvious disease of mind' to feature in ancient Greek medicine, citing among other evidence the name's etymology: the ancient Greek

[15] Robert L. Martensen, 'Willis, Thomas (1621–1675), Physician and Natural Philosopher', *ODNB*, 4 October 2007, https://doi.org/10.1093/ref:odnb/29587.

[16] Later published in English as 'The Anatomy of the Brain', in Pordage (trans.), *The remaining medical works*, Part VI, pp. 50–192.

[17] Glenda C. McDonald, 'Concepts and Treatments of Phrenetis in Ancient Medicine' (PhD thesis, University of Newcastle, 2009), pp. 15–16.

[18] Thumiger, *Phrenitis*, pp. 24–30.

phrēn – the nexus of memory, thought, and feeling animating Homer's fictional heroes – would later be translated as 'mind'.[19] This translation is not a one-to-one match, but it will serve our purposes for now.

One point on which the Hippocratic authors could not agree was the precise location of this *phrēn*. The prevailing view in ancient Greece was that it was situated somewhere in the thoracic cavity – either in the heart, the lungs, the diaphragm, or its membranes.[20] The association was so firm that, at some point, the word *phrēn* came to signify *both* the diaphragm *and* the thinking, feeling mind. A lone objector to this view was the author of the Hippocratic fragment *On the Sacred Disease*.[21] Although the many vessels and nerves connected to the thoracic cavity made it especially sensitive to stimuli, so that 'the heart and the *phrēn* feel things especially', in fact, this author insisted, neither had 'a share in thinking, but of all these things the brain is the cause'.[22]

The question of where the mind and its diseases were located in the body was still unsettled in the common era. When the Roman medical encyclopaedist Aulus Cornelius Celsus (c. 25–50 CE) set about composing a book on 'Specific Diseases', he decided to start with a list of whole-body diseases, before running through the localized ones from head to toe. Following his Greek sources, Celsus listed three species of *insania* (madness): *phrenitis* (now Latinized as *phrenesis*), *melancholia*, and an unnamed type which roughly corresponded to the ancient Greek *mania*. Yet it was in the first section of his book – and not among the diseases of the head – that Celsus placed these diseases. In his view, neither *phrenesis* nor any other type of *insania* could be 'assigned to a specific part of the body'.[23]

The imperial physician Claudius Galen (129–216 CE) had no time for such fence-sitting: the only proper way to understand a disease, he declared, was to identify the anatomical location of the activity which it had disrupted.[24] The Hippocratic authors had at least hazarded a guess as

[19] Peter Singer and Chiara Thumiger, 'Introduction. Disease Classification and Mental Illness: Ancient and Modern Perspectives', in Thumiger and Singer (eds.), *Mental Illness in Ancient Medicine*, p. 2.

[20] Chiara Thumiger, 'Mental Disorder and History: Methodological and General Issues', in *A History of the Mind and Mental Health in Classical Greek Medical Thought*, p. 38.

[21] McDonald, 'Concepts and Treatments', p. 24.

[22] 'On the Sacred Disease', trans. McDonald, in 'Concepts and Treatments', p. 27.

[23] Celsus, 'On Medicine', in W. G. Spencer (trans.), *On Medicine. Volume I, Books 1–4*, LCL 292 (Cambridge, MA: Harvard University Press, 1935), p. 289.

[24] McDonald, 'Concepts and Treatments', pp. 82–83.

to that location, albeit a wrong one: only the author of *On the Sacred Disease* had hit the mark. The activities of the *phrēn* (Galen preferred to call it the *hēgemonikon psychēs*, the 'ruling part of the soul') happened in the brain. He heaped scorn on his contemporaries who – in the face of all the evidence – continued to believe that these activities were located in the thorax. Didn't they know this doctrine had been disproved by 'all the anatomists'? Besides, 'they must have seen that it was rejected for many other [reasons], not least because of the cure of phrenetics'.[25] They knew from experience to apply rose water and vinegar to the head of a phrenetic; if they truly believed in their own doctrines, would they not do better to 'anoint the chest?'[26] No. Only cooling the head would help to alleviate the mental alienation of these patients; ergo, *phrenitis* was a disease of the brain.[27]

Determined to redeem the reliability of Hippocrates himself, Galen explained the confusion which had arisen as follows: true *phrenitis* was an inflammation of the brain causing mental alienation (*paraphrosynē*). But mental alienation was not unique to brain disease: it could also be caused by heat and corruption arising anywhere in the body. It was especially severe in cases of diaphragmatic inflammation. In these cases, however, the brain was affected secondarily and only by its connectedness – its 'sympathy' or 'consent' – with the rest of the body. However much the patient's speech and behaviour resembled that of a phrenetic, to diagnose him or her as such would be a mistake. This was not true *phrenitis*, but a clever impersonator, easily exposed by therapeutic intervention: cool the diaphragm, and the mental alienation would vanish along with the fever.[28]

From late antiquity to early modernity, as Galen's authority steadily grew, the contributions of other ancient and late antique authors were either overshadowed or absorbed into the Western medical canon under his name. In thirteenth-century Europe, it was a Latinized, Christianized version of Galenism which formed the foundation of the new European medical faculties' curricula. Unsurprisingly, then, it was

25 '[hanc opinionem] omnes anatomici iam damnarunt … cum per alia multa, tum maxime in phreniticorum lethargicorumque curationibus'. Galen, 'De locis affectis', lib. 1, cap. 1, p. 19.

26 'si hoc praesidio phrenitidis causa sanari possit, not capiti, sed thoraci ipsum adhibere'. Galen, 'De locis affectis', lib. 2, cap. 10, pp. 130–131.

27 Julien Devinant, 'Mental Disorders and Psychological Suffering in Galen's Cases', in Thumiger and Singer (eds.), *Mental Illness in Ancient Medicine*, p. 201, n. 8.

28 Galen, 'De locis affectis', lib. 3, cap. 9, p. 178; Bartholomaeus Anglicus, *De proprietatibus rerum* (London, 1535), ff. 86r–v.

Galen's brain-based understanding of the mind and its diseases which won out over its competitors.[29] Any medieval physician worth his salt knew the difference between 'true' and 'false' *phrenitis*, or – to give them their Latin names – *phrenesis* and *paraphrenesis*. In sixteenth-century England, it was these names which populated the pages of emerging print genres like the vernacularized encyclopaedia and the diagnostic *practica*.

The translators of these works found themselves faced with the unenviable task of explaining the ancient disease and its complications to lay readers. One of them was the Elizabethan polymath Stephen Bateman, whose 1582 translation of the classic thirteenth-century mendicant encyclopaedia *De proprietatibus rerum* soon graced bookshelves across the land.[30] Arriving at *phrenitis*, Bateman did his best:

> the barbarous word is *Frenesis*, or in English, a phrensie or madnesse: an impostumation [abscess] bread [bred] & ingendered in the Pellycles [membranes] of the braine, named in Latine *Pia mater*, the which Apostumation, doth make alienation of mans mind and memorie. There is another accident Phrenyse [sic], the which is ioyned with another sicknesse, as a Phrensie with a Feaver, or with a Pleurisie.[31]

As *phrenitis* and its lookalike *paraphrenitis* (translated by Bateman as 'accident Phrenyse') entered the vernacular, they were kneaded, stretched, reshaped, and – increasingly frequently – rolled into one. At the start of the seventeenth century, the difference between *phrenitis* and *paraphrenitis* was still clear to a university-educated physician like Hall – but to a self-taught practitioner like Mildmay, it was not.[32] As we move forward, it will be important for us to keep in mind *both* the academic distinction between the two conditions, and the widespread conflation of the two.

To complicate matters further, by the seventeenth century, even the academic distinction had started to change. Medical specialists were starting to favour a new term for the accident state of mental alienation which accompanied fevers: *delirium*. *Delirium* had been used to describe states of unreason since antiquity, but its meanings had never been narrow;

29 See Singer and Thumiger, 'Introduction', pp. 1, 8, 23; Thumiger, 'Mental Disorder and History', pp. 32–33.

30 Bartholomaeus Anglicus, *De proprietatibus rerum*, in Stephen Bateman (trans.), *Batman vppon Bartholome, his booke De proprietatibus rerum* (London, 1582).

31 Ibid., lib. 7, cap. 5, fol. 88v.

32 John Hall, 'Curationum Historicarum et Empiricarum' (1635), in Wells (trans.), *John Hall*, p. 142. All further quotations from Hall are from Wells's translation. Linda Pollock (ed.), *With Faith and Physic: The Life of a Tudor Gentlewoman Lady Grace Mildmay, 1552–1620* (London: Collins & Brown, 1993), pp. 119–121.

for most Latin-speakers, it was simply a synonym for madness.[33] Now, it was being superimposed on the symptomatic state which Galen had once called *paraphrosynē*. Thus, in his 1672 *De anima brutorum*, Thomas Willis declared that

> The *Delirium* is not a Disease of it self, but only a *symptom* proceeding from other Distempers . . . This word taken after an especial manner, is the same with *paraphrosynē* or a going crooked, or out of the right or straight way, and denotes an hurt of the same Animal Function such as ariseth in fits of the Feavour.[34]

Although Willis did make a passing mention of *paraphrenitis* in *De anima brutorum*, he titled the chapter in which it appeared 'On Delirium and Phrensie'.[35] This was not just a rebranding exercise; if Willis was quietly phasing out *paraphrenitis*, it was because he had real doubts about its existence. In the series of lectures on which the book was based, given at Oxford in the early 1660s, he had noted

> That paraphrenzy does not arise from an inflammation of the diaphragm, as is commonly believed, is proved by the case of an academic suffering from pleurisy . . . The purulent matter had extravasated [leaked out] from his side and had poured into his thorax covering the diaphragm: indeed this venemous matter had perforated the diaphragm in its fleshy part but he never suffered from paraphrenzy.[36]

After several such autopsies, Willis had rejected the traditional Galenic definition of *paraphrenitis* as a form of mental alienation arising from an inflamed diaphragm. The lack of correspondence between the presence or absence of the symptom and the subsequent post-mortem findings did not lead him to instantly disown *paraphrenitis*. But – in Willis's book, at least – it had dwindled to the size of a problematic footnote. It was hard to see what exactly the diagnosis did that *delirium* could not do better.

Likewise, although he knew the definition of *paraphrenitis* by rote, the court surgeon Richard Wiseman does not seem to have encountered a single case.[37] This was not for a want of patients suffering from inflammation, fever, and mental alienation; he must have seen hundreds

33 According to Robert Burton, '*Delirium*, Dotage . . . is a common name to all the following species [of madness]'. Robert Burton, *The anatomy of melancholy* (Oxford, 1621), p. 8.

34 Thomas Willis, *Two discourses concerning the soul of brutes*, trans. Samuel Pordage (London, 1683), p. 179.

35 Ibid.

36 Thomas Willis, *Thomas Willis's Oxford Lectures*, trans. Kenneth Dewhurst (Oxford: Sandford, 1980), p. 120. All further quotations are from Dewhurst's translation.

37 Richard Wiseman, *Severall chirurgicall treatises by Richard Wiseman* (London, 1676), p. 14.

if not thousands over the course of the civil wars. But he had given them one of two diagnoses: *delirium* or *phrenitis*.[38] Cast adrift from its moorings in the body, *paraphrenitis* was losing its explanatory power. Its displacement by *delirium* left no room for ambiguity: frenzy could no longer slip back and forth over the conceptual borderline between symptom (Bateman's 'accident Phrenyse') and disease. Of course, for orthodox academic physicians, this slippage should never have happened in the first place: the whole point of maintaining the distinction between *phrenitis* and *paraphrenitis* had been to keep that barrier in place. But Galen's theories were no longer gospel in post-war England; in fact, his once unquestioned hegemony was facing resistance from multiple quarters. The reconfiguration of humoral physiology by Willis and his peers presented one such threat. Another quite different challenge came from England's so-called Neo-Hippocratic physicians, chief among them Thomas Sydenham.

Abandoning high politics, in 1660 Sydenham had embarked on a new, less explicitly political campaign: he would restore the art of medicine to its former Hippocratic glory.[39] Unfortunately, when it came to classifying states of mental alienation, it was post-Hippocratic medical theorists like Celsus and Galen who had done most of the heavy lifting.[40] This created something of a problem for Sydenham, for – working with the sufferers of smallpox and fever – he saw cases of mental alienation all the time. Fortunately, the Hippocratic authors did have one working diagnosis for use in such cases: *phrenitis*. But *paraphrenitis* – that meaningless piece of Galenic paraphernalia – had to go. The best witness here is Sydenham's silence: *paraphrenitis* is nowhere to be seen in his writings, and where a substitute is needed, *phrenitis* stands in. Describing 'the Continual Fever of the Year 1661', for example, he warned that 'if the blood ferments . . . we may reasonably fear the sick is in danger of a Phrensy, or some other ill symptom'.[41] In cases of smallpox, too, sometimes 'the patient through the too intense ebullition of his bloud from cordials and hot keepeing becomes

[38] Ibid., pp. 302–303 (*phrenitis*); pp. 40, 128, 391–392, 400, 430, 447 (*delirium*).

[39] Cunningham has argued argued that Sydenham's Sydenham's reputation as 'the English Hippocrates' was in large part 'laundered' by his self-identified successor, the Leiden physician Herman Boerhaave (1668–1738). See Cunningham, 'Sydenham', pp. 188–190. Nonetheless, Hippocrates was one of the very few ancient medical authorities whom Sydenham took seriously, and the influence of the Corpus can be seen in his terminological choices as well as in his much-touted empiricism.

[40] See Thumiger and Singer, *Mental Illness in Ancient Medicine*, chs. 4–6, 10, 11, 14.

[41] Thomas Sydenham, in John Pechey (trans.), *The whole works of that excellent practical physician Dr. Thomas Sydenham* (London, 1696), p. 22.

phreneticall'.[42] This is the only form in which *phrenitis* ever appears in Sydenham's writings: as a symptom or complication of another disease.

Training his gaze on the epidemics of his own day, Sydenham was tailoring the Hippocratic *phrenitis* to size. Of course, he might well have countered that the only tailoring involved was unstitching, for it was *his* usage which was faithful to the original. To his critics, however, this was yet another example of Sydenham's wilful ignorance of the medical canon. How 'many *scruples* is this Doctor *Sydenham* freed from, by suffering our best *Writers* to remain *untouched, unconsulted!*', a fellow of the Royal College of Physicians jeered in 1671.[43] Sydenham's self-appointed editor, the ex-mountebank William Salmon, was determined to spare his hero from further embarrassment. In his English translation of Sydenham's *Processus integri*, Salmon noted reproachfully that, 'besides those diseases our Author has here treated of, there were several other very common Maladies, and which were the almost every day practice of physicians, of which he had not taken the least notice'.[44] Sydenham had probably forgotten to mention them, Salmon concluded, but it was no trouble for him to correct the oversight. Amongst Salmon's insertions was an entirely conventional chapter 'Of Frenzy and Delirium'.[45] It is hard to imagine Sydenham acknowledging the kindness with anything other than a sharp turn in his grave. His iconoclastic writings had been made conformable to learned medicine – by a quack.

Sydenham's redefinition of *phrenitis* did not catch on, not even after his posthumous canonization as the 'English Hippocrates'.[46] In late eighteenth-century Edinburgh, the School of Medicine's leading professor William Cullen was still pausing his lectures to tut at 'what he [Sydenham] improperly calls *phrenitis*'.[47] But, in attacking the academic physicians' stronghold, Sydenham may have forced them to test the robustness of their own classificatory system. Perhaps, on closer inspection, the distinction between *phrenitis* and *paraphrenitis* did seem too flimsy to be worth keeping. Or perhaps Sydenham had nothing to do with it; perhaps pillars of the establishment like Willis and Wiseman had reached this conclusion

[42] Thomas Sydenham, 'Smallpox [dedicated to the first Earl of Shaftesbury]', in Kenneth Dewhurst (trans.), *Dr Thomas Sydenham (1624–1689), His Life and Original Writings* (London: Wellcome Historical Medical Library, 1966), p. 113.

[43] Henry Stubbe, *The Lord Bacons relation to the sweating-sickness examined* (London, 1671), p. 222.

[44] William Salmon (trans.), *Praxis medica. The practice of physick, or Dr Sydenham's Processus integri*, 3rd ed. (London, 1716), preface, item VII.

[45] Ibid., p. 173. [46] Cunningham, 'Sydenham', pp. 188–190.

[47] William Cullen, *Lectures on the Materia Medica*, 2nd ed. (Dublin, 1781), p. 286.

independently. Whatever the cause, *paraphrenitis* was on its way out. A hundred years later, Cullen did not even consider it: what Sydenham should have said – he instructed his students – was *delirium*.[48] Throughout the seventeenth century, this newly standardized symptom had been steadily encroaching on ground once occupied by *paraphrenitis*; now, the usurpation was complete.

The result, as we will see, was a narrowing of frenzy's affordances as a diagnosis. Of course, the academic Galenists' definition of *phrenitis* had always been narrow. What had changed, in the second half of the seventeenth century, was the sheer number of self-educated, scientifically literate readers keeping track of these new developments.[49] The new vernacular translations of Latin medical treatises appearing in English bookshops in these decades had been produced just for them.[50] Now, any interested coffeehouse patron could learn that whereas delirium was 'only a *symptom*', frenzy was a 'continual dotage, or deprivation of the principal faculties of the Brain, arising from an Inflammation of the *Meninges*, with a continual Feavour'.[51] For Elizabethan autodidacts like Mildmay, Forman, and Napier, the diagnosis had been capable of doing a lot more work (albeit with less precision). We now return to their more capacious understanding of frenzy, to consider some of its possible causes: fluids, fumes, wounds, and passions.

Causes

Humours

For most of sixteenth-century England's medical thinkers, the key to preserving human health lay in four vital fluids known as the humours: blood, phlegm, yellow bile (choler), and black bile (melancholy). Each of these fluids also had its own unique combination of *qualities*: colour, weight, viscosity, and – most importantly – temperature and moisture.

48 Ibid.

49 See, e.g., Robert G. Frank, *Harvey and the Oxford Physiologists: A Study of Scientific Ideas and Social Interaction* (Los Angeles: University of California Press, 1978); Mary Fissell, 'Readers, Texts, and Contexts: Vernacular Medical Works in Early Modern England', in Roy Porter (ed.), *The Popularization of Medicine, 1650–1850* (London: Routledge, 1992), pp. 72–96.

50 To give just one example, the first English edition of William Harvey's *De motu cordis* (Frankfurt, 1628) appeared in the mid-century, entitled *The anatomical exercises of Dr. William Harvey ... concerning the motion of the heart and blood* (London, 1653). At the time, no member of the academic medical community would have been expected to need a vernacular translation.

51 Willis, *Two discourses*, pp. 179, 181.

Blood was hot and wet, phlegm cold and wet, choler hot and dry, and melancholy cold and dry. The mixture of humours within a body (its *complexion*) thus automatically determined its *qualitative* condition (its *temperament*). Temperamental differences amongst individuals explained aspects of their being which we would now place under several different headings: the temperature of their skin; the size, texture, and appearance of their flesh, hair, veins, and muscles; their appetite, digestion, energy, quality of sleep, memory, personality, and mood. An imbalance of the humours *distempered* the body, and this distemper could throw any or all of these aspects into disarray.

The temperamental body possessed its own delicate system of self-regulation: in health, it could quickly correct any imbalances by repleting and excreting humours as required. But the system was not failsafe. Early modern humoral theorists liked to describe the body as an oven, fired by the 'hearthstone' of the heart. It was the body's 'vital heat' which 'concocted' the four humours out of the first product of digestion (chyle). Temperature control was crucial, for like the food from which they came, the humours could end up either rotten or burnt. It was these 'corrupt' or 'adust' (burnt) humours which created the right conditions for *phrenitis*. In Galen's account, the distemper began with an accumulation of yellow bile in the brain, which began to overheat that organ's naturally cold, moist substance. The darker this bile, the more violent the derangement it caused: 'the type of phrenitis is milder ... when it originates from a pale yellow bile, but the type caused by dark yellow bile is more violent. And above and beyond these is the melancholic and bestial madness generated by burnt yellow bile.'[52] As a quick thumbnail sketch, the theory of the 'four humours' can seem naïve in its simplicity. But it was the simplicity of its broad outlines which allowed it to accommodate screeds of complex and sometimes contradictory small print. Galen had added one such clause: alongside the four naturally occurring humours, he counted four arising 'contrary to nature'.[53] The worst 'melancholic and bestial' *phrenitis* was caused, he explained, not by 'natural' black bile, but by the 'unnatural' kind: that is, not by melancholy, but by the charred remains of burnt choler.

52 'Atque hanc ob causam phrenitis nonnunquam mitior est, quum a pallida bile ortum contraxit; interdum vehementior, quum flava bilis eam peperit; atque insuper alia nonnunquam desipientia occurrit ferina et melancholica, flava bile praeassata.' Galen, 'De locis affectis', lib. 3, cap. 9, pp. 177–178.

53 'praeter naturam'. See ibid., pp. 177–178, 195; Galen, 'De humoribus', pp. 490–491.

This minor clause in Galen's writings was to cause protracted headaches for his early modern readers. Overactive bile was implicated in all three of the species of madness which they had inherited from antiquity: melancholia, mania, and frenzy. Each of these diseases caused its sufferers to behave in distinct ways, and the differences between them were usually explained with reference to the qualities of the bile at work. Melancholy – the cold, leaden bile – caused the coldness and heaviness of heart suffered by melancholics. Choler – the hot, inflammable bile – was to blame for the raging, raving, and violent agitation seen in mania and frenzy. Mania, like melancholy, was chronic and non-febrile, while frenzy was acute and always accompanied by a fever. The process of differential diagnosis could not have been simpler – except, that is, when it came to unnatural black bile.[54] Was the hot, 'bestial' madness which this humour produced a melancholic frenzy, or was it an uncharacteristically frenzied melancholia?

The overlap between these three species of madness remained a nagging concern in early modern England. But on one point everyone could agree: whether black or yellow, burnt or raw, choler was the primary culprit in cases of frenzy. As Forman put it, the disease was 'caused of too moch burnte collor [choler] which is hote and dri . . . and by reason of his heate it doth overheat and dry the brain, infecting the naturall and vital blod'.[55] 'And the more adust [burnt] the choler is, the more pernicious is the disease', added Mildmay.[56] A surfeit of choler was like a heap of hot, dry tinder: it was only a matter of time before it burned. Once burnt, it tainted the blood, and the corrupt blood inflamed the tissues of the brain. There were variations on this theme; sometimes the blood overheated of its own accord, sometimes it bled out into the brain. But the humours at fault were usually the same (blood and choler), and so too were the basic processes (burning, corruption, and inflammation).

This also had implications for the gender prevalence of the disease. An average man tended towards a more choleric complexion (hot and dry), and vice versa, an average woman tended towards a phlegmatic one (cold and wet). This gave women a greater natural resistance to frenzy, for – of all four humours – phlegm was the only one that did not burn. When, in 1615, the London College of Physicians had asked 'a quack practising on

54 On the presentation of 'natural' versus 'unnatural' melancholy, see Burton, *The anatomy*, pp. 37–38, 181–183. Even Burton admitted that he found 'the matter . . . divers and confused' (p. 37).

55 Forman, 'Liber Juditiorum Morborum' (c. 1600), Oxford, Bodleian Library, MS Ashmole 355, p. 133.

56 Pollock, *With Faith and Physic*, p. 119.

mad people ... for a distinction between mad men', the 'quack' had replied that 'they are not all of one kinde, but of all the foure humours, and those burnt'. His interrogators leapt on the opportunity to catch him out: 'But how is flegme burnt? ... and what author hath he for it?'[57] The man declined 'to dispute', and this was probably for the best: he was not about to change their minds. While all men had some phlegm in their bodies – and a particularly phlegmatic man could have more than a particularly choleric woman – on average, men's hotter, drier temperaments put them at greater risk of succumbing to this quintessentially hot, dry disease.

This traditional humoral account still had currency in 1700. In the section on frenzy which he had added to Sydenham's *Processus integri*, Salmon summarized: 'The cause of this Disease may be from a Discrasy [imbalance] of the blood inflamed, or from Choler enraged, causing an inflammation in the brain or its membranes; or from adust Choler carried to the *Brain*.'[58] This account was faithful enough to Galen (if not to Sydenham), but Salmon's medical contemporaries would have seen it as hopelessly out of date. Over the course of the seventeenth century, new rivals to the Hippocratic-Galenic model of human physiology had been capturing the imaginations of European medical readers. One was the model endorsed by the advocates of chemical medicine (also known as iatrochemistry). Chemical medicine was not new to England: it had flourished in English friaries in the centuries before the Reformation, and had re-emerged in the 1570s under the banner of 'Paracelsianism'.[59] Named after its author, the cantankerous Swiss-born metallurgist Paracelsus (1493–1541), this was a mystical, anti-Galenic, anti-intellectualist reinvention of the old alchemical tradition. Paracelsianism had posed no real threat to the Hippocratic-Galenic hegemony in the reigns of Elizabeth I and James VI and I. But the outbreak of the first civil war had changed everything: the collapse of old institutions and the suspension of censorship had made heterodox ideas simultaneously more thinkable and more available. The time was ripe for chemical medicine. This time, it entered common currency via the writings of the Flemish physician Jan Baptist van Helmont (1580–1644), who had revised and expanded

[57] London, Royal College of Physicians, *Annals*, MS 43144, vol. 3, f. 19v.

[58] Salmon, *Praxis medica*, p. 174.

[59] Peter Murray Jones, *The Medicine of the Friars in Medieval England* (York: Boydell & Brewer, 2024), esp. pp. 121–129, 135–137; Charles Webster, 'Alchemical and Paracelsian Medicine', in Charles Webster (ed.), *Health, Medicine and Mortality in the Sixteenth Century* (Cambridge: Cambridge University Press, 1979), pp. 313–334.

Paracelsus's chemical philosophy in the early decades of the seventeenth century.[60]

The Helmontian vision of human physiology differed from that of the Galenists in two important respects. In the traditional humoral account, bodily fluids consisted of a mixture of the four elements – air, fire, earth, and water – and it was this elemental make-up which determined their qualities (melancholy's earthiness made it cold and dry, phlegm's wateriness made it cold and wet, and so on). For the chemists, this was only half the story.[61] The doctrine of the elements was of some 'help for the unfolding the Phaenomena of Nature', Willis admitted, but it only got a physician so far: it was 'almost the same thing, to say an House consists of Wood and Stone, as a Body of four Elements'.[62] The elements had to be broken down even further to be understood. At the most fundamental level, they were composed of three chemical principles: salt, sulphur, and mercury.[63] Thus, where Galenists described the bodily fluids principally in terms of heat and moisture, the chemists described them as 'volatile' or 'fixed', 'sulphureous', 'sweet', or 'saline'.

Secondly, and relatedly, the model of the body looked different: the oven had become a brewer's vat. Just as 'Must, or new Wine, or new Ale or Beer, be closely Bottled up, or put into Vessels of small vent . . . will grow so very hot, [so] that often the Vessels are in danger of breaking', Willis explained, so too the juices of 'Animals, as also all Liquors Concreted, and compounded of many things quickly Ferment'.[64] The language was now not of cooking but of chemistry: 'concoction' was being replaced by 'fermentation', 'ebullition' (boiling), and 'explosion'.[65] It is in this light that we can make sense of Sydenham's warnings about the dangers of giving 'cordials and hot keepeing' to feverish patients, for, 'if the Blood Ferments so violently . . . we may yet reasonably suspect that the Patient is either obnoxious [vulnerable] to a Phrensie, or any other troublesom Symptom proceeding from too great an Ebullition of the Blood'.[66]

60 The drive for medical reform did not arise in a vacuum, but the precise nature of its alignment with the religious and political reform movements of these decades has been disputed. See Charles Webster, *The Great Instauration: Science, Medicine and Reform, 1626–1660* (London: Duckworth, 1975); Peter Elmer, 'Medicine, Religion, and the Puritan Revolution', in French and Wear (eds.), *Medical Revolution*, pp. 10–45.

61 Andrew Wear, *Knowledge and Practice in English Medicine, 1550–1680* (Cambridge: Cambridge University Press, 2000), pp. 37–40.

62 Thomas Willis, *A medical-philosophical discourse of fermentation* (London, 1681), p. 2.

63 Willis added earth and water back into the mix, but this was unconventional. Ibid.

64 Ibid., pp. 1–2. 65 Ibid., sig. A3r, pp. 1, 10, 46.

66 Thomas Sydenham, *Collections of acute diseases. The second and third part* (London, 1688), pp. 40–41.

No wonder that fevers ended in this way, Sydenham lamented, when physicians insisted on making their patients' blood boil.

For others of Sydenham's generation, the iatrochemical model worked best when combined with another recently resurrected ancient philosophy: atomism. Long tarnished by the ill repute of its ancient advocates, the theory that everything was made up of minute 'atoms' or 'corpuscles' had been freshly sanitized in the 1640s by the French philosopher Pierre Gassendi (1592–1655).[67] Gassendi's brand of atomism was palatable even to a sober Anglican like Willis. Up close, Willis declared, the humours were mere conglomerations of 'heterogeneous Particles', and it was the chemical interactions of these tiny bodies which quickened – and sickened – the body.[68] Thus, some individuals were predisposed 'to the *Phrensie*' by 'the previous disposition of the Blood . . . that contains very many sulphureous Particles in it self, which are apt to inflame the Blood in a Feavour more than ought to be, and to insinuate its burning into the Brain'.[69] There were other predisposing factors, too, but the immediate cause was always the same: 'the boiling blood doth transfer its adust or burnt recrements to the Head', driving 'the Feavourish matter into the Brain'.[70] These recrements in the brain consisted not of yellow bile, but 'the burnt-up matter or waste products of the blood'. At the macro level, then, Willis's chemical account of frenzy sounded remarkably similar to the humoral one. The old organic pathways of the disease remained more or less unchanged. The blood boiled or burned; sulphur deposited itself in the brain, and 'there heaped up, and stagnating' produced 'an inflamed tumor, or a serous deluge'. Willis had done little more than pour new wine into old wineskins.

Fumes

These two rival physiological models also offered remarkably similar accounts of *paraphrenitis*. Galen, the chief architect of the traditional humoral account, had followed the ancient Greek philosopher Aristotle (384–322 BCE) in dividing the human soul (*psychē*) into three hierarchical tiers: the vegetative (common to all living beings), the sensitive (common to all animals), and the rational (unique to humans). Each of these souls kept office in a particular organ: the vegetative in the liver, the sensitive in

[67] John Henry, 'The Matter of Souls: Medical Theory and Theology in Seventeenth-Century England', in French and Wear (eds.), *Medical Revolution*, p. 98, n. 26.

[68] Willis, *Two discourses*, p. 180. [69] Ibid., p. 183. [70] Ibid., p. 181.

the heart, and the rational in the brain. But a soul needed more than an office to do its work; it needed a conductive *medium*, a fast-flowing current which kept it connected to the whole body. In ancient Greek medicine, the role was allocated to *pneuma* – an invisible breath of life, more like fire or air than liquid.[71] It was *pneuma*, Galen decided, which travelled through the brain and nerves as the conduit of sensation and motion.[72]

Galen's *pneuma* was later to be translated as *spiritus*, or (in English) *spirits*.[73] For Galenists, these spirits came in three degrees of purity, each progressively distilled from the last. The liver produced the venous blood and its 'natural' spirit, which powered the vegetative faculties (e.g. nutrition, excretion, growth). Passing into the heart, some of this blood was aerated and transformed into the lighter, hotter 'vital spirits', which performed the operations of the sensitive soul (e.g. motion, sensation, reaction to stimuli). Lastly, a small fraction of these vitalized spirits was carried by the arterial blood to an ultrafine tracery of capillaries (the *rete mirabile* or 'marvellous net') located at the base of the skull. Passing into the brain via these capillaries, it was changed into the purer, hotter 'animal spirits' (the name derived from *animus*, the Latin word for 'rational soul' or 'mind'). The animal spirits were so rarefied that they scarcely merited the name of fluids at all: they were better compared to fumes, light, or heat. Leaving the brain via the spinal cord, they flooded the hollow channels of the nerves, delivering the soul's instructions to the body and the body's sensations back to the soul. The animal spirits served as the rational soul's 'material instrument' – or at least they did when they were working properly. Their efficacy depended entirely on their quantity and quality, and their quality depended on the condition of the humours from which they had been distilled. When choler burned in the stomach, Galen had

[71] On medical understandings of *pneuma*, see Roger French, *Robert Whytt, The Soul, and Medicine* (London: Wellcome Institute of the History of Medicine, 1969), pp. 94–107; Fabrizio Bigotti, *Physiology of the Soul: Mind, Body and Matter in the Galenic Tradition of the Late Renaissance (1550–1630)* (Turnhout: Brepols, 2019), pp. 87–89; D. P. Walker, 'Medical Spirits in Philosophy and Theology from Ficino to Newton', in Jean Jacquot (ed.), *Arts du Spectacle et Histoire des Idées: Recueil Offert en Hommage à Jean Jacquot* (Tours: Centre d'Études Supérieures de la Renaissance, 1984), pp. 287–300; John Henry, 'Medicine and Pneumatology: Henry More, Richard Baxter, and Francis Glisson's *Treatise on the Energetic Nature of Substance*', *Medical History* 31 (1987), 15–40.

[72] Edwin Clarke and C. D. O'Malley, *The Human Brain and Spinal Cord: A Historical Study Illustrated by Writings from Antiquity to the Twentieth Century* (Berkeley, CA: University of California Press, 1968), pp. 141–146.

[73] This translation would come to furnish early modern Christians with endless opportunities for confusion, conflation, and equivocation. See Henry, 'The Matter of Souls', pp. 104–105; Sachiko Kusukawa, *The Transformation of Natural Philosophy: The Case of Philip Melanchthon* (Cambridge: Cambridge University Press, 1995), pp. 93–120.

explained, it produced not a bright, enlivening spirit but a 'smoky or sooty' sort, which soon rose to the head.[74] The brain was affected by 'consent' or 'sympathy' because of the density of the nerves connecting the two areas. Or, as Bateman neatly put it, 'the accident Phrensie commeth . . . through hot fume ascending from the stomacke to the braine', and 'through colligation [connectedness] of the nerues . . . which the braine hath with the midriffe'.[75]

The old animal spirits were nicely compatible with the new chemical model; after all, these substances had long been compared to the distilled spirits of wine. Of course – the iatrochemists agreed – the Galenists' understanding of these substances was woefully lacking. Fortunately, Willis had conducted his own chemical analyses, and stood ready to enlighten them: 'Animal spirits, rightly constituted, should consist of spirits with volatile salt. But if they contain sulphur rather than volatile salts (as in spirits of wine) then they are extremely ebullient and excite a phrenzy'.[76] The winemaker's vat was now a chemist's alembic: 'I have oftentimes compared the production of the Spirits from the Blood into the Brain, to a Chymical Distillation; of which it is observed, if the spirituous sulphureous liquor be provoked with too strong fire, that in Distilling it sometimes takes fire, and ascends in the *Alembick* with a very great flame.'[77]

If the chemical composition of the animal spirits had changed, in practice, their actions had remained much the same. This hot sulphureous serum, Willis explained, 'arouses the spirits to fury, moves them from their place, and agitates them so that they are driven tumultuously rendering the whole man furious'.[78] Or, as Salmon put it, 'the blood is ascended and boils . . . whereby which preternatural Effervescence, and spumeous Rarefaction of the Blood and Juices, Heterogenous and sharp Particles of Choler and other Humours are carried up, and penetrating the Pores of the Brain, put the Animal Spirits into this frantick Commotion'.[79] Whether explained in terms of soot, smoke, or sulphur, the combination of direct pipelines and poor ventilation was every bit as dangerous as it sounds.

Burnt matter was not the only hazard, for even well-concocted humours had an expiry date. If retained in the body for too long, they would eventually start to putrefy, releasing noxious fumes into the delicate

74 'reliquis delirium supervenit, ascendente ad caput . . . interdum vero spiritu vaporoso vel fumoso ant fuliginoso' Galen, 'De locis affectis', lib. 3, cap. 9, p. 179.

75 Bateman, *Batman vppon Bartholome*, f. 88v.

76 Willis, *Oxford Lectures*, pp. 120–121.

77 Willis, *Two discourses*, p. 183.

78 Willis, *Oxford Lectures*, p. 120.

79 Salmon, *Praxis medica*, p. 175.

passageways of the brain. This was why, for Galenists, any hiatus in the body's customary cycles of evacuation – especially defecation, urination and bleeding – was bad news. Recording her treatment of 'a maid that was so outrageous for a quarter of a year, that her friends were making means to send her to Bedlam', Mildmay noted that the patient had been 'exceeding costive [constipated] and had other unnatural stoppings in her body'.[80] It was only after a course of laxatives had 'opened her obstructions . . . that she began to be a little more quiet'.[81]

Alongside the bladder and the guts, female bodies could also evacuate humours via the womb. This was a positive asset, in humoral terms; in fact, the menstruating body was often described as the gold standard in efficient evacuation.[82] But when this system went wrong, it went badly wrong. According to Forman, frenzy often developed 'in those who haue not their Courses [menses] well. but stopt on them and then their matrix [womb] is ful of melancoly and burnte blod the fumosity wherof ascendeth to the braine'.[83] Willis, of course, reframed the process in Helmontian terms: given that the 'blood of females is richer in fermentative particles than that of males', 'if this kind of matter is not completely expelled . . . it is regurgitated into the blood and deposited with the nervous liquor in the brain'.[84] This was why these conditions occurred 'in women and virgins who suffer from suppressed menses', Willis explained. A failure to bleed after giving birth was even more perilous: 'indeed if the lochia are suppressed women rarely escape'.[85] This much was common knowledge: if any part of the afterbirth was retained in the body, it would corrupt at a terrifying speed.[86] In 1630, John Hall wrote of his twenty-four-year-old patient Anne Jackson: 'after childbirth, as she was not well purged, she fell suddenly into a severe *phrenitis* with no other illness appearing'.[87]

80 Pollock, *With Faith and Physic*, p. 120. 81 Ibid.

82 Gianna Pomata, 'Menstruating Men: Similarity and Difference of the Sexes in Early Modern Medicine', in Valeria Finucci and Kevin Brownlee (eds.), *Generation and Degeneration: Tropes of Reproduction in Literature and History from Antiquity to Early Modern Europe* (Durham, NC: Duke University Press, 2001), pp. 109–152.

83 Oxford, Bodleian Library, MS Ashmole 355, p. 133. 84 Willis, *Oxford Lectures*, p. 89.

85 Ibid.

86 Leah Astbury, 'Being Well, Looking Ill: Childbirth and the Return to Health in Seventeenth-Century England', *Social History of Medicine* 30(3) (2017), 509–510.

87 Hall, 'Curationum', p. 142. Hall borrowed this phrasing from the *observationes* of the Swiss physician Felix Platter. Platter had treated the original case of postpartum *phrenitis* in January 1593. 'Pverpera iuuencula, non bene post partũ purgata, in graue delirium subitò [incidit] . . . Phrenetidem veram esse statim iudicaui'. Felix Platter, *Observationes* (Basel, 1614), lib. 1, p. 86.

Richard Napier saw at least fifty such cases of postpartum frenzy between 1596 and his death in 1634.[88]

Wounds

In its textbook Galenic definition, *phrenitis* had never been a strongly age- or gender-related disease. Being naturally hot-blooded and choleric, men below the age of fifty were more 'subiect to hot feuers, frenzies, and diuers other diseases' than any other group.[89] But that was as far as it went; whereas *melancholia* went on to spawn gendered variants, frenzy did not.[90] But one consequence of rolling *phrenitis* and *paraphrenitis* together into one catch-all diagnosis was that the disease *did* end up with distinctly gendered lines of causation. Menstrual obstructions and obstetric complications were risk factors only for women; for men, on the other hand, frenzy was likelier to arise in the wake of a cut or a blow. And, despite Willis's insistence that 'the blood of females is richer in fermentative particles than that of males', men's wounds seemed to fester all the same.

Head injuries were known to be especially dangerous. One of Napier's frantic patients, the thirty-three-year-old Thomas Stiles, had been 'frighted with 2 fellows that fell vppon him & wounded him in the head . . . with a long staffe & felled him & [he] bled abundantly'.[91] Seven years had passed since the attack, but Stiles was still 'mutch amiss'.[92] A similar case had been reported in East Suffolk some sixty years earlier: a fishmonger's servant named Andrew Prince had been struck 'so sore and grievous stroke upon the head that the same stripe did perish and . . . the same Andrew became frantic therewith'.[93] When, around 1671, the civil war veteran Rowland Hughes had his stipend stopped on report that he had 'abused and rayled at the Justices of the Peace', his neighbours begged for pardon on account of his 'Phrenzy'. They explained that

> dureing the sayd warres [he had] been sorely bruised and wounded in severall parts of his body and especially the head to the brackeing and

[88] Philippa Carter, 'Childbirth, Madness, and Bodies in History', *History Workshop Journal* 91(1) (2021), 31.

[89] Peter Lowe, *The whole course of chirurgerie* (London, 1597), sig. D3v.

[90] See Burton, *The anatomy*, pp. 193–195.

[91] Lauren Kassell et al. (eds.), *The Casebooks of Simon Forman and Richard Napier, 1596–1634: A Digital Edition*, https://casebooks.lib.cam.ac.uk, case 53649.

[92] Ibid., cases 53649, 55170, 58292.

[93] Kew, The National Archives (hereafter TNA), C 1/1344/51.

> crushing of his scull-bone whereby he is not onely becomen in the nature of a Lunaticke, insensible of reason or understanding but very prone at severall tymes to scowle, rayle and rave.[94]

That frenzy could follow in the wake of such an injury was apparently too self-evident to need much explaining. 'For such is the formation of the head', Salmon explained, 'that whatsoever Wound happen in its Skinny or Carnous Substance, it may easily, by a Fracture of the Skull, be communicated to the *Meninges*, and the Brain itself.'[95] When 'you are call'd to such a Patient', Wiseman advised, 'you shall enquire . . . whether he vomited, or was stupified at the first receipt of the Blow or Fall, or a Resolution of the Nerves followed . . . or *delirium*, or raving; these shew the Membrane of the brain affected, and the Patient in great danger'.[96]

Wiseman's junior colleague at the Restoration court, the surgeon-in-ordinary John Brown (1642–1702), had heard of many such cases. He recounted the case of a 'Lad of 15 years of age' who

> having received a Contused Wound about his *Bregma* [top of the skull], with Fracture, the Wound being at first dilated, and the pieces of bones extracted, it was brought to a happy suppuration, and all evil Symptomes disappeared. The Eleventh day being past, the Child being vexed, and moved to Anger, suddainly fell into a Fever, and Phrensie, so that in four dayes after he dyed; he being dissected, the Membranes of the Brain were found inflamed, and both the Ramifications of Veins and Arteries much tumified with blood.[97]

The story went to show, Brown concluded sadly, 'what strength Passion is in young Children'. What decided the difference between life and death was not necessarily the severity of the wound, or the success of the surgery, but the capacity of the patient to manage his or her own passions.

Passions

That a fit of anger had ended in frenzy would have surprised none of Brown's predecessors. For those well read in medicine, it would have belonged to a set of health-related factors known as the 'six non-naturals': sleep, exercise, environment, repletion/evacuation, diet, and – last but not

94 'The petition of Rowland Hughes of Rhiw, Carnarvonshire, c. 1671–1673', in Andrew Hopper et al. (eds.), *Civil War Petitions* (2017–2022), www.civilwarpetitions.ac.uk/petition/the-petition-of-rowland-hughes-of-rhiw-carnarvonshire-c-1671-to-1673/.

95 William Salmon, *Ars chirurgica* (London, 1698), p. 151.

96 Richard Wiseman, *A treatise of wounds* (London, 1672), p. 84.

97 John Brown, *A compleat discourse of wounds* (London, 1678), p. 148.

least – the passions. The 'non-naturals' had earned their somewhat awkward name because they were not strictly *of* the body, or not in the way that humours were; the passions, for example, were technically actions of the 'soul'.[98] Yet this did nothing to diminish the force of their effects upon the body. As the surgeon Peter Lowe reminded his readers, 'the motion and perturbations of the minde, bringeth great motions and mutations to the naturall heate' and thus 'many die by the motions and perturbations of the minde'.[99]

Among all the passions, the most notorious inciter of frenzy was anger, for it was simultaneously

> an ardent heat or ebulission of bloud done in the heart, with desire of vengeance: whereof come euill accidentes, this inflameth the whole habitude of the body, causeth feuer, because by the inflamation of the heart, the spirit and bloud are troubled, likewise the braines and nerues, of the which commeth Frenzie and diuers other accidents.[100]

Napier attended just as closely to his patients' passions as he did to their bodies. And, although he did judge some cases of frenzy to have been brought on by anger, he was not simply deferring to the ancients. In plenty of cases, he decided that the ruling passion was not anger, but grief, fear, or disappointment. Of his nineteen-year-old patient Harry Peace, for example, he wrote that the young man had 'growen starke mad by meanes of a cruelle Aunte that whipped him naked with a carte whippe in the night & threatened agayne by her ranne out at night in his sherte to the minister of that towne & since is growen starke mad & cryeth out agaynst his Aunt'.[101] Harry was 'frenticke with grefe', Napier concluded. This was not a figure of speech; the distress caused by his aunt had sickened Harry, body and mind. This notion was still feasible sixty years later. Frenzy, Willis wrote, was often incited by 'violent passions, as of Love, hatred, envie, indignation or sadness; or immoderate studies: for these kind of occasions render the Blood and Animal Spirits, growing Feavourishly hot, very propense to the frantick Distemper'.[102]

Although Willis had ditched the Galenic 'non-naturals', he knew from experience that passions were among the 'evident causes of the *Phrensie*'.[103] Despite all the changes to humoral physiology ushered in by men like

98 See Elena Carrera, 'Anger and the Mind–Body Connection in Medieval and Early Modern Medicine', in Elena Carrera (ed.), *Emotions and Health 1200–1700* (Leiden: Brill, 2013), pp. 95–146.

99 Lowe, *The whole course of chirurgerie*, sig. F4v.

100 Ibid., sig. G1v.

101 Kassell et al., *Casebooks*, case 19336.

102 Willis, *Two discourses*, p. 184.

103 Ibid.

Willis, there was enough continuity of thought about the mediating role of the animal spirits to sustain the belief that extreme passions could cause disease.

Signs

Behaviour

The relationship between the passions and disease was a two-way street: a fit of extreme passion could be a cause of frenzy, but it could also be a sign of the disease. Of course, this was a symptom which could be detected only in proxy signs: crying, laughing, shouting, blushing, and so on. As historians of emotion have long argued, all such displays were acts of communication, and their recipients were as quick as anyone alive today to detect someone going off script.[104] There seem to have been several criteria for identifying a fit of passion as madness: its duration, intensity, and tone were all subject to careful scrutiny. Most fundamental, however, was its aptness to the circumstances. For, as the English apothecary Thomas Johnson put it, 'what man that was well in his wits, did ever fall into a laughter, unlesse he formerly knew, or saw somewhat said or done, which might yeeld occasion of laughter?'[105] Laughter was sane when it was merited by laughable events, and this was a fundamentally collective verdict. Failing to adhere to it showed a fault in the faculty of reason; and this failure could mark out any show of emotion as madness.

Learned medicine was nothing if not systematic, and its theorists could not resist the urge to code these behavioural signs in humoral terms. The passions caused by the disease, they decided, differed according to the mixture of blood or choler at fault. Mildmay wrote out the standard Galenic line into her notes: frenzy was caused 'either by abundance of blood, and then they will be subject to laugh and to conceive pleasant objects, or blood mixed with choler, and then they will be furious and

[104] See Rosenwein, *Anger's Past*; Rosenwein, *Emotional Communities*; William Reddy, *The Navigation of Feeling: A Framework for the History of Emotions* (Cambridge: Cambridge University Press, 2001); Monique Scheer, 'Are Emotions a Kind of Practice (and Is That What Makes Them Have a History)?', *History and Theory* 51 (2012), 193–220.

[105] Ambroise Paré, in Thomas Johnson (trans.), *The workes of that famous chirurgion Ambrose Parey* (London, 1634), p. 39. The original author of this rhetorical question seems to have been Paré's son-in-law, pupil, and translator Jacques Guillemeau, for it does not appear in the original French *Oeuvres* (Paris, 1575). Johnson relied chiefly on Guillemeau's Latin translation, the *Opera Ambrosii Parei* (Paris, 1582).

angry'.[106] A century later, Salmon echoed the old refrain: 'If it is from adust choler, the Sick is raving Mad, and fit to be bound'; if 'from Blood ... then it is observed that the Sick is affected with a foolish laughter'. Choler, as we have seen, was the hot, dry, combustible bile; even in good health, an individual whose humoral complexion was dominated by choler was liable to be hot-tempered. Blood, on the other hand, made for a sanguine temperament: cheerful, easily amused, amorous, and sociable. Frenzy took these natural tendencies and amplified them to the point of social aberration.

Of course, what counted as socially aberrant behaviour depended on a particular set of social norms, and those norms were always gendered. 'I have seene many both men and women in this disease', Forman claimed, and he marked a difference between the two. Whereas 'the men will saie what art thou a Constable or iustice what woldeste thou haue whie comeste thou hether', the women would become 'over lecherouse'. In both cases, this was a sign that the sufferer's body had departed from its 'natural', sex-determined temperamental range. As we have seen, the humoral difference between men and women had consequences not only for bodily health but also for mood, personality, and behaviour. A naturally phlegmatic woman whose body was suddenly inundated with burning blood or choler would develop 'hot stones', shown in her increased boldness and 'lechery'. Under the same conditions, a man would be likelier to start a fight. This, at least, was Forman's experience. Why the same humoral change should produce such different behaviours in men and women was a question he did not attempt to answer.

The identification of these temperament-specific behavioural signs was in large part the work of medieval and early modern medical theorists. They had not had much to work with, for the definitive signs of *phrenitis* listed by the ancients were surprisingly few: fever, mental alienation, wheyish urine. The only behaviour which pointed unambiguously to *phrenitis* was the plucking motion of the fingers variously referred to as 'picking at straw' (*karphologia*) and 'pulling at wool' (*krokydism*). Galen had described these phrenetic hand gestures in three different books, and his words were dutifully paraphrased by his early modern readers.[107]

[106] Pollock, *With Faith and Physic*, p. 119.

[107] McDonald, 'Concepts and Treatments', pp. 133–135; Galen, 'De locis affectis', lib. 4, cap. 2, pp. 226–227; Galen, 'On the Differentiae of Symptoms', in Ian Johnston (trans.), *Galen: On Diseases and Symptoms* (Cambridge: Cambridge University Press, 2006), pp. 191–192. For a few early modern paraphrases, see Andreas Hyperius, *Two common places taken out of Andreas Hyperius* (London, 1581), sigs. F6r–F6v; John Cotta, *A short discouerie* (London, 1612), pp. 61,

Sufferers of frenzy, Salmon noted, were 'apt to . . . pick Straws, play with Feathers, and sometimes pull the Sheets, but with a trembling hand'.[108] Returning to the self-taught medicine of Mildmay, Forman, and Napier, however, this gesture is nowhere to be found. If it appears once in their notes on frenzy, it is lost in a thicket of description. According to Forman,

> they that haue this kind of madnes or frensy will singe and Rime. and never leaue talkinge and playing with their handes and whirring them Round aboute on another. & will laugh moch and will out of the bed naked and about the house and clymb up to the top of the house. yf they get loose and will teare their apparrelle and kerchefes . . . and many tymes they wil sodeinly catch them that stand by. and bite them by the Arms or handes and knawe the shites [sheets] and sing baudy songes and Rimes and say come Kisse me or come to bed to me which is a signe of moch lechery and that yt comes by a Reuoltion of Nature.[109]

Despite its lack of learned citations, Forman's list of signs has its own distinct logic: all of these behaviours conform either to the classic 'sanguine' and 'choleric' subtype: laughter, boldness, unbridled physicality. Although in this instance Forman had neglected to sort these behaviours either by ruling humour or by sex, his other comments (quoted above) suggest that he would have had no trouble doing so. What counted as a 'Reuoltion of Nature' depended on what was 'natural' to the temperament in question, and – in humoral theory – that specific nature was always inflected by sex.

As Galenism began to lose its hold, this list of signs grew shorter and simpler. In the 1660s, Willis was still asserting that '[t]he Phrensie is distinguished into Sanguineous, Cholerick, Phlegmatick, or Melancholick . . . for the Animal Spirits are wont to grow hot and burning, after a diverse manner, in this Disease, according to their various dispositions'.[110] Although the signs of frenzy still varied according to 'disposition', the humours which had once determined that temperament were becoming increasingly denatured. For Willis, as we have seen, this language was already a convenient shorthand: phlegm, properly speaking, was the 'watery' part of the blood, choler its 'saline-sulphureous' part, and melancholy the latter's 'earthy', 'feculent' dregs.[111] It was due to the high proportion of 'inflameable' sulphur and 'sharp' salt in their blood,

69; Lazare Rivière, in Nicholas Culpeper and Abdiah Cole (trans.), *The practice of physick* (London, 1655), p. 38.

[108] Salmon, *Praxis medica*, p. 174.

[109] MS Ashmole 355, p. 134.

[110] Willis, *Two discourses*, p. 184.

[111] Willis, *A medical-philosophical discourse*, pp. 58–59.

respectively, that 'Cholerick and Melancholic persons . . . are more prone to become furious'.[112] Yet, this comment aside, Willis was silent on what these 'diverse' presentations might look like. Unlike his predecessors, and unlike Salmon, he did not sketch out a 'Sanguineous' version of the disease.

There was a reason for this silence: a merry frenzy had no clear place in Willis's medical philosophy. At some point in the Interregnum period, he had been exposed to the ideas of the French philosopher René Descartes, who had lambasted the Aristotelians for their fanciful talk of 'sensitive souls' and 'attractive faculties'.[113] Living bodies, Descartes had declared, consisted of matter in motion. He had explained the organic functions once attributed to 'faculties' in mechanical terms, inspired by the hydraulic water-clocks, fountains, and automata which he had seen in his princely patrons' courts and gardens.[114] Willis was wary of the metaphysical implications of Descartes's philosophy, but his reinvention of physiology left a lasting impression. It was important for Willis to be able to account for the gestures of the body not only in corpuscular terms, but also in mechanistic ones.

And there was little in Willis's mechanistic account of frenzy that lent itself to expression in 'sanguine' or 'phlegmatic' modes. The disease mechanisms modelled in his writings varied little: the overheating of the blood volatized and bound together its 'saline' and 'sulphureous' particles; this burning, biting saline-sulphureous matter then infiltrated and inflamed the animal spirits.[115] The spirits, in turn,

> being struck as it were with madness, tumultuate not only in the Brain, but also in the *Cerebel*, and every where in the nervous Stock; wherefore, *Frantick* people not only talk idly, but breath unequally, speak aloud, strike with their fists, fling about their hands and feet, yea and stretch forth all their members with a mighty strength, and a most strong force.[116]

When the 'Saline-sulphureous Recrements of the Blood and Humours are precipitated into the Brain or its Membranes', ran Salmon's paraphrase, 'Sometimes the Sick jumps suddenly out of Bed, according as the raging

112 Willis, *Two discourses*, p. 184.

113 Robert G. Frank, 'Thomas Willis and His Circle: Brain and Mind in Seventeenth-Century Medicine', in G. S. Rousseau (ed.), *The Languages of the Psyche: Mind and Body in Enlightenment Thought* (Berkeley: University of California Press, 1996), pp. 117–118.

114 See Simon Werrett, 'Wonders Never Cease: Descartes's *Météores* and the Rainbow Fountain', *British Journal for the History of Science* 34(2) (2001), 129–147; Dennis Des Chene, *Spirits and Clocks: Machine and Organism in Descartes* (Ithaca, NY: Cornell University Press, 2001).

115 Willis, *Two discourses*, pp. 183–184.

116 Ibid., p. 182.

Animal Spirits rush violently into this or that Part or Muscle'. The spirits 'make them furious and bold, [ready] to attempt the most desperate things; [they] are apt to fight, tho' unfit for it'.[117] Given that frenzy depended more on the animal spirits 'than upon the Humors or solid parts being distemper'd, its kinds and differences are neither various nor manifold', Willis declared.[118] What could enraged, agitated spirits produce other than enraged, agitated behaviour? These signs had always been essential to the stereotype of the 'frantic' madman, but never to the exclusion of all others. Now, increasingly, the 'raging' stereotype was the only one in stock.

Speech

Alongside 'wild or frantick gestures' – Salmon continued – a key sign of frenzy was 'incongruous speech'.[119] Most medical authors described the quality of this speech in a word – 'incoherent', 'raving', 'idle' – without detailing its content. Forman, on the other hand, was characteristically fulsome. The frantic, he wrote, will 'say they see dyvells and sprites', or conversely they will

> talke moch of god & of the holy goste and sai they be or haue byne in heauen. and then they talke of witches coniurors & Juglers and then they will say: loe, wher he or they do com, or how they doe tormente them & crie out sodenly & wepe saying they pintch them or hurt them: loke sai they doe youe not see them. and haue moch ydell talke.[120]

The 'idle speeches' of Napier's frantic patients centred on all the same themes. Some described being troubled by 'ill spirits' or forsaken by good ones; the traumatized nineteen-year-old Harry Peache would cry out that his 'good spirite is gone & that he is haunted'.[121] A second theme was witchcraft. Napier's patient Sibill Fisher had begun talking 'idley' soon after she had given birth:

> She had 2 midwives the first unskilfull the 2nd froward & would not meddle with her because she was not first sent, her suspected to be a witch, the woman well laid but a weeke after fell into these fittes & at first speaking of her 2nd midwife said, what doest thou there with thy black hen & such like speeches.[122]

[117] Salmon, *Praxis medica*, p. 174. [118] Willis, *Two discourses*, p. 182.
[119] Salmon, *Praxis medica*, p. 174. [120] MS Ashmole 355, p. 134.
[121] Kassell et al., *Casebooks*, case 19336. [122] Ibid., case 15411.

Other victims accused themselves. The 'frantick' new mother Mary Boddington, Napier reported, 'speaketh she knoweth not what. Sayeth of her self that she is a witch & sayeth the devill tempted her to kill her self . . . she sayeth that the devill entred into her mouth'.[123] Napier showed no sign of taking these childbed accusations seriously. Nor did he react as we might expect an orthodox churchman would to his 'frantic' patient George Baker's claims 'that god is in him' and 'that if he be borne of the spirite he cannot synne'.[124] Only rarely did he neglect to preface these 'idle' speeches with the qualification 'sayeth that'; usually, he took care to confine all such unexpected visitations to his patients' diseased imaginations.

The frantic talk heard by Napier and Forman was surprisingly predictable: it centred on God, the Devil, witches, and spirits of variable theological pedigree. It is worth reminding ourselves that, for most of the inhabitants of sixteenth- and seventeenth-century England, the existence of some or all of these beings was nothing less than a dread-inducing reality. Dwelling excessively upon it could signal madness, but then so too could indifference. It is unclear, then, what it was about this talk that made it self-evidently 'frantic'. Sometimes, there are obvious departures from orthodox doctrine; George Baker's talk was variously blasphemous and heretical. At other times, it seems to have been the immanent presence of these beings which raised eyebrows: it was very common to believe in malevolent spirits, but not to see them or feel their pinches when others did not.

Whatever had given the game away, these practitioners and their fellow observers had detected a misalignment between the collective consensus on reality and the world experienced by the sufferer. Just as laughing or grimacing were proxy signs of disordered passions, 'idle talk' and 'frantick gestures' were proxy signs of a disordered 'phantasy' or 'imagination'. These were faculties of the sensitive soul: the 'phantasy' cobbled together new figments from old sense memories, and the 'imagination' presented them to the mind's eye. When these faculties were compromised by disease, the sufferer could see, hear, or feel anything at all – from hairs poking out of the bedsheets to devils hiding under the bed. It was *possible*, of course, that an immaterial being had made itself visible to his or her eyes only, but it was far likelier that these were the 'fantasies' (or 'fancies') of a diseased brain.

[123] Ibid., case 45836. [124] Ibid., case 70048.

Not one of the post-1640 cohort recorded the 'idle talk' of their patients in anything like the same detail as Forman and Napier. It is tempting to read this silence as a sign of the times: in the traditional timeline, the years after 1660 saw the first bloom of the 'Enlightenment' and the 'Disenchantment of the World'.[125] Whatever we make of these narratives, the tenor and pitch of polite conversation *was* changing in England in these decades. It was becoming increasingly distasteful to talk too fervently about the upcoming war in heaven – about God, the Devil, their ghostly foot soldiers, or their human recruits. In some circles, this was a deliberate policy: in post-war Oxford, for example, Willis and his fellow experimentalists had agreed to preserve a diplomatic silence on all things supernatural.

For some, the policy went beyond self-censorship. In fact, Michael MacDonald argued that it was Restoration Anglicans like Willis who deliberately reallocated delusionality – traditionally a symptom of *melancholia* – to the violent, raging sort of madness.[126] This particular claim does not stand up to scrutiny; as we have seen, seeing things that no-one else saw had been a symptom of *phrenitis* since Galen's day. There is nonetheless truth to MacDonald's conclusion: England's educated elites were making a concerted effort to pathologize religious 'enthusiasm'. Anyone who saw the Devil or heard his voice was now – by definition – mad. This is one way to interpret the apparent lack of such 'idle talk' among the patients of Wiseman, Willis, Sydenham, and Salmon. Yet it is not the only possible interpretation. Napier and Forman were not only more explicit about the content of their frantic patients' talk than these four practitioners; they were also more explicit than their academic peers. In the case of his phrenetic patient Anne Jackson, Hall had copied out a pertinent line from an earlier medical authority: 'She was enraged, chiefly with those whom previously she had most loved, though she spoke much about religion.'[127] Unlike Napier and Forman – whose working notes happen to have been preserved for posterity – Hall had compiled his manuscript with an eye to publication. Drawing a veil over the more lurid, gossip-worthy details of a patient's history was what was expected of any professional physician – not least one who had chosen to put his bedside observations in print. Hall's late seventeenth-century successors may

[125] Alexandra Walsham, 'The Reformation and the "Disenchantment of the World" Reassessed', *The Historical Journal* 51(2) (2008), 497–528.

[126] MacDonald, 'Insanity and the Realities of History'.

[127] Hall, 'Curationum', p. 142.

simply have been holding themselves to the same standard. Certainly, the fact that none of these practitioners repeated their frantic patients' words does not mean that Satan had stopped visiting diseased imaginations. Satan still loomed large in the minds of Hannah Allen (c. 1638–1668) and George Trosse (1631–1713), both of whom wrote intimate accounts of their experiences of madness in the last third of the century.[128]

Prognosis

Of all frenzy's signs and symptoms, few boded well. A typical case history of *phrenitis* in the Hippocratic *Epidemics* had ended 'Third day. General exacerbation. Fourth day. Death'.[129] None of the Hippocratic physicians' patients had survived more than eleven days. This was the logic underpinning the ancient Greek categorization of *phrenitis* as an acute rather than a chronic disease: the patient deteriorated rapidly, reached crisis point, and then either died or recovered. In cases of *phrenitis*, death was likelier.[130] An early modern physician who predicted any happier outcome was not merely making himself a hostage to fortune; he was flaunting the authority of the ancients. Most dared not. 'A Phrensie is a very acute and dangerous Disease', Salmon warned his readers, and 'for the most part it kills in seven Days time'.[131] 'The Prognostick in this Disease is always doubtful, and the event is to be instituted with an evil suspicion', Willis warned his readers.

The doctor's worst suspicions were easily confirmed by 'evil Signs'.[132] Among the most certain was the characteristic plucking motion of the fingers recorded by the ancients.[133] If the patient 'seekes haire, and there about below & vpon the bed, as threds, and haeres of the face, also feathers, or filth of the couerings, also straw, rushes, and other thinges', the surgeon Peter Lowe warned his readers, '[these] are al mortall signes'.[134] White urine or stools also foretold death, for – as Salmon explained – they signalled 'that the Choler is not carried to the Intestines to tinge the Excrements, but to the brain'.[135] Willis repeated the same list of humoral signs: 'if the Feavour be not cured and carries still the Morbific

128 Hannah Allen, *A narrative of God's gracious dealings with that choice Christian Mrs Hannah Allen* (London, 1683); George Trosse, *The Life of the Reverend Mr Geo. Trosse, later minister of the gospel* (Exeter, 1714).

129 Hippocrates (attrib.), *Epidemics*, 3.17, case 4, in W. H. S. Jones (trans.), *Airs, Waters, Places. Epidemics 1 and 3. The Oath. Precepts. Nutriment*, LCL 147 (Cambridge, MA: Harvard University Press, 1923), pp. 265–267.

130 Thumiger, *Phrenitis*, pp. 22–30.

131 Salmon, *Praxis medica*, p. 175.

132 Ibid.

133 Thumiger, *Phrenitis*, pp. 26–27.

134 Lowe, *The whole practice of chirurgerie*, sig. B2r.

135 Salmon, *Praxis medica*, p. 175.

matter to the Head . . . if the Urine be pale, if that frequent bleeding at the Nose, if Vomiting, and Convulsion happen, the *Physician* concludes death to be at hand'.[136]

The case histories recounted by the practitioners in this sample suggest that the ancients' pessimism was warranted: Hall had judged one of his newly delivered patients to be in 'great danger of death'.[137] Neither Wiseman nor Brown had succeeded in saving their phrenetic patients' lives. Returning to the case histories recorded by Forman, Napier, and Mildmay, on the other hand, the standard disease profile starts to refract back into a kaleidoscope. Some patients diagnosed with frenzy *did* die within days. Yet these were the exceptions: most of their frantic patients seem to have lived with frenzy for months, years, or decades. Some reported recovery; some lapsed in and out of episodes of illness; some seem never to have experienced relief at all. None of these three practitioners concluded that those who died had been suffering from an inflammation of the brain, and those who lived had been suffering only from a troubled mind. For them, it was not this sort of fine-tuned differentiation which made the diagnosis useful.

This is not to say that an academic physician like Hall would have approved of these practitioners' grouping together of the chronically and acutely ill under the same conceptual umbrella. The whole point of prognosis was that the rational physician was supposed to get it right; if frenzy could kill in three days or three decades, this was no use at all. If frenzy lasted for years, this meant that the initial diagnosis should have been mania. If a diagnostician *did* make this mistake, however, there was at least a plausible get-out clause: what had started as frenzy could end as mania. This was a believable enough prognostic pathway, for the two diseases were very alike. Mania 'differeth from the frenesie, because in that there is a feuer. But *Mania* commeth without a feuer', wrote Philip Barrough, the author of the bestselling medical compendium *The methode of phisicke* (1583).[138] But mania, too, was 'caused of much bloud, flowing vp to the braine ... sometime only the aboundance of it doth hurt, sometime of sharpe and hote cholericke humours, or of a hote distempure [sic] of the braine'.[139] Sometimes, the deadly fever passed without the brain ever recovering its former balance. Napier had seen such cases: when he had first encountered the 'frentick' Anne Syred in the summer of 1614, he had described her as 'very hot inward in her chest & soarli distracted in

136 Willis, *Two discourses*, p. 185. 137 Hall, 'Curationum', pp. 145–146.
138 Philip Barrough, *The methode of phisicke* (London, 1583), p. 34. 139 Ibid.

her brayne'.[140] Three years later, he made no mention of bodily heat: she was now simply 'a strange mad filthy creature'.[141]

Once again, Thomas Willis managed to preserve the phenomenon while reinventing the disease mechanism. Mania could succeed 'a long *Phrensie*', he explained, because

> the Animal Spirits (though their burning should cease) contract a vicious nature, or that the passages and Pores of the Brain are perverted, a perpetual raving oftentimes succeeds . . . Wherefore it is vulgarly said of those that are *Frantick,* and not soon Cured, that their Brains are crack'd or broken, so that after that, they are always Mad or raving.[142]

Frenzy arose when the animal spirits became 'too sulphurous'; if 'the particles of sulphur . . . joined with the salty and vinegary ones', it would degenerate into mania.[143] Like 'Stygian waters' (*aqua stygia*, a mixture of nitric and hydrochloric acid), the force of these saline-sulphurous spirits was 'corrosive' and 'most defuse [diffuse]', penetrating 'deeply' into the marrow of the brain.[144] This was why the madness became chronic: the spirits 'carve out other paths for themselves, and it is difficult for them to leave and return to their former ones'.[145] Salmon echoed Willis: 'the old Impressions of the Brain' – the ones imprinted before the disease's onset – are 'worn out', and 'the inflamed spirits being degenerated from their natural Temper, are scarcely ever reduced to their former State'.[146] If the likeliest outcome of frenzy was death, the next likeliest was lifelong madness.

Conclusion

This prognostic patchwork confirms the impression given throughout this chapter: the diagnosis available to the self-taught lay practitioner was far more elastic than the one available to the university graduate. By 1700, both these diagnoses – the lay and the academic – had narrowed in scope.

140 Kassell et al., *Casebooks*, cases 23738, 23753. 141 Ibid., case 44800.

142 Willis, *Two discourses*, p. 185. That changes to the brain could outlast the febrile diseases which had caused them was not just 'vulgarly said'. The ancient Greek historian Thucydides had observed that the survivors of the plague of Athens (430 BCE) had been 'unable to recognize either themselves or their relatives', and Galen had taken note. See Ricardo Julião, 'Galen on Memory, Forgetting and Memory Loss', in Thumiger and Singer (eds.), *Mental Illness in Ancient Medicine*, pp. 222–244. Classically educated readers knew this episode well; see, e.g., John Edwards, *The plague of the heart its nature and quality* (Cambridge, 1665), p. 8; Thomas Sprat, *The plague of Athens* (London, 1667), p. 3.

143 Willis, *Oxford Lectures*, pp. 120–121, 130. 144 Ibid., pp. 130–131. 145 Ibid., p. 120.

146 Salmon, *Praxis medica*, p. 189.

Most of the types of patients which lay practitioners had once diagnosed as 'frantic' – the victims of pox, fever, retained placentas, tumours, ulcers, contusions, concussions, and wounds – were now simply 'delirious'. Those who lived with chronic mental alienation were now likelier to be described as 'mad', 'melancholy', or both. Yet this new diagnostic precision was bought at the cost of a loss of flexibility: it was no longer possible to explain injuries to the passions, the faculties, the organs, the humours, and the spirits with the invocation of a single word.

Even the learned physicians' *phrenitis* had been put to the test, as successive waves of theoretical innovation presented new threats to its integrity. But, in the end, frenzy emerged from these intellectual revolutions more or less intact. Like the humoral framework which had given it birth, its flexibility was key to its success. It had long hovered somewhere between a disease and a symptom; Sydenham's insistence that it was only ever a symptom or complication of febrile illness did it no lasting harm. It was just as easily translatable into the terms of the new chemical, corpuscular, and mechanical physiologies. In 1746, its onset was still being blamed on 'nitro-sulphureous, salt, sharp, or pungent Particles', which 'being mixed together . . . disturb the whole Mass of Blood, which they inflame by Means of a quick Circulation'.[147] The core physiological processes driving the distemper – heat, corruption, inflammation – could be explained in any number of ways. If frenzy had long been associated with one or two humours, it had never been defined by them. The demise of humoralism was no great blow; the models changed, the basic diagnosis did not. Frenzy had outlived the very framework which had brought it into being.

[147] Peter Frings, *A Treatise on phrensy* (London, 1746), p. 22.

CHAPTER 2

Anatomizing the Mind

Introduction

Frenzy was a disorder of the fluid economy of the body; it was caused by burnt or corrupted bile or blood. But to speak of fluids is to tell only half the story, for – as we saw in the last chapter – the disease was also supposed to have a particular anatomical seat: the brain and its meninges. Yet early modern medical theorists' understandings of these body parts and their functions were no more static than their understandings of the disease; in fact, over the course of the fifteenth and sixteenth centuries, the anatomy of the human body was undergoing transformations every bit as radical as its physiology. At the same time as frenzy was being reconfigured to fit new physiological models, it was also being folded into a newly articulated brain. In this chapter, we will look at how the relationship between brain structure, function, and disease was puzzled out by early modern anatomists, focusing in particular on the work of Thomas Willis. Willis and his contemporaries could boast of having the edge on their Renaissance forebears: they were able to conduct post-mortem dissections not just on criminals, but on their own deceased patients. The new acceptability of private autopsy among the elites of Restoration England allowed these physician-anatomists to systematically correlate the behavioural signs of brain disease with the appearance of the organ at death.[1] Yet, despite their empiricist rhetoric, these anatomists' models were 'never pure': they were

[1] Robert L. Martensen, '"Habit of Reason": Anatomy and Anglicanism in Restoration England', *Bulletin of the History of Medicine* 66(4) (1992), 518–524. The practice of private autopsy was already common in Renaissance France and Italy. According to David Harley, a series of high-profile forensic investigations introduced it to England in the 1610s, and paved the way for its more widespread uptake. This did not happen overnight; William Harvey managed to autopsy more friends, relatives, and fellow academics (presumably considered fair game) than private patients. Only in the 1650s did English physicians start to enjoy steady success in patient recruitment. See David Harley, 'Political Post-Mortems and Morbid Anatomy in Seventeenth-Century England', *Social History of Medicine* 7 (1994), 1–28.

never fashioned only from the raw materials proffered by the dissected brain.[2] They were built from many other materials too – whether memories of frantic patients, observations of non-human behaviour, or verses from scripture – and they were also designed to accommodate what *those* data suggested about the nature of the human mind. The totalizing effects of frenzy upon the mind, I argue, was a particularly urgent stimulus to Willis. It drove him to puzzle out a model of brain–mind relations which would simultaneously explain the effects of brain disease *and* preserve his most deep-seated beliefs: in the pre-eminence of the human being above all other creatures, and the untraversable ontological divide which separated the rational soul from all other souls.

Anatomical Localization

To 'Physicians conversant about diseases of the Head', the Restoration physician Walter Charleton (1619–1707) wrote in 1669, it was 'evident . . . that the Seat and principal Organ of the *Intellectual Faculties* is the *Brain*; and that they are more or less perfect in their Operations, according to the divers temperament, magnitude, figure and schematism of that Noblest Organ'.[3] Anatomy, physiology, and pathology were closely intertwined in Charleton's mind, and no wonder: these areas of medical knowledge had long been mutually co-productive.[4] The definition of the disease known as *phrenitis* had long depended on where one believed the mind sat in the body, and the disease, in turn, had always furnished the best proof of that location.[5] For most of the ancient Greek physicians, the seat of both the *phrēn* and *phrenitis* had been the diaphragm. Only with the triumph of Galenism in late antiquity and (in the Latinate world) the Middle Ages had the brain-based nature of both phenomena become self-evident.[6]

Galen's understanding of brain–mind relations had been profoundly informed by his experiences with 'diseases of the Head', and especially by

[2] Steven Shapin, *Never Pure: Historical Studies of Science as if it was Produced by People with Bodies, Situated in Time, Space, Culture, and Society, and Struggling for Credibility and Authority* (Baltimore, MD: Johns Hopkins University Press, 2010).

[3] Walter Charleton, *Two discourses* (London, 1669), pp. 40–41.

[4] 'Physiology' and 'pathology' (in the narrowest sense of these words) did not gain currency until the seventeenth century, but – as names for distinct branches of medical knowledge – they would not have been completely unintelligible to earlier thinkers.

[5] McDonald, 'Concepts and Treatments', pp. 100–120, 139–141; Thumiger, *Phrenitis*, pp. 95–110.

[6] Singer and Thumiger, 'Introduction', p. 1.

his clinical encounters with *phrenitis*.[7] One of those encounters had been too close for comfort. As a young man, he recounted,

> [when] stricken by a burning fever in summer, I thought that little sticks of dark straw were protruding from my mattress, as well as pieces of wool from my gown. I attempted to pull these out . . . When I heard two friends that were present telling each other 'he is pulling wool and plucking straw', I understood that I had the affection of which they spoke, but I realized that I was not deranged in my reasoning faculties and said 'What you say is right, but help me that I should not suffer from phrenitis'.[8]

Elsewhere, Galen recounted the history of an anonymous patient who had begun to throw household utensils from his window, pausing with each one to ask

> those passing if they would order him to throw. He spoke the name of each of the utensils quite precisely, from which it was clear that he was neither damaged in the imagination about these things nor in the memory of their names. Why then did he wish to throw all these things from a high place and shatter them? This he was no longer able to understand, but by the act itself he was manifestly delirious.[9]

For Galen, the disease had deranged the imaginative faculty and yet left the reason intact: he had soon grasped that the straw sticking out of his mattress was unreal. The anonymous patient had been in precisely the opposite condition: everything had been left intact *except* for his reason.

There was no question, then, that the presentation of *phrenitis* depended on which of the 'ruling powers' (*hēgemonikon*) had been affected. For Galen, however, clinical observation alone was not enough; the proof of the pudding lay on the dissecting table. Human heads were strictly off-limits in imperial Rome, but the heads of goats, oxen, and sheep were fair game, and Galen cut open hundreds of them, both dead and alive. It was on this raw evidence that he built his working model of the brain. Although for Galen no part of the organ was without a function, in his view, its solid structures served primarily as the scaffolding for the corridors of power within: a series of interconnected cavities known today as the ventricular system. He counted four ventricles (as neuroanatomists

[7] Thumiger, *Phrenitis*, pp. 95–117.

[8] Galen, 'On the Affected Parts', in Rudolf Siegel (trans.), *Galen on the Affected Parts* (Basel: Karger, 1976), p. 108; in 'De locis affectis', lib. 4, cap. 2, pp. 226–227.

[9] Galen, 'De locis affectis', lib. 4, cap. 2, pp. 226–227; 'On the Differentiae of Symptoms', in Ian Johnston (trans.), *Galen: On Diseases and Symptoms* (Cambridge: Cambridge University Press, 2006), pp. 191–192; Siegel (trans.), *Galen on the Affected Parts*, p. 108.

still do), two anterior, one middle, and one posterior. These were the flow channels of the *pneuma*, Galen concluded, and this was why their injury instantly impaired the ruling powers of the *psychē*. He proved this claim on the exposed brains of still-living animals (mostly pigs and oxen), compressing the two front ventricles would send the animal into a light stupor, compressing the middle would send it into a deep stupor, and compressing the rear brought about 'a very heavy and pronounced' stupor.[10]

Although Galen was certain that the flow of *pneuma* through the ventricular system was crucial to the workings of the *hēgemonikon*, he categorically refused to localize its various operations (reasoning, etc.) within that architecture. None of the many brains he had cut open, he believed, had yielded sufficient evidence to merit this sort of speculation.[11] But Galen's late antique followers could not resist the urge to fill in the blanks. And, just as *phrenitis* had prompted Galen to disaggregate the faculties of the *hēgemonikon*, so too it seems to have prompted these later Galenists to allocate each faculty its own seat within the brain. The earliest surviving account of 'ventricular localization', attributed to the fourth-century physician Posidonius of Byzantium, survives in a later Byzantine medical encyclopaedia.[12] And it appears not in a section on normative anatomy, but in the chapter on *phrenitis*:

> There are many different forms of *phrenitis*, but three are most important: . . . If the front part of the brain is harmed, only the *phantastikon* (imagination) is damaged; in cases where the middle ventricle of the brain is harmed, a derangement of the *logistikon* (reason) occurs, but if the hinder part of the brain in the occiput is harmed, the *mnēmoneutikon* (memory) perishes, but together with it generally also the other two.[13]

Posidonius had taken two different sets of observations which Galen had made – his anecdotes about the diverse clinical presentations of *phrenitis*, and his descriptions of dissected quadruped brains – and superimposed the one onto the other. When Galen had pressed down on each ventricle in turn, the only difference in function which he had noticed was the depth of the animal's stupor. But combining Galen's anatomy of the ventricular

[10] Galen, 'Book IX: On the Brain', in Wynfrid Laurence Henry Duckworth (trans.), *Galen on Anatomical Procedures: The Later Books* (Cambridge: Cambridge University Press, 1962), pp. 17–19; Julius Rocca, *Galen on the Brain: Anatomical Knowledge and Physiological Speculation in the Second Century A.D.* (Leiden: Brill, 2003), ch. 5.

[11] Rocca, *Galen on the Brain*, pp. 196–199, 245–247.

[12] Ricarda Gäbel, 'Mental Illnesses in the Medical Compilations of Late Antiquity: The Case of Aëtius of Amida', in Thumiger and Singer (eds.), *Mental Illness in Ancient Medicine*, pp. 315–340.

[13] Aëtius of Amida, *Libri medicinales*, trans. Gäbel, in ibid., pp. 326–327.

system with his clinical observations allowed Posidonius to go one step further: it allowed him to offer a full explanation of the diverse manifestations of *phrenitis*. When the inflammation reached one of these three parts of the ventricular system, it disrupted or corrupted the *pneuma* flowing through it, and thus disturbed the faculty located in that part.

By 400 CE, the Christian bishops Nemesius of Emesa and Augustine of Hippo were producing their own versions of this brain–mind map.[14] By the thirteenth century, there were so many variants circulating in the Greek-, Latin-, and Arabic-speaking worlds that it would be impossible to do them all justice here.[15] But the textbook version inherited by sixteenth-century English readers was at least relatively straightforward. It ran as follows: the organ of the brain was covered by two membranes (the *meninges*); the outer, harder meninx was known as the *dura mater* (the 'tough mother') and the inner, softer one as the *pia mater* (the tender mother). Under the *pia mater* lay the brain, which was solid except for the three hollow cells (often called 'ventricles') at its core. For followers of Galen, the *pia mater* also reached down into the substance of the brain to line the walls of each ventricle.[16] Thus, in Stephen Bateman's 1587 translation of Bartholomaeus Anglicus, the *pia mater* not only 'keepeth & knitteth the brain togethers, that it flow not neither fail by the fleeting and softness thereof', but also 'departeth [parts] asunder the foresaid cells'.[17] Or, as the sixteenth-century surgeon Thomas Vicary put it, the 'Piamater deuideth the substaunce of the Brayne, and lappeth it into certen selles or diuisions, . . . or ventrikles'.[18]

The *pia mater* did not just form the cubicle partitions of the ventricular system; it also gave 'the brayne both spirite and lyfe'. Galen had noticed tiny webs of capillaries (*plexus choroïdes*) lining the walls of the four ventricles, and had identified them as extensions of the *pia mater*.[19] From this inner membrane, Vicary glossed, sprang 'a great number' of

[14] See Jessica Wright, *The Care of the Brain in Early Christianity* (Oakland: University of California Press, 2022).

[15] For a sense of this diversity, see Edwin Clarke and Kenneth Dewhurst (eds.), *An Illustrated History of Brain Function* (Oxford: Sandford, 1972), pp. 10–48; Ynez Violé O'Neill, 'Meningeal Localization: A New Key to Some Medical Texts, Diagrams and Practices of the Middle Ages', *Mediaevistik* 6 (1993), 211–238; Christopher D. Green, 'Where Did the Ventricular Localization of Mental Faculties Come From?', *Journal of History of the Behavioural Sciences* 39(2) (2003), 131–142; William MacLehose, 'The Pathological and the Normal: Mapping the Brain in Medieval Medicine', *Progress in Brain Research* 243 (2018), 23–53.

[16] Galen, 'De usu partium', in Kühn (ed.), *Claudii Galeni Opera Omnia*, vol. 3, book 8, pp. 656–657.

[17] Bateman, *Batman vppon Bartholome*, f. 37r.

[18] Thomas Vicary, *A profitable treatise of the anatomie of mans body* (London, 1577), sig. D2v.

[19] Galen, 'De usu partium', in Kühn (ed.), *Claudii Galeni Opera Omnia*, vol. 4, ch. 16, pp. 331–335.

veins and arteries, which 'ramefying throughout al his substaunce . . . goo foorth of him, and enter into the diuisions of the brayne, and there drinketh of the brayne substaunce'.[20] This was why the *pia mater* had earned the name of the 'tender mother', Vicary explained: 'it is so softe and tender ouer the brayne, that it nourisheth the brayne and feedeth it, as doth a louing mother vnto her tender childe or babe'.[21] And this was not the only reason why these membranes were known as 'mothers'. According to Galen, they also reached out to cover the whole nervous system: first descending from the base of the brain down the spinal column, and then branching off to coat each individual nerve.[22] The marrow at the core of each nerve was like the pith of a tree; the *pia mater* like the soft inner rind, and the *dura* like the outer protective coat.[23]

The development of this ventricular theory has sometimes been depicted as an attempt to relocate the 'rational soul' from the solid parts of the brain to the breath-like animal spirits.[24] But, as Jessica Wright has shown, this is an oversimplification. The advocates of ventricular localization had always stressed that all parts of the brain – the solid parts, cavities, humours, *and* spirits – had to be in good working order for the soul to be able to exercise its powers properly. The dominant conceptual metaphor, Wright suggests, was the musical instrument: 'ventricular localization signalled not the displacement of rational faculties from the brain substance to the pneuma, but, as in a lyre, the collaboration between structure, air, and strings'.[25] It took a terrible discord between these parts to produce a true *phrenitis*.

The complexity and diversity of these early models of ventricular localization inevitably complicated the question of where the disease took hold. The Byzantine medical encyclopaedists had settled on the meninges as the site of the characteristic 'aposteme' (abscess).[26] But at some point in

[20] Vicary, *A profitable treatise*, sigs. D1v–D2r. [21] Ibid., sig. D1v.

[22] Galen, 'De Hippocrat. et Platonis decretis libri IX', in Kühn (ed.), *Claudii Galeni Opera Omnia*, vol. 5, pp. 602–604.

[23] Ibid., p. 602.

[24] Walter Pagel, 'Medieval and Renaissance Contributions to Knowledge of the Brain and Its Functions', in F. N. L. Poynter (ed.), *The History and Philosophy of Knowledge of the Brain and Its Functions* (Oxford: Blackwell, 1958), pp. 97–100; Stanley Finger, *Minds Behind the Brain: A History of the Pioneers and Their Discoveries* (Oxford: Oxford University Press, 2000), p. 53; Tullio Manzoni, 'The Cerebral Ventricles, the Animal Spirits, and the Dawn of Brain Localization of Function', *Archives Italiennes de Biologie* 136 (1998), 103–152.

[25] Jessica Wright, 'Ventricular Localization in Late Antiquity: The Philosophical and Theological Roots of Enduring Model of Brain Function', *Progress in Brain Research* 243 (2018), 3–22, quotation on p. 18.

[26] Gäbel, 'Mental Illnesses in the Medical Compilations', pp. 315–340.

the disease's passage into the Arabo-Islamic medical canon, it seems to have spread to the brain. Thus, in his *Canon of Medicine*, the tenth-century Galenist Ibn Sīnā (known in Latin as Avicenna) wrote that while *karabitus* (*phrenitis*) was the proper name for a hot 'aposteme in the coverings of the brain', it was also thought 'acceptable in some places sometimes to use it to refer to an aposteme in the substance of the brain'.[27] The steady expansion of frenzy's intracranial coordinates over the centuries helps us to understand the ambivalence of early modern medical authors on the subject. For Bateman, following Bartholomaeus, it was an 'impostumation bread [bred] & ingendered' in the *pia mater*; for Lady Grace Mildmay, it was simply an 'inflammation of the phlegms [films] of the brain'.[28] Others preferred to hedge their bets: 'the frenisy is an inflammacion of the brain or the filmes therof', declared Barrough in 1587.[29] Most later English medical authors followed suit.[30]

As vernacular medicine continued to expand alongside the learned tradition, some linguistically amphibious authors began to depart even from Barrough's open-ended definition. One fascinating example can be found in the medical astrologer Simon Forman's unpublished manuscript, his 'book of the judgement of diseases' (c. 1600). He began the chapter on frenzy with a (fairly) standard Latin definition: '*Frenesis* is an abscess which occurs in the anterior cell of the head. It is called *frenesis* after the *phrenes* or membranes which encircle the brain, where this abscess occurs'.[31] But mid-way through this discussion, he paused to add: 'and somtyme yt taketh the Newek of the back and then they ar hard to be Cured'.[32] The 'newek' or 'nuke' (in Latin, *nucha*) referred to the spinal cord, and particularly to the part contained by the seven cervical vertebrae – in other words, the area corresponding to the nape of the neck.[33] Given what has been said about the Galenic belief that the inner sheath coating the spinal marrow was an outgrowth of the *pia mater*, it made sense that an inflammation of the 'mother' might affect the whole. In fact, given that

[27] 'karabitus, & sirsen est nomen proprium apostematis velaminis cerebri, quum est calidum, licet in quibusdam locis quandoque concedatur etiam dici de apostemate substantiae cerebri'. Avicenna [Ibn Sīnā], *al-Qānūn*, lib. 3, fen 1, tract. 3, cap. 1, in *Arabum medicorum principis*, p. 468.

[28] Bateman, *Batman vppon Bartholome*, f. 88v; Pollock, *With Faith and Physic*, p. 119.

[29] Barrough, *The methode*, p. 17.

[30] See, e.g., London, British Library, Sloane MS 640, f. 64v; Robert Bayfield, *Enchiridion Medicum* (London, 1655), p. 6; Salmon, *Praxis medica*, p. 173.

[31] 'Liber juditiorum morborum', Oxford, Bodleian Library, MS Ashmole 355, p. 133.

[32] Ibid.

[33] Juhani Norri, *Dictionary of Medical Vocabulary in English, 1375–1500* (Abingdon: Ashgate, 2016), s. v. 'nucha'.

Galen had found that the fourth ventricle sat much lower down than the first three – adjacent to the base of the skull – neck problems might have been positively expected.

And yet (to the best of my knowledge), 'taking' of the neck was not a sign of frenzy discussed by any of the authors of the *practica*. Nonetheless, Forman wrote, 'I have seen many of these [frantic patients]'.[34] Even Napier, Forman's unlikely protégé, had seen at least one. On 4 July 1597, the husband of a local charwoman named Alice Scot came to consult with the rector on behalf of his sick wife. The disease 'tooke her in the neck in the morning as she was charring at Rawson', he reported. Napier's verdict was grim: '*phrenesis*. death'. He seems to have been right; he later wrote that Scot had died 'about a week after'.[35] Forman was more of a copyist than an innovator, and – if his reference to the 'Newek' looks novel – it may be simply that I have not managed to trace its source. Yet it may also afford us a rare glimpse of bedside experience deviating from book learning. If so, it is no less remarkable for the fact that – unlike most of the signs in the learned *practica* – a seized-up neck is still legible as a sign of meningeal inflammation today.

The precise location of frenzy was still up for debate at the beginning of the seventeenth century, as indeed was the map of the ventricular system. Forman counted 'but 3 Ventrikells, yet the formost is diuided into 2 partes. and soe som call them 4'.[36] In 1616, the London College of Physicians' newly appointed lecturer in anatomy, William Harvey (1578–1657), counted four, but noted of the fourth: 'Some deny that it is a ventricle.' This aside was immediately followed by another: '[There are] those who dispose the faculties according to the ventricles, like [Michael] Scot, Thomas [Aquinas], Albertus [Magnus], &c., [who] locate memory here.'[37] The juxtaposition of these two lecture notes hints at why many early modern thinkers had trouble believing in a fourth ventricle (despite its identification by Galen and his successors). The brain needed three rooms (and not four) because it still had to accommodate the triad of faculties possessed by the Byzantine *hēgemonikon psychēs*: *phantastikon* (imagination), *logistikon* (reason), and *mnēmoneutikon* (memory). The fact that the list of cognitive faculties had grown quite a lot longer since Posidonius's day was irrelevant: there was no reason to change the basic

[34] MS Ashmole 355, p. 133. [35] Kassell et al., *Casebooks*, case 13210.

[36] MS Ashmole 355, p. 135.

[37] William Harvey, in C. D. O'Malley, F. N. L. Poynter, and K. F. Russell (trans.), *Lectures on the Whole of Anatomy: An Annotated Translation of* Prelectiones Anatomine Universalis (Oakland: University of California Press, 1961), p. 222.

seating plan. The front cell was still the work station of the faculties involved in sense perception: the 'common sense', which processed and compiled the raw data received from the sense organs; the 'imagination', which displayed the results to the mind's eye; and the 'phantasy', which cut up those sense impressions and rearranged them into more fanciful forms (e.g., collaging a horse and a narwhal horn into a unicorn).[38] The middle cell housed the 'reason' (or, in non-human brains, the 'estimation'), and the posterior cell, near the back of the skull, still housed the 'memory'.[39]

In a state of health, the front-to-back flow of spirits through these ventricles could be discerned – perhaps even physically felt – in the process of knowledge acquisition: fresh information entered the common sensorium via the external sense organs; once processed and packaged, it was sent to the middle cell for assessment, and lastly, to the memory for storage. In dreaming, fantasizing, or remembering, the process worked in reverse: sense impressions were extracted from the posterior cell and sent back to the anterior.[40] All of this required a well-nourished, well-tempered brain, an unimpeded, uninflamed network of cells and corridors, and a steady supply of pure, uncorrupted animal spirits. This was why, as the medical popularizer William Salmon put it, 'If the whole Brain is inflamed, the Sick quite loses his Reason and Understanding: If it is the Fore part only which is Inflamed, the *Imagination* is more disturbed than the Reason; but if the Back-part is only affected, the *Memory* is then lost in a great measure'.[41]

At the end of the seventeenth century, Salmon was still following his Galenic predecessors in mapping out the variant presentations of *phrenitis* onto these discrete parts of the ventricular system. Learned theorists had done the same for other diseases of mind – although there was still plenty of disagreement, both over the reliability of the map, and the question of which disease affected which part.[42] Still, there were

38 E. R. Harvey, *The Inward Wits: Psychological Theory in the Middle Ages and the Renaissance* (London: Warburg Institute, 1975); Katharine Park, 'Psychology: The Organic Soul', in C. B. Schmitt et al. (eds.), *The Cambridge History of Renaissance Philosophy* (Cambridge: Cambridge University Press, 1988), pp. 464–484.

39 See Clarke and Dewhurst, *An Illustrated History*, pp. 10–39.

40 Vesalius, *De fabrica*, 7.1, p. 623, in William Frank Richardson and John Burd Carman (trans.), *On the Fabric of the Human Body, Volume 5: Book VI: The Heart and Associated Organs, Book VII: The Brain* (San Francisco, CA: Norman Publishing, 2009), p. 164. Vesalius was not endorsing this theory, but making fun of the lecturers at Louvain who had taught it to him.

41 Salmon, *Praxis medica*, p. 174.

42 As Francis Bacon put it, 'the placing of the *Intellectuall Faculties* . . . according to the ventricles of the Braine, is not without error'. Francis Bacon, *The advancement and proficiency of learning* (Oxford, 1640), p. 185. I owe this point to Reader C.

some points of consensus: melancholia had a reputation for disordering the imagination (in the front cell); lethargy the memory (in the anterior).[43] What was different about *phrenitis* was that it could attack any and all of these parts, and thus any combination of the faculties. This was why the disease had become the classic case study of brain–mind relations. For Galen, it had served to prove that this organ (and not the heart or diaphragm) was the seat of the 'ruling powers'. For later brain cartographers, it showed that each faculty of the mind had its own dedicated room within its recesses.

Rebuilding the Brain

Salmon's 1707 description of frenzy might have passed muster with Forman, Napier, or Mildmay, but it would not have earned him much credit amongst his medical peers. Once again, he had blithely overlooked the theoretical developments of the last two centuries. From the mid-sixteenth century, a new generation of medical humanists – literate not just in Latin but in Greek – had sought to purge Hippocratic-Galenic medicine of its medieval accretions. Leading the way in human anatomy was Andreas Vesalius (1514–1564), whose magnum opus *De humani corporis fabrica libres* (1543) was in its day the most detailed and comprehensive study of human anatomy ever produced.[44]

Realizing that Galen's anatomical project had been held back by his lack of access to human cadavers, Vesalius had decided to finish it for him. And his dissections of the human brain had revealed some surprises. First, the so-called *rete mirabile* – the production site of the animal spirits – was nowhere to be found. Galen must have found the feature in ruminant brains, Vesalius inferred, and wrongly assumed its presence in human ones. His predecessor at Bologna, the cranial surgeon Jacopo Berengario da Carpi (c. 1460–1530), had in fact noted Galen's error some twenty years earlier, but had been reluctant to make a public spectacle of the ancient anatomist. As we saw, Galen had also thought that further refinement of the animal spirits would happen within the choroid plexuses, the parts of the *pia mater* which lined the walls of the cerebral ventricles; Berengario discreetly suggested that – given the absence of the *rete* in

[43] MacLehose, 'Mapping the Brain in Medieval Medicine', pp. 38–42.
[44] See Sachiko Kusukawa, *Andreas Vesalius: Anatomy and the World of Books* (London: Reaktion Press, 2024).

humans – it was the *pia mater* which served as the sole factory for the animal spirits.[45]

Vesalius, by contrast, had built his career on his capacity to make a public spectacle (even in this he was following Galen's example; his urge to share a pedestal with his ancient hero was just as strong as his urge to take him down a peg or two).[46] He scoffed at Galen for thinking that

> the cerebral substance is so soft that the ventricles carved into it would have collapsed if they were not lined on the inside by the thin membrane [the *pia mater*] . . . In fact the ventricles are not lined by membranes, for this would prevent the cerebral substance from transforming into animal spirits the material that is conveyed to the ventricles.[47]

Having loudly denounced Galen's mistaken extrapolation of the *rete mirabile* to the human brain, Vesalius refused to accept the alternative proposed by Berengario (the *pia mater*). It was nothing other than the 'cerebral substance', he claimed, which transformed 'the material that is conveyed to the ventricles' into spirits. This did not mean that the ventricles had no role to play in the production of spirits. On the contrary, Vesalius insisted,

> I have no hesitation at all in saying that the ventricles produce animal spirit, but I cannot say anything about the areas in the brain occupied by the faculties of the soul-in-chief (though the people who nowadays like to be called theologians and consequently think there are no limits to their powers allot these as well).[48]

The ventricles continually fed the cerebrum with the 'material' which it would transform into spirit. This was why the notion that they were lined by foldings of the *pia mater* was so absurd: impermeability was entirely contrary to their function. If the ventricular system still had an ancillary role in producing animal spirits, it was not the seat of the 'soul-in-chief', for the spirits sprang into action only when they reached the substance of the cerebrum. And as for localizing the soul's faculties – the evidence was too thin to warrant the attempt, and anyone who claimed otherwise was a fool (or a theologian). This was an emphatic break with the late antique brain–mind model, which at this point had held sway in Christendom for

45 Andrew Cunningham, *The Anatomical Renaissance: The Resurrection of the Anatomical Projects of the Ancients* (Aldershot: Scolar Press, 1997), p. 128.
46 Ibid., pp. 182–190.
47 Vesalius, *De fabrica*, 7.6, p. 635, in Richardson and Carman (trans.), *On the Fabric of the Human Body*, vol. 5, pp. 197–198.
48 Ibid., p. 198.

over a millennium. For those who accepted Vesalius's new brain, the standard map of ventricular localization was now as good as useless.

Brute Comparisons

A resurrected Galen might reasonably have objected that he had called ventricular localization a fool's errand back in the second century. Vesalius's attack on those who 'like to be called theologians' was probably better justified: after all, two of the three brain–mind maps surviving from late antiquity had been drawn up by bishops (Nemesius and Augustine). The fact that Harvey's 1616 list of 'those who dispose the faculties according to the ventricles' ran to three thirteenth-century scholastics – and he would have known full well that 'Scot, Thomas, [and] Albertus' were not the last to make the attempt – suggests that Vesalius's attitude may have rubbed off on him. But Vesalius and Harvey were right: theologians had had as much of a hand in developing the brain–mind map as had anatomists. No surprise, then, that the results had long been shaped by theological imperatives as well as medical ones.[49]

One was the requirement that human nature be utterly distinct from the natures of all other animals. In the Book of Genesis, the Creator God had declared: 'Let us make man in our image, after our likeness: and let them have dominion over the fish of the sea, and over the fowl of the air, and over the cattle, and over all the earth, and over every creeping thing that creepeth upon the earth.'[50] From the thirteenth century onwards, Aristotle's Christian readers had carefully integrated this ancient Hebrew account of Creation with the ancient Greek philosopher's hierarchy of souls. The 'image of God' in man, they agreed, was his most noble part: his rational soul.[51] A creature's rationality (or lack thereof) determined its place on the cosmic 'ladder of nature' (*scala naturae*), sometimes also described as 'the great chain of being'.[52] Adam was famously created

[49] Wright, 'Ventricular Localization in Late Antiquity', pp. 5–7, 12–18. For early modern theologians' engagements with anatomy, see Dennis Des Chene, *Life's Form: Late Aristotelian Conceptions of the Soul* (Ithaca, NY: Cornell University Press, 2000), pp. 45–52; Kusukawa, *Transformation of Natural Philosophy*, esp. pp. 83–107; Michael Edwards, 'Body, Soul and Anatomy in Late Aristotelian Psychology', in Gideon Manning (ed.), *Matter and Form in Early Modern Science and Philosophy* (Leiden: Brill, 2012), pp. 33–75; Davide Cellamare, 'Anatomy and the Body in Renaissance Protestant Psychology', *Early Science and Medicine* 19 (2014), 341–364.

[50] KJV, Genesis 1:26–28.

[51] See, e.g., Sir John Davies, *Nosce teipsum* (London, 1599), pp. 22, 54.

[52] See Raymond Sebond, *La Theologie naturelle de Raymond Sebon*, trans. Michel de Montaigne (Paris, 1569), chs. 1–5. Eustace M. W. Tillyard, *The Elizabethan World Picture: A Study on the Idea of Order in the Age of Shakespeare, Donne, and Milton* (New York: Knopf Doubleday, 1961); Arthur

'a little lower than the angels', but his rational soul set him well above the 'brutes'.[53] If God had declined to bestow the faculty of reason on the other species, this was because he had intended human beings to 'subdue' and 'have dominion' over them.[54]

Surely, the scholastics reasoned, God must have furnished his noblest creature with a brain of greater complexity than any of the rest. This was the conclusion reached by one thirteenth-century physician named Richard the Englishman: midway through his description of the ventricular system, he paused to remind his readers: 'this is the anatomy of the human brain and of its cells, not of brutes, because they are not believed to possess all the cells, because they do not have the middle one, just as they do not have all the faculties of the soul'.[55] Other medieval brain cartographers were more generous to their fellow creatures: rather than draw up a second map of a two-celled brain, they added an extra animal-friendly faculty to the map they already had. Whereas in humans the middle cell housed 'reason' or 'cogitation' (*cogitatio* or *vis cogitativa*), in 'brutes' it was allocated to the lesser faculty of 'estimation' (*estimatio* or *vis estimativa*).[56] The estimative faculty plugged the gap left by the absence of reason: it assessed new sense impressions, cross-referenced them with old ones, and instructed the body on how to respond. Thus, when a sheep caught sight of a wolf, the estimation – confronted with memories of danger – issued the instruction to flee.[57]

A stopgap of this sort was badly needed, for examples of beasts discerning and learning were not in short supply. As the English naturalist John Maplet wrote in his *Greene forest, or a naturall Historie* (1567),

> in some there is a certain kind of perceiueraunce [perception] and adiudging or esteeming what is what (but the same spoken of vs by resemblance and vnproperly) which we may perceive they haue through their care in

O. Lovejoy, *The Great Chain of Being: A Study of the History of an Idea* (Cambridge, MA: Harvard University Press, 1963); Marion Leathers Kuntz and Paul Grimley Kuntz (eds.), *Jacob's Ladder and the Tree of Life: Concepts of Hierarchy and the Great Chain of Being* (New York: Peter Lang, 1987).

53 KJV, Hebrews 2:7–9.

54 The landmark study remains Erica Fudge, *Brutal Reasoning: Animals, Rationality and Humanity in Early Modern England* (Ithaca, NY: Cornell University Press, 2006).

55 'et nota quod hec est anathomia cerebri humani et cellularum eius, non brutorum, quia non creduntur omnes cellulas habere, quia nec mediam sicut nec habent omnes anime operaciones'. Karl Sudhoff, 'Der "Micrologus" Text der "Anatomia" Richards des Englanders', *Archiv für Geschichte der Medizin* 19 (1927), 217.

56 Park, 'Psychology: The Organic Soul', pp. 466–473. For illustrations, see Clarke and Dewhurst, *An Illustrated History*, pp. 30–39.

57 Park, 'Psychology: The Organic Soul', p. 471; Jörg Alejandro Tellkamp, '*Vis aestimativa* and *vis cogitativa* in Thomas Aquinas's *Commentary on the Sentences*', *The Thomist* 76 (2012), 611–640.

> bringing vp & tendring their yong: as also in artificiall maner of building their Nest, in hunting and seeking after their pray, in remedying and curing woundes.[58]

Despite Maplet's insistence that he was speaking of animal judgement only by its 'resemblance' to the human faculty, and thus 'vnproperly', many of the anecdotes in his natural history seem to belie this claim. One told of 'a King in the North', who decided to breed a 'very faire Fole' with the foal's own mother. To this end,

> he seperated them the one from the other: Insomuch that one mought forget the other. And after such time had, and the Dam so attired & vsed, that the Colt should espie no apparant signe that she should be his Dam, was brought to the Mare thus vsed, frollick and lustie, and he not knowing of this, and vnwitting, fell anone to coniunction [copulation], and ere he had ended (the Dams face by chaunce discouered) he was by and by at this daunted, departing as it were in a *frensie*, and running vp vppon a certaine Mountaine, threw downe himselfe headlong, and dyed.[59]

Maplet offered no account of the thoughts and feelings which had 'daunted' this equine Oedipus, and it is hard to imagine how he would have managed one with the limited tools at his disposal. The estimative faculty was supposed to be limited to the basic kind of cost–benefit calculation described above. Subscribing to moral taboos, registering their violation, self-recognition, self-disgust – all of this should have been well beyond its compass. And yet Maplet's foal, torn from his state of 'vnwitting', apparently had wits to lose.

Nor was the notion of a horse suffering from frenzy merely the stuff of legend. In *Cauelarice, or The English horseman* (1607), Gervase Markham described the telltale signs of the disease:

> they wil haue heauy countenances, but fiery eyes, they will beat their owne heads against the walles, bite at any thing sodeenly, and as they stand they will gnawe vpon the manger; . . . and now and then beate their heads with their legs, they will forsake all foode, or if they do eate, they will snatch their meate hastily, and seldome chew it.[60]

This passage bears a distinct resemblance to the descriptions of human sufferers which we encountered in the last chapter. And the experts on equine medicine seem to have assumed that frenzy attacked all of its victims' brains in the same way, regardless of species. As Markham

[58] John Maplet, *A greene forest, or A naturall historie* (London, 1567), p. 68. [59] Ibid., pp. 89–90.
[60] Gervase Markham, *Cauelarice, or The English horseman* (London, 1607), p. 22.

explained, '*Frenzie* . . . is a fault very much incident to horses, and I haue had much experience thereof, and as farre as I can coniecture it proceeds only from the torment of the brain or pannickle, when they are either corrupted with naughty bloud, or inflamed with the heate of poisonous humors'.[61] The exact translatability of frenzy between different species does not seem to have bothered Markham. His guides to horsemanship are full of references to horses' minds; it can hardly have come as a surprise to him that they sometimes suffered from diseases of mind. But he was writing neither as a philosopher nor as a theologian: he was writing as a man who spent his days working with horses.

So, too, was the Duke of Newcastle, William Cavendish, who declared in 1658 that the fact that horses had minds was 'so well known to a complete horseman, that it is needless to say more on this subject'.[62] 'What makes scholasticks degrade horses so much', he went on,

> proceeds (I believe) from nothing else, but the small knowledge they have of them, and from a persuasion that they themselves know everything. They fancy they talk pertinently about them, whereas they know no more than they learn by riding a hackney-horse from the University to LONDON, and back again. If they studied them as horsemen do, they would talk otherwise.[63]

Not only were horses capable of thought, understanding, and memory, but sometimes they exceeded their riders in their use of these faculties: 'if a man has lost his way, let him leave the horse to himself, and the horse will find the way . . . This is fact, for I have been in the same circumstances; and I believe I should have lost my way, had it not been for my horse'.[64]

Unfortunately, anecdotes like this one had never been much help in persuading the 'scholasticks' that animals had minds. Similar accounts had been cited in the preceding century by the humanist scholars Girolamo Rorario (1485–1556), Michel de Montaigne (1533–1592), and Pierre Charron (1541–1603), who – like Cavendish – had insisted that the scholastics had vastly underestimated their fellow creatures' capacity for reason, understanding, and will.[65] These authors were writing in a moral philosophical vein, and, as such, their reflections on the nobility of the 'brutes' were really reflections on the ignobility of which human beings

[61] Ibid., p. 22. [62] William Cavendish, *A general system of horsemanship* (London, 1743), p. 12.
[63] Ibid., p. 13. [64] Ibid.
[65] See Girolamo Rorario, *Quod animalia bruta ratione utantur melius homine* (Paris, 1648); Michel de Montaigne, 'Apologie de Raimond Sebond', in *Livre des essais* (Lyon, 1593), pp. 431–626; Pierre Charron, *Le thresor de la sagesse, compris en trois livres* (Lyon, 1606), book 1, esp. pp. 67–84.

were capable.[66] At the turn of the century, however, the physician Hieronymus Fabricius (1533–1619) took this animal-positive tradition in a new direction: he rested his high estimation of animals' cognitive faculties not on the authority of the ancients, but on his own natural philosophical observations.[67] Watching and listening to animals had been enough to convince him that they were capable of complex communication, whether via gesture, facial expression, or vocalization (*loquela*).[68] For those who still embraced Thomist Aristotelianism, however, it was impossible to admit this much: using signs to signify things called for abstraction, and this was supposed to be a power unique to the rational soul.[69]

By Cavendish's day, the rise of Cartesianism had both reinvigorated and permanently altered the terms of this debate. The scholastics had thought that brutes were incapable of reason because they possessed merely sensitive souls; Descartes's claim was that they did not possess souls *at all.* The only entity which merited the name 'soul' (*l'âme, animus*), he insisted, was the human mind (*l'ésprit, mens*). Non-human animals were automata, devoid not just of reason but of conscious awareness.[70] Of all of Descartes's radical new ideas, this was the one which prompted the most immediate critical backlash. Some of his critics turned to the sixteenth-century humanists for support; others – like Cavendish – appealed to everyday experience: 'If he [the horse] does not think (as the famous philosopher Des Cartes affirms of all beasts) it would be impossible to teach him what he should do', the duke declared.[71]

Others looked for answers on the dissecting table. An avid dissector in his own right, Descartes had suggested that the pineal gland in the brain was the control centre of the rational soul, and the site of all its commerce with the body. The suggestion had been met with widespread scepticism, but it had also stimulated fresh attempts to identify a likelier alternative.[72]

66 Richard Serjeantson, 'The Passions and Animal Language', *Journal of the History of Ideas* 62(3) (2001), 436–437.
67 Ibid., pp. 438–441. 68 Hieronymus Fabricius, *De brutorum loquela* (Padua, 1603).
69 Richard Serjeantson, 'The Soul', in Desmond M. Clarke and Catherine Wilson (eds.), *The Oxford Handbook of Philosophy in Early Modern Europe* (Oxford: Oxford University Press, 2011), p. 124. For a seventeenth-century Thomist account, see Francisco Suárez, 'Tractatus de anima', in *Partis secundae summae theologiae tomus alter complectans tractatus secundum ... et tertium de anima* (Lyon, 1621), tract. 3, esp. cap. 4, pp. 21–26.
70 René Descartes, *Discours de la méthode pour bien conduire sa raison et chercher la vérité dans les sciences* (Leiden, 1637), pp. 56–60; Des Chene, *Spirits and Clocks*, pp. 93–94.
71 Cavendish, *A general system of horsemanship*, p. 12.
72 See Robert L. Martensen, *The Brain Takes Shape: An Early History* (Oxford: Oxford University Press, 2004), chs. 3–4.

What these post-Cartesian anatomists were looking for was a divine hallmark – ideally, one unique to the human brain – which would serve as both philosophical proof and physiological explanation for the superiority of the human soul to all others.[73] The trouble was that Vesalius had already made this search more than 100 years before, and had found no such structural anomaly. In his *De fabrica*, he had announced with characteristic certitude that '[i]t is a fact that the brain of a sheep, a goat, an ox, a cat, an ape, a dog and even of certain birds that I have dissected shows virtually no difference from the human brain in respect of the conformation of the parts, and especially in respect of the ventricles'.[74]

There was no structural difference significant enough to account for the supposed incommensurability of human and non-human souls. Given that the 'brains of quadrupeds ... resemble men in all of their parts', the Flemish anatomist mused, the unschooled could be forgiven for ascribing to them 'every power of reason, and even a rational soul, contrary to the doctrines of the theologians'.[75] The number and form of the cerebral ventricles was the same. If there *was* a correlation between the organ and the soul, Vesalius concluded, it was not in its shape but in its proportions: 'We do, however, know that there is a difference in size according to the amount of reason that they seem to possess: man's brain is the largest, followed by the ape's, the dog's, and so on, corresponding to the amount of rational force that we deduce each animal to have.'[76] This was not a solution which would have satisfied many theologians (as Vesalius was well aware). Rationality was not supposed to be meted out on a sliding scale, and certainly not by the square inch. Animals were not supposed to have a certain 'amount of reason'; they were not supposed to possess the faculty at all.

In 1669, Charleton was still marvelling at Vesalius's boldness: 'the Prince of Anatomists in the last age, expresly, not without derision of those who believed and taught the contrary, affirms, that the Fabrick of Mans Brain is not in the least different from that of the Brains of Brutes'. The English physician found this passage from *De fabrica* so 'remarkable,

[73] William F. Bynum, 'The Anatomical Method, Natural Theology, and the Functions of the Brain', *Isis* 64(4) (1973), 466.

[74] Andreas Vesalius, *De humani corporis fabrica libri septem* (Basel, 1543), 7.1, p. 624, in William Frank Richardson and John Burd Carman (trans.), *On the Fabric of the Human Body, Volume 5: Book VI: The Heart and Associated Organs, Book VII: The Brain* (San Francisco, CA: Norman Publishing, 2009), p. 165. All further quotations from Vesalius's *De fabrica* are taken from Richardson and Carman's English edition.

[75] Vesalius, *On the Fabric of the Human Body, Volume 5*, trans. Richardson and Carman, p. 165.

[76] Ibid.

the great Authority of the man considered', that he decided to quote it in full.[77] 'To this You'l answer perhaps', he continued,

> that such indeed was the judgement of Vesalius; but You are not obliged to acquiesce therein, because You have lately not only read a certain Book, *de Proprietatibus Cerebri Humani*, wherein the Author observes many considerable Differences betwixt the Humane Brain, and those of all other Animals; but also with Your own eyes behold those Differences demonstrated by the same Author, in some Dissections for that end made by him at the command of the Royal Society.[78]

Yet, even granting 'that there really are those Differences betwixt Man and all other Animals', Charleton went on, nobody was any better equipped than before to explain the nature of the interface between the rational soul and the brain. Even 'the Author of that Treatise' had been obliged to admit 'that notwithstanding his frequent observation of those Differences, he was still as ignorant of the principal seat of the soul, and what parts she made use of in her several Functions, as before he first entred into the Anatomick Theatre'.[79]

The author to whom Charleton referred was, of course, Thomas Willis. The irony was that – although Willis certainly had been looking for these 'Differences betwixt Man and all other Animals' – he was far from satisfied that he had found them. He had apparently succeeded in concealing his disappointment in the *Cerebri anatome* (or at least he had concealed it from Charleton), but it came through eight years later in the preface to *De anima brutorum* (1672). Given that he had 'shewn, by comparing the Corporeal Soul of the Brute, with the Rational of Man, what vast difference there is between them', Willis pre-empted his reader, it might seem 'to the purpose, to compare the Brains of either, and to observe their differences. But this Anatomy being elsewhere made [in the *Cerebri anatome*], we have noted little or no difference, in the Head of either, as to the Figures and Exterior Conformations of the Parts, the Bulk only excepted'.[80]

Vesalius had been right (although Willis did not once mention him by name), no ventricle, gland, or structural configuration was missing or deficient in the non-human brain. With all due respect to Descartes, the pineal gland could not possibly be the seat of the rational soul, for 'Animals, which seem to be almost quite destitute of Imagination, Memory, and other superior Powers of the Soul, have this glandula or

77 Charleton, *Two discourses*, p. 41. 78 Ibid., pp. 43–44. 79 Ibid., pp. 45–46.
80 Willis, *Two discourses*, p. 44.

kernel large and fair enough'.[81] Despite this unpromising start, Willis persevered in his search for a hallmark of human difference in the fabric of the brain.[82] There was little interspecies variation to be found in the hard cerebellum sitting at the base of the skull; thus, Willis concluded, it had to be responsible 'for certain necessary offices, which are performed in all after the same manner ... [e.g.] the motions of the Heart and Respiration'.[83] Willis took the opportunity to cluster all the 'brute' faculties in this lower tier of the brain: thus, the adjacent *corpus striatum* (the 'streaked body') was assigned sense perception and motion, while the surrounding nerves served 'the Functions, wont to be performed by the Instinct of Nature, or the force of the Passions, rather than by the beck of the Will'.[84]

It was the 'Bulk' of the cerebrum, Willis declared – Vesalius would doubtless have rolled his eyes – which varied noticeably between species. Not only was its proportionate size larger in man, but its

> folds or rollings about are far more and greater in a man than in any other living Creature, to wit, for the various and manifold actings of the superior Faculties ... Those Gyrations of Turnings about in four footed beasts are fewer, and in some, as in a Cat, they are found to be in a certain figure and order.[85]

If the cerebrum varied from species to species, it *had* to be the home of the faculties which had been unequally endowed by God. *This*, then, was the 'region of the Brain where the principle [sic] faculties of the knowing or understanding soul reside'.[86] The fewer the folds and the more predictable their pattern, the simpler and more predictable the brain-based operations of the soul. Of course humans had been given the most intricately folded cerebrum, for what other creature was capable of such 'various and manifold actings of the superior faculties'?[87] After their winding journey through the cortex, the next stop for the spirits was the *corpus callosum* (the harder white matter). As the common 'Mart or Exchange of the Spirits', this 'callous body' had to serve as the site of the 'Imagination'. Finally, funnelled through the narrow passageway of the fornix, the spirits were 'made more subtil', and there performed the 'more subtil acts of the Phantasie'.[88] Despite all the alterations, Willis's brain still resembled the old Aristotelian version in some respects: 'common sense', 'imagination', and 'phantasie' had changed room, but they were still bedfellows.

81 Willis, 'Anatomy', p. 106. 82 Willis, *Two discourses*, p. 44. 83 Willis, 'Anatomy', p. 112.
84 Ibid., pp. 102–103, 111–112. 85 Ibid., p. 92. 86 Willis, *Two discourses*, p. 153.
87 Willis, 'Anatomy', p. 92. 88 Ibid., p. 93.

Willis was very ready to admit that his new blueprint of anatomical localization was mostly speculation, and his peers did not let him forget the fact.[89] Only a year after the publication of the *Cerebri anatome*, the Danish polymath Nicolaus Steno (1638–1686) damned Willis with faint praise: 'We know so little of the true structure of the *corpus callosum* that a reasonably intelligent person may say about it whatever he likes'.[90] But if Willis's new model was speculative, it was not arbitrary. This was a carefully stratified brain. The basic autonomic functions – formerly the 'vegetative' faculties – sat at the very bottom, in the hindbrain. The following layers gradually advanced from the 'instinctive' or passion-driven functions (in the mid-brain) to the imagination (in the *corpus callosum*), through to 'knowing and understanding' (in the uppermost cerebral hemispheres). Willis had built Aristotle's bottom-up ladder of souls into the bottom-up structure of the brain. In quadrupeds, the order was reversed. This was why,

> The figure of the Skull in four-footed beasts is narrow and prest down, but in man, . . . his face is erect or lifted up: so the brain it self is placed in a more eminent place, to wit, above the Cerebel and all the Sensories. But in Brutes, and such whose faces are prone towards the Earth, and have a brain unfit for speculation, the Cerebel, however serving to the more noted action and office of the Praecordia, is placed in the highest seat to which the mole [mass] of the brain is subjected.[91]

The notion that the 'dignity of man' was evidenced by his upright posture and the angle of his gaze had been a staple of renaissance humanism.[92] But it also fit nicely with Willis's new cerebral materialization of the scale of nature. In a human brain, the rational soul sat in the throne room of the cerebrum, elevated above its inferiors. In a non-human brain, the centre of autonomic functions took precedence, and the cerebrum was 'subjected' to its directives.

The task of differentiating between 'man' and 'brute' was especially imperative for Willis, for he was unwilling to follow Descartes in denying them souls. He had been persuaded instead by Descartes's friend and

89 Bynum, 'The Anatomical Method', p. 452.

90 'Certes, le corps calleux nous est si inconnu, que pour peu qu'on ayt d'esprit, on en peut dire tout ce qu'on veut'. Nicolaus Steno, *Discours de Monsieur Stenon, sur l'anatomie du cerveau* (Paris, 1669), p. 12.

91 Willis, 'Anatomy', p. 78.

92 See, e.g., Maurice Scève, *Microcosme* (Lyon, 1562), pp. 7–8; Guillaume du Bartas, *La sepmaine, ou creation du monde* (Antwerp, 1579), p. 184; Constantinos A. Patrides, *Premises and Motifs in Renaissance Thought and Literature* (Princeton, NJ: Princeton University Press, 1982), ch. 5.

intellectual opponent Pierre Gassendi, who 'in his late Experimental Philosophy'

> had enumerated very many Instances, by which the Cunning and Wonderful Sagacity of brute Animals were declared; and also the Epithets, whereby these kind of Animals are noted by Philosophers, to wit, that some are called *Excelling in Knowledg*; others *Artificial*, these Dexterous and Compleat, or Crafty and Wise, at length the Author adds, that, *These things could not deservedly be attributed to them, unless they granted them a certain kind of Reason*.[93]

Willis himself had heard many such 'admirable Histories', especially of 'the Subtilties and Craft of the Fox', who – it was said – 'might allure the Hens within the Compass of his Chain, with which he was tyed, lying all along, his legs stretched forth, feigns as if he were dead, then they coming near him, he readily leaps upon them'.[94] This behaviour could not be explained without resort to premeditation: 'notions so arising from one faculty or power, answer to Actions drawn from another, from thence is produced a certain Kind of Discourse or Ratiocination, and often times it is continued by a certain Series or Thrid [thread] of Argumentation'.[95]

The low, 'subjected' position of quadruped cerebrum made it 'unfit for speculation', but it did not make it unfit for remembering, or even (in some animals) for thinking. The larger and more complex the brain, the more complex the train of thought it could sustain. This was why 'in a Man, Dog, Fox, and other more sagacious Creatures', the mid-brain protuberances known as the *nates* (today known as the inferior colliculi) were 'marrowy thorow the whole'. Other less 'sagacious' creatures – 'Sheep, Ox, and many four-footed Beasts' – had a less extensive distribution of 'marrow'.[96] The same was true of the folds of the cerebrum. 'A cat thinks on, or remembers scarce any thing but what the instincts and needs of Nature suggest', he declared, and this simplicity was reflected in the simple, regular gyri of its brain.[97]

On the face of it, Willis had made an advance on Vesalius's comparative anatomy: in the greater complexity of the human brain's gyri, he had identified a key structural variance which preserved the category difference between 'man' and 'brute'. Yet, from a theological perspective, this explanation was no more satisfactory than those offered by his Renaissance predecessors. As Bynum argued in 1985, Willis and his fellow natural

[93] Willis, *Two discourses*, p. 4. [94] Ibid., p. 37. [95] Ibid., p. 37. [96] Ibid., p. 27.
[97] Willis, 'Anatomy', p. 92.

theologians wanted to have their cake and eat it: they argued that the minor structural differences which they found in human brains reflected the superiority of 'Man' to all other species, but – at the same time – they continued to insist that the fundamental likeness of human and non-human brains was proof that the difference was not one of bare anatomy but of ensoulment.[98] Human beings possessed reason not because they had more folds in their brains than any other species, but because God had endowed them – and them alone – with rational souls.

Ultimately, Willis had not succeeded in finding incontrovertible anatomical proof for this insurmountable metaphysical boundary. If brains differed only by degree of complexity, then it was all too easy to infer that cognition, too, differed only by degree and not by kind.[99] Vesalius had teased 'the theologians' by dangling this prospect under their noses, but, for Willis, this was no laughing matter.[100] The study of nature *was* theology, and – as one of its faithful students – it was his duty to nip heterodoxy in the bud.[101] This was why he was at pains to stress that what Gassendi had called '*a certain kind of Reason*' was only a faculty *like* reason. Even in the subtlest of beasts, 'the most Intricate Actions of Brutes, which seem to contain Ratiocination, may be explained, and reduced into Competent notions of the sensitive Soul'.[102] What *seemed* like ratiocination could in fact be reduced down to simpler operations: memory, 'Natural Instinct', 'Phantasy', and 'Sense'.[103]

To say that animals could 'think' in this limited way was far from radical; these faculties had belonged to the old scholastic 'sensitive soul' too, and 'estimation' had plugged the gap between them. But, given the profound influence which Gassendi had on Willis's thinking, the latter's insistence on the old category difference between human reason and non-human estimation is significant. Although Gassendi had been right in saying that animals were capable of thought, he had overstepped the mark in saying that 'the difference seems merely to be

[98] Bynum, 'The Anatomical Method', esp. pp. 454–477.

[99] For later expressions of this idea, see Pierre Bayle, 'Pereira', in *Dictionnaire historique et critique* (Rotterdam, 1697), vol. 2, part 2, p. 785; Joseph Priestley, *Disquisitions Relating to Matter and Spirit* (London, 1777), p. 235, cited in Charles T. Wolfe, 'Boundary Crossings: The Blurring of the Human/Animal Divide as Naturalization of the Soul in Early Modern Philosophy', in Stephanie Buchenau and Roberto Lo Presti (eds.), *Human and Animal Cognition in Early Modern Philosophy and Medicine* (Pittsburgh, PA: University of Pittsburgh Press, 2017), pp. 147–172.

[100] Vesalius, *De fabrica*, 7.1, p. 624, in Richardson and Carman (trans.), *On the Fabric of the Human Body*, vol. 5, p. 165.

[101] Bynum, 'The Anatomical Method', pp. 444–468.

[102] Willis, *Two discourses*, p. 38.

[103] Ibid., pp. 38–39.

one of degree'.[104] The French philosopher, like Fabricius before him, had pointed to animal language in support of this claim:

> You say they do not speak ... You may say that even a delirious man can still string words together to express his meaning, which even the wisest of the brutes cannot do. But surely you are not being fair if you expect the brutes to employ human language and are not prepared to consider their own kind of language.[105]

Self-expression through language was not the sole prerogative of humanity, and it, too, came in degrees of perfection. A delirious man could become less capable of coherence (in his own tongue) than 'the wisest of the brutes' in theirs. Although Willis's comparative anatomy – with its subtle gradations of cerebral complexity – seemed like the ideal support for Gassendi's claim, he refused to lend it to the cause. 'Brutes' and 'men' could not be permitted to sit at two different points on the same sliding scale of rationality.

And yet brain disease did nothing to lessen the disconcerting impression that the difference between animal and human reason was one of degree and not of kind. It seemed to shove its human and non-human sufferers from their rungs on the ladder of nature with the same terrible ease. Some kinds could even hop species; the catching nature of 'canine madness' (known to learned physicians as *hydrophobia*) was all too familiar to the inhabitants of early modern England.[106] Frenzy was not catching, at least, but it inflamed non-human brains in just the same way as it did human ones. Perhaps horses and dogs – possessing only an ersatz 'estimation' in place of reason – were thought to have less far to fall than their human counterparts. But, if so, this metaphysical difference produced no discernible difference in the behaviour of sufferers.

Relocating the Disease

Willis had been pondering these problems long before he had started opening heads. On his appointment as Oxford's Sedleian Professor of Natural Philosophy in 1660, he was asked to lecture on the same subject as his predecessors: 'the Offices of the Senses, both external and also internal, and of the Faculties and Affections of the Soul, as also of

[104] 'nihil videtur discriminis, nisi secundum magis & minus'. Pierre Gassendi, 'Objectiones quintae', in Charles Adam and Paul Tannery (eds.), *Oeuvres de Descartes* (Paris: L. Cerf, 1904), vol. VII, p. 271.

[105] Ibid. [106] See Burton, *The anatomy*, pp. 9–10.

the Organs and various provisions of all these'.[107] These lectures were supposed to introduce students to the time-honoured primer on the subject: Aristotle's treatise *On the soul* (*De anima*).[108] But Willis's syllabus took an unexpected turn: after a brief introduction to 'the Faculties and Affections of the Soul', he spent the rest of the lecture series discussing their catastrophic malfunctions: 'Delirium', 'Phrenzy', 'Mania', and 'Stupidity'.[109] At this point, Willis had spent around fourteen years making his living as a physician; he must have ministered to many mentally disturbed patients in that time. For some reason – whether because he had found these cases clinically puzzling, personally taxing, or both – the memories had stayed with him.

None of the available accounts of brain–soul relations had been able to provide him with a satisfactory explanation of what had being happening in these patients' heads. This was why, Willis explained,

> thenceforward I betook myself wholly to the study of Anatomy: and as I did chiefly inquire into the offices and uses of the Brain and its nervous Appendix, I addicted my self to the opening of Heads especially, and of every kind, and to inspect as much as I was able frequently and seriously the Contents; that . . . some truth might at length be drawn forth concerning the exercise, defects, and irregularities of the Animal Government; and so a firm and stable Basis might be laid, on which not only a more certain Physiologie than I had gained in the Schools, but what I had long thought upon, the Pathologie of the Brain and nervous stock, might be built.[110]

It was his preoccupation with 'the Pathologie of the Brain and nervous stock' which had spurred him to anatomize those parts in such exhaustive detail.[111] The *Cerebri anatome* promised to 'declare more aptly the Causes of the Symptoms, and shew the Reasons of Curing more accommodate to every Disease. I doubt not that this way may be an help . . . for the more happy Curing of Cephalick [head] diseases'.[112] Anatomy was to give rise to a new, 'more certain Physiologie'; 'Physiologie' to 'Pathologie', and that, in turn, to more certain cures.

Willis had an edge on his predecessors in being able to join the dots between anatomy, physiology, and pathology. In England, the notion that a private physician might cut open his deceased patient's diseased body after death – under completely unsuspicious circumstances – had only

107 Willis, 'Anatomy', sig. H4r.
108 Louis Caron, 'Thomas Willis, the Restoration, and the First Works of Neurology', *Medical History* 59(4) (2015), 541–542.
109 Willis, *Oxford Lectures*, pp. 118–122, 130–138.
110 Willis, 'Anatomy', sig. H4r.
111 Ibid.
112 Willis, *Two discourses*, sig. A4v.

recently gained acceptance.[113] For the first time, a request for a post-mortem autopsy was not only a sane directive for an English patient to make – it was a positively forward-thinking one.[114] The fact that so many of Willis's elite clients *did* consent to being autopsied was crucial to his achievements. It allowed him to correlate external observations with interior lesions, with an exactitude which the haphazard dissection of criminal bodies had never allowed. Just as importantly, it meant that he was able to base his claims on the bodies of former organs of church and state: clergymen, statesmen, scholars, and aristocrats. Willis was at pains to stress not only the high status of his autopsied patients, but also their moral excellence: one 'very noble Lady' had been 'highly indued with a virtuous disposition, of minde and manners' before the onset of her disease.[115] This was more than just namedropping on Willis's part: the status of Willis's dissected subjects was vital to the validity of his arguments.[116] In the hierarchical world of Restoration England – one in which nobility of soul, mind, and status were still expected to dovetail – a general model of brain–mind relations could never have rested squarely on the heads of criminals.

We saw in Chapter 1 how the practice of post-mortem autopsy had led Willis to doubt the validity of *paraphrenitis*: he had seen patients die sound in mind only to discover their gruesome chest infections. The practice also confirmed his doubts about *phrenitis*. After all, he declared in 1683,

> I have often seen in Anatomical Dissections, the *Meninges*, yea sometimes also the exterior compass of the Brain, beset with an inflamed tumor, and the sick not distemper'd with a *Phrensie*, but on the contrary with a stupidity, and have dyed with a *Carus*, or some other sleepy Diseases. And truly, that it is so, reason plainly declares; for the *Meninges* being inflamed, and by that made more tumid, press together the Brain very much, and about its compass shut up the ways and passages of the Spirits; . . . far otherways in the *Phrensie*, all the passages and Pores of the Brain, for the excursions of the Spirits, seem to be too largely open, because the Images hidden or laid up, are raised all at once, out of the utmost, and all the places of the memory, which together with others, suggested from the Phantasie to the common sensory, tumultuously, bring forth such manifold and highly confused notions.[117]

Frenzy could not be an inflammation of the meninges, or of any other solid part of the brain. For one thing, there was no discernible correlation

[113] Martensen, '"Habit of Reason"', pp. 518–524; Harley, 'Political Post-Mortems', pp. 1–28.
[114] Plenty of moribund patients – not to mention their friends and relatives – begged to differ.
[115] Willis, 'Of convulsive diseases', in *The remaining medical works*, p. 83.
[116] Martensen, '"Habit of Reason"', pp. 519–521. [117] Willis, *Two discourses*, p. 181.

between the clinical signs observed in life and the pathological ones observed after death. For another, the notion made no conceptual sense: 'tumid' matter could only constrict the 'passages and Pores of the Brain', the resulting blockage of the spirits would – and did – result in a stuporous, coma-like state.[118]

There was only one viable solution: the inflammation had to be moved from the solid substance of the brain to the fluids running through its cavities. Thus, Willis explained,

> the blood burning Feavourishly, doth pour forth on the Brain sometimes sulphureous Particles, ... [which] immediately entring into all the marrowy and nervous passages, adhere everywhere to the spirits, and so render them being inflamed, highly rageing and implacable. Certainly it is more likely, that the *Phrensie* is rather excited after this manner, by an inflammation of the Spirits, than from that of the *Meninges*or of the Brain, which more surely causes an Headach or Lethargy, than a Fury, as we have frequently found by *Anatomy*.[119]

For this explanation to work, Willis had to shake loose from his readers' imaginations the common-sense assumption that 'inflammation' was something that happened to the solid parts of the body. This was not the familiar state change heralded by pain, swelling, and redness of the flesh. The word needed to be taken at face value: like any inflammable gas, the volatile spirits could literally ignite.

This great conflagration of spirits took place, not in the ventricles, but in the substance of the brain. The ventricles could not even be credited with supplying the cerebrum with pre-spiritous 'material' (*pace* a still-unnamed Vesalius); the 'yellow and salt *Serum*' which Willis had found pooling in these cavities was far too viscous and unpleasant for that.[120] It was the *arteries* which supplied the brain with the 'material' it needed; the spirits were distilled directly from the arterial blood into the 'marrowy and nervous passages' of the cerebrum.[121] The ventricular system was simply 'a drain for clearing away the serous filth' that remained.[122]

Frenzy was nothing less than a 'burning or inflammation of the whole sensitive soul, or animal spirits', Willis insisted.[123] But if the 'rageing and implacable' motions of those spirits continued long enough, they would ultimately leave their marks on the marrow of the brain. Whereas in 'delirium the spirits are only lightly irritated and traverse and disturb only

[118] Ibid., p. 182. [119] Ibid., p. 183. [120] Willis, 'Of convulsive diseases', p. 33.
[121] Willis, *Two discourses*, p. 183; Willis, *Oxford Lectures*, p. 138.
[122] Willis, *Oxford Lectures*, pp. 139–140. [123] Willis, *Two discourses*, p. 183.

their own paths', he explained, in frenzy, '[they] are driven tumultuously rendering the whole man furious: they continue to do so until the matter is completely blown away and dissipated, which does not happen quickly'.[124] After a while, 'on account of their violent motion, [the spirits] carve out other paths for themselves, and it is difficult for them to leave and return to their former ones'.[125] This was why, after 'a long *Phrensie*', because

> the passages and Pores of the Brain are perverted, a perpetual raving oftentimes succeeds, the former Disease passing into Madness, or Melancholy ... Wherefore it is vulgarly said of those that are *Frantick*, and not soon Cured, that their Brains are crack'd or broken, so that after that, they are always Mad or raving.[126]

Sulphurated spirits bit new grooves in the soft copperplate of the marrow; the deeper those tracks, the harder they became to undo. This idea seems to have been Willis's invention (although it probably owed something to Descartes's model of brain function). It remains strikingly consonant with twenty-first-century notions of neuroplasticity.

And yet it did not catch on. Perhaps, in reframing frenzy as an inflammation of the 'sensitive soul', he was simply asking too much of his seventeenth-century readers. Inflammations were fleshy phenomena – everyone knew that. Inflamed membranes were easily observed, and inflamed blood was imaginable (dark blood was understood to be its burnt recrements). Visualizing the inflammation of invisible, intangible 'souls' or 'spirits' was a much harder ask.[127] Most of Willis's readers seem to have preferred to base their understandings of frenzy on firmer foundations. As we saw, an autodidact like Salmon was still embracing the old cellular model at the end of the century.

Even the cutting-edge comparative anatomist Samuel Collins begged to differ with his Oxford colleague. 'While Dr. *Willis* is of an Opinion, that a *Phrenitis* doth proceed from an inflammation of the Animal Spirits, and not from the coats of the Brain', Collins ventured in 1685,

> I humbly conceive (with the leave of this Learned Physician) That the Phrensie is not only deducible from an effervescence of the nervous Liquor, and Animal Spirits, but from an inflammation of the Membranes of the

124 Ibid., p. 183; Willis, *Oxford Lectures*, p. 120. 125 Willis, *Oxford Lectures*, p. 120.
126 Willis, *Two discourses*, p. 185.
127 This is not to say that the idea was implausible to everyone but Willis. On the contrary, Neoplatonist and Paracelsian thinkers had long held that *spiritus*, communing with and partaking of both the immaterial and the material, could become infused with the latter's qualities (including heat).

> Brain, proceeding from an extravasated Blood, lodged in the Interstices of the Vessels, seated in the substance, belonging to the Membranes, encircling the ambient parts of the Brain, by reason the putrid indisposition of the Blood.[128]

Collins could meet Willis on his own turf, for he too had conducted 'Dissections of the Heads of Persons dying of Phrensies', and had found the *pia mater* 'often inflamed without the tumor of the substance of the Brain'.[129] Thus, in one patient, 'the Brain was bespecked with Red spots, derived from extravasated Blood; And the Membranes, and especially the Pia mater was tumefied, being distended with blackish Blood and the Branches transmitted through the substance of the Brain, did seem to be swelled and inflamed, which were imparted from the *Pia mater*'.[130] The root of the disease was in once again in the *pia mater*: the inflamed vessels reaching out from that membrane down into the 'substance of the Brain' had bled out onto the marrow.

Despite his polite amendments, Collins was evidently deeply influenced by Willis: he still gave the 'effervescence of the nervous Liquor, and animal Spirits' a lead role in causing the disease.[131] And yet, in moving the inflammation back to the familiar terrain of the meninges, Collins had more in common with pre-Vesalian brain cartographers than with Willis. And – although it was Willis who would be remembered as the father of neurology – on this point, history was on Collins's side. *Phrenitis* was still being used to describe an inflammation of the *pia mater* at the turn of the nineteenth century. It was retired only after the coinage of two new clinical diagnoses: 'encephalitis' (1798), and 'meningitis' (c. 1828).[132]

Conclusion

Willis has gone down in history as the discoverer of the nerves, the man who turned the brain from an unknown 'bowl of curds' into the solid structure we recognize today.[133] This story is not altogether without

[128] Samuel Collins, *A systeme of anatomy* (London, 1685), p. 1141. [129] Ibid.
[130] Ibid., p. 1142. [131] Ibid., p. 1141.
[132] Conrad George Ontijd, *A treatise on mortal diseases* (London, 1798), p. 223; John Abercrombie, *Pathological and Practical Researches on Diseases of the Brain and the Spinal Cord* (Edinburgh, 1828), p. 51.
[133] Zoltán Mólnar, 'Thomas Willis (1621–1675), The Founder of Clinical Neuroscience', *Nature Reviews Neuroscience* 5 (2004), 329–335; Carl Zimmer, *Soul Made Flesh: How the Secrets of the Brain Were Discovered in Seventeenth-Century England* (London: Penguin, 2005); Katie Birkwood, 'Thomas Willis: The Father of Neurology', *Royal College of Physicians Online*, 20 May 2016,

substance; he and his collaborators did identify several new anatomical structures in the brain, and depicted their findings in a series of extraordinarily detailed and persuasive images.[134] Yet one consequence of Willis's entry into the annals of history as 'the founder of clinical neuroscience' has been a tendency to downplay the centrality of fluids to his understanding of the brain and its diseases. Focusing on frenzy has told another sort of story about this seventeenth-century anatomist: in fact, it has turned the traditional story on its head. The traditional Galenic accounts of the disease had centred on some decidedly solid parts – whether the meninges, the brain, or the ventricular system. Willis went further than any of his predecessors – and most of his successors – in moving the inflammation from the solids found inside the head to the spirits running through them.

His account did not catch on. But then, as we have seen, the question of where frenzy took its anatomical 'seat' – and how it did its damage – had never remained settled for long. And the basic account of the disease's actions did not require an answer. For this much was clear: for the brain to perform its duties as the mind's instrument, what was required was an unbroken exchange between fluids (humours, spirits) and solids (membranes, nerves, vessels). The mental alienation seen in victims of frenzy could stem from any disruption to that exchange. And, as we saw in Chapter 1, this story of brain–soul communications – and how they failed – was robust enough to endure any number of edits. Frenzy had endured several physiological regime changes; it was not about to be made redundant by a simple restructuring of the brain. When Willis decided that the 'superior faculties' had to be moved out of the ventricular system and into the cerebrum, the disease came along with them. When he found no sign of meningeal inflammation at autopsy, he shifted the inflammatory load onto the animal spirits. *Of course* there was no inflammation to be seen: the spirits were not visible to the naked eye, and – in any case – they had evaporated as soon as the brain was opened.

The arch-empiricist Thomas Sydenham had nothing but scorn for this brand of speculative anatomy. To talk of 'nervous juice' was all very well, Sydenham declared, but 'tis certaine the anatomist of all men, if he be true to his principles, should not suppose it, since he ought not to believe anything but what he sees, and when he makes it visible others may believe

https://history.rcplondon.ac.uk/blog/thomas-willis-father-neurology. Note that these authors were not necessarily writing with a readership of academic historians in mind, and I do not wish to criticize them for prioritizing interest and narrative coherence over the nitty-gritty.

[134] Alexander Wragge-Morley, 'Imagining the Soul: Thomas Willis (1621–1675) on the Anatomy of the Brain and Nerves', *Progress in Brain Research* 243 (2018), 55–56.

it too'.[135] Sydenham, for one, was not holding his breath. It was a fair criticism: arguing from an absence of evidence – in this case, an absence of inflammation – was hardly best practice for a supposed advocate of Baconian empiricism.

But there is no reason to think that Willis was not in earnest in reconfiguring frenzy as an inflammation of the spirits. It would have served neither the advancement of 'Medical Science' nor the 'Curing of Cephalick Diseases' for him to make up a novel disease mechanism just for the sake of it.[136] Besides, it was not just the look and feel of autopsied tissues that had led Willis to rethink the 'Pathology of the Brain and Nervous Stock'.[137] It was his clinical observations of his patients – and of the violent changes that 'irregularities of the Animal Government' had wrought in their speech and behaviour – which had made him a brain anatomist in the first place.[138] It was his realization – after years of comparative dissection – that no structure in the brain *except* for the cerebrum could possibly hope to account for the psychic difference between 'man' and 'brute' which had forced him to move the 'superior faculties' there.

It was no small task for Willis to line up his observations of his disturbed patients, his findings on the dissection table, and his knowledge of the nature of the soul. His model of frenzy was carefully engineered to save these disparate phenomena. The disease was easily localized to the cerebrum, for this was the site of the 'superior faculties' whose impairment signalled its onset. It inflamed the spirits, for only 'rageing and implacable' spirits could produce such 'rageing and implacable' patients.[139] If the frenzy continued after the spirits had calmed, this was a sign that they had carved out new tracks in the brain marrow.

And yet, for all its ingenuity, this account of brain–mind relations had not solved all of Willis's problems. It had not done away with one inconvenient truth: in practice, frenzy rarely limited its range of fire to the imagination, the fantasy, the memory, or the passions. It could produce permanent unreason, even in the supposed possessors of rational souls. The faculty of the reason – the 'image of God in man' – was not supposed to be something its owners could easily lose. It was certainly not supposed to be vulnerable to brain disease. It is to this problem which we now turn.

[135] Thomas Sydenham, 'Anatomie, 1668', in Kenneth Dewhurst (trans.), *Dr Thomas Sydenham (1624 –1689), His Life and Original Writings* (London: Wellcome Historical Medical Library, 1966), p. 90.

[136] Willis, *Two discourses*, sig. A4v. [137] Ibid., sig. A3v. [138] Willis, 'Anatomy', sig. H4r.

[139] Willis, *Two discourses*, p. 183.

CHAPTER 3

Saving the Soul

Introduction

In 1599, the poet Sir John Davies (1569–1626) published a verse poem entitled *Nosce teipsum* ('Know yourself'). The 'self' which Davies wanted his readers to recognize would not have come as too much of a shock. It consisted of a body and a soul, and that soul was an immaterial, immortal spirit, closer in nature to the angels than the 'brutes'. The 'reason', the 'understanding', and the 'will' were its noblest possessions. But Davies cannot have felt that he was simply preaching to the choir, for he devoted several stanzas to shooting down possible objections to his claims. Headlining the list of his fictive opponents were the 'Epicures', who (in Davies's telling) seized on every instance of cognitive impairment – whether a consequence of infancy, old age, heredity, disease, or intoxication – as a proof of the soul's mortality. 'How is it that some wits are interrupted, That now they dazled are, now clearely see?' these 'Epicures' demanded to know if souls 'are not ... within themselues corrupted?' Davies was not wrong to anticipate this question. It had been asked a decade earlier by the writer Ludowick Bryskett, this time voiced not by an anonymous Epicure but by his deceased friend, the poet Edmund Spenser: 'how cometh it to passe (replied Maister *Spenser*) that the soule being immortall and impassible, yet by experience we see dayly, that she is troubled with Lethargies, Phrensies, Melancholie, drunkennesse, and such other passions[?]'. This was a very real doubt in early modern England. It was not the notion that the soul could sicken the body which caused problems; it was the thought that the traffic could go in the other direction – that the body could sicken the soul. For daily experience said that it could. Fortunately, Davies had a response at the ready:

> if a Phrensie do possesse the braine,
> It so disturbes and blots the formes of things,
> As phantasie proues altogether vaine,

And to the wit no true relation brings.
Then doth the wit admitting all for true,
Build fond conclusions on those idle grounds.[1]

Contrary to appearances, no faculty of the rational soul was touched by the disease. The 'wit' had only been misinformed by the 'phantasie', which had in turn been misled by 'the tender braine'. Nothing had been damaged by the disease except the organ itself. The dispute between Davies and his phantom opponents was not new: it echoed a debate on the soul's immortality which had rumbled on in Latin Christendom since at least the thirteenth century. Davies was one of the earliest English authors to enter the fray in print, but he would not be the last. Nor would he be the last to invoke 'Phrensie' to make his case. The brain disease seems to have become an edge case for combatants on both sides of the debate; for body/soul dualists, it showed that it was possible for the immortal soul to outlive the brain; for their opponents, it proved that it was not. Before we turn to the debate as it played out in early modern England, it is worth taking a brief look at its origins.

Christianizing the *Psychē*

The first chapter gave a thumbnail sketch of the Aristotelian tripartite *psychē*: the vegetative (common to all living beings), the sensitive (common to all sensate beings), and the rational (unique to humans). In the early Middle Ages, Aristotle's writings on the *psychē* had shared the same fortunes as Galen's on the *hēgemonikon*: Latin Christendom – that is, the former western half of the Roman Empire – had lost access to them. It was not until the thirteenth century that Aristotle's full oeuvre became available to Latin readers. Sensing the immense potential of his philosophy, Christendom's theologians immediately set to work reconciling it with the doctrines of their faith. The most influential among them was the Dominican friar Thomas Aquinas (1225–1274), who adapted Aristotle's carefully ordered cosmos to the requirements of Christian divinity. Long into the sixteenth century, the teaching of natural philosophy at the European universities rested on this distinctly Thomist Aristotelian foundation.[2] Progressing through Aristotle's

[1] Davies, *Nosce teipsum*, p. 90.

[2] Emily Michael, 'Renaissance Theories of Body, Soul, and Mind', in John P. Wright and Paul Potter (eds.), *Psyche and Soma: Physicians and Metaphysicians on the Mind–Body Problem from Antiquity to Enlightenment* (Oxford: Oxford University Press, 2000), pp. 147–148; Serjeantson, 'The Soul', p. 123.

works on natural phenomena, the syllabus culminated with his book on the soul, *De anima*.[3]

Yet, despite Aquinas's best efforts, some aspects of Aristotle's philosophy proved resistant to synthesis, and his account of the *psychē* was a particularly stubborn case. Part of the problem probably lay in Aristotle's own ambivalence on the subject. In life, he had been a physician's son, and a devoted dissector of frogs. But he had also spent several years studying philosophy under Plato, for whom the body was a prison for the soul, and the contemplation of dead frogs a definite red herring. When writing about the *psychē*, as Philip van der Eijk puts it, Aristotle was not always 'wearing the same hat'.[4] Certain passages in his *Nicomachean Ethics* describe the *psychē* in terms which would have made Plato proud: as something godlike, unique to humans, and perfected only by contemplation, union with the divine, and separation from the natural body.[5]

But Aristotle's fullest articulation of a theory of *psychē* was to be found, not in the *Nicomachean Ethics*, but in *De anima*.[6] And the soul described in *De anima* was characterized not by antipathy towards matter, but by total complementarity and interdependence with it. Every physical thing possessed its own distinctive immaterial *form*, which gave shape, extension, and function to the undifferentiated potentiality of *matter*. In the case of living things, their forms *were* their souls. As we have seen in the last two chapters, plants, humans, and beasts all possessed distinctive types of soul; the more faculties possessed by the soul, the greater the complexity of the organism. Plato had sought to locate the powers possessed by the human soul within the body, suggesting – as would Galen – that rational activity happened in the head, vital activity in the thorax, and vegetative in the liver.[7] Aristotle was less interested in this question: as the body's 'form', the soul was both unextended and present in every feature of its structure.[8]

Like the other scholastic brain cartographers whom we met in the last chapter, Thomas Aquinas had been obliged to give this Aristotelian soul a stiff massage to get it into a theologically acceptable shape.[9] When Aristotle

[3] See Des Chene, *Life's Form*; Paul Mengal, *La naissance de la psychologie* (Paris: L'Harmattan, 2005).

[4] Philip J. van der Eijk, 'Aristotle's Psycho-physiological Account of the Soul–Body Relationship', in Wright and Potter (eds.), *Psyche and Soma*, pp. 58–63, quote on p. 62.

[5] Aristotle, 'Nicomachean Ethics', in H. Rackham (trans.), *Nicomachean Ethics*, LCL 73 (Cambridge, MA: Harvard University Press, 1934), book 10, pp. 612–613, 617–619.

[6] Van der Eijk, 'Aristotle's Psycho-physiological Account', p. 62.

[7] Ibid., p. 69; T. M. Robinson, 'The Defining Features of Mind–Body Dualism in the Writings of Plato', in Wright and Potter (eds.), *Psyche and Soma*, p. 47.

[8] Van der Eijk, 'Aristotle's Psycho-physiological Account', pp. 68–69.

[9] T. H. Irwin, 'Who Discovered the Will?', *Philosophical Perspectives* 6 (1992), 453–455.

had divided the rational from the sensitive soul, he had attributed to the latter two kinds of instinctive drive: *epithumia* ('appetite', 'desire') and *thumos* ('passion', 'spirit').[10] *Epithumia* sought pleasure; *thumos* dignity and the avoidance of shame. Aristotle's thirteenth-century translator William of Moerbeke had rendered *epithumia* and *thumos* as the 'concupiscible' and 'irascible' appetites: the former drove the soul to embrace a perceived good, the latter to overcome obstacles to its attainment. This was the terminology taken up by Aquinas.[11]

Unfortunately, Aristotle had failed to furnish the rational *psychē* with its own rational appetite. In his ethical works, however, he had occasionally spoken of *boulēsis*: this was a deliberative, intentional wishing, apparently quite distinct from *epithumia* and *thumos*.[12] Aristotle had never situated *boulēsis* within his hierarchy of psychic faculties, but Aquinas took the liberty of doing it for him. The pagan philosopher, he decided, was talking about what the church father Augustine of Hippo had called the 'will'.[13] The will was the rational appetite unique to the immortal human soul; it was (in principle) free to choose between good and evil.[14] In its unfallen state, it naturally strove towards the ultimate good, and this was God. It still yearned for the same end after the Fall, but it was also fatally weakened by sin. As such, it was easily bent to the whims of its baser cousins, the passional appetites. This was what made human efforts to seek God so futile, for the rational will was in thrall to 'concupiscence', a word which encompassed all self-serving and sensitive desires.[15]

The Immortality Problem

Aquinas had equipped the newly Christianized Aristotelian soul with its necessary attributes: reason, understanding, and will. But the Bible's promise of resurrection and eternal life required more of the soul than

10 Ibid., p. 457; Victor Saenz, 'Shame and Honor: Aristotle's *Thumos* as a Basic Desire', *Apeiron* 51(1) (2018), 73–95; Giles Pearson, *Aristotle on Desire* (Cambridge: Cambridge University Press, 2012), chs. 4, 5.

11 Robert Miner, *Thomas Aquinas on the Passions* (Cambridge: Cambridge University Press, 2009), p. 47; Thomas Dixon, *From Passions to Emotions: The Creation of a Secular Psychological Category* (Cambridge: Cambridge University Press, 2006), p. 42.

12 Irwin, 'Who Discovered the Will?', p. 456.

13 Ibid., pp. 453–468.

14 Peter King, 'Aquinas on the Passions', in Scott MacDonald and Eleonore Stump (eds.), *Aquinas's Moral Theory: Essays in Honor of Norman Kretzmann* (Ithaca, NY: Cornell University Press, 1999), p. 101.

15 Christian Tornau, 'Augustine of Hippo', in Edward N. Zalta and Uri Nodelman (eds.), *The Stanford Encyclopedia of Philosophy*, 26 April 2024, https://plato.stanford.edu/archives/sum2024/entries/augustine.

'noble' faculties: it required its immortality. Unfortunately, the *psychē* of *De anima* had not been purpose-built to furnish proof of human immortality; it had been designed to explain what made living beings tick. When an animal died, Aristotle seemed to imply, both matter and form would cease to be, for the one had no actuality without the other. As the human being's substantial form, the *psychē* would not outlive the body. This was to prove a longstanding headache for his Christian readers. Augustine had played a major role in shaping orthodox Christian doctrine, and he in turn had been influenced by Platonic and Neoplatonic writings on the soul.[16] For the bishop of Hippo, the human soul was nothing less than the 'image of God' in man: an immortal, immaterial intelligence.[17] It was single, unified, and co-extensive with the body, through which it spread 'not by a local diffusion' – for in that case cutting off a limb would also sever some part of it – 'but by a certain vital intention'.[18] This meant that it was also indivisible: 'the whole is in all the parts, and in every part it is whole'.[19] The soul animated the body, but was also superior to and fully separable from it. And indeed at the moment of death the soul *would* separate from the body, and would survive without it until a final reunion at the end of days.[20]

The problem, for Aquinas, was that the Platonic overtones of Augustine's body/soul dualism brought it a little too close for comfort to the dualism of the heretics of his own day, who were said to see the physical world as a trap which the soul was duty-bound to escape. For Aquinas and his fellow Dominicans, this was an insult to the divine creator, who had created that world and called it good.[21] Aristotle's body–soul composite seemed like a good antidote to this heresy; but then it also sounded worryingly perishable. Aquinas's solution was to Christianize the Aristotelian *psychē*, bringing it in line with Augustine's

[16] Ibid.

[17] See Bruno Niederbacher, 'The Human Soul: Augustine's Case for Soul–Body Dualism', in David Vincent Meconi and Eleanore Stump (eds.), *The Cambridge Companion to Augustine*, 2nd ed. (Cambridge: Cambridge University Press, 2014), pp. 125–141; Gareth Matthews, 'Internalist Reasoning in Augustine for Mind–Body Dualism', in Wright and Potter (eds.), *Psyche and Soma*, pp. 133–146.

[18] 'Per totum quippe corpus quod animat, non locali diffusione, sed quadam vitali intentione porrigitur'. Augustine, 'De origine animae hominis liber, seu Epistola CLXVI', ch. 2, sect. 4, in Jacques-Paul Migne (ed.), *Patrologia Latina* (Paris: Migne, 1841–1857), vol. 33, col. 0721.

[19] 'in omnibus tota, et in singulis tota est'. Ibid.

[20] See Niederbacher, 'The Human Soul', pp. 127–129.

[21] This was Catharism, a heretical movement which, in the twelfth and thirteenth centuries, was seen as a major threat to orthodox Christendom. See Roger French and Andrew Cunningham, *Before Science: The Invention of the Friars' Natural Philosophy* (Abingdon: Ashgate, 1996), pp. 180–192.

teachings. The result was a soul–body composite, made up of one soul (now also its Aristotelian 'form') and one body (furnishing its 'matter'). Although this soul was still recognizably Augustinian (it was single, indivisible, immaterial, and immortal), it also possessed the full spectrum of Aristotelian faculties (rational, sensitive, and vegetative). Like any lesser soul, this human soul used each of its tailormade organs to exercise a specific faculty: the ears to hear, the stomach to digest, and so on. Apart, that is, from one exception: the rational (or intellective) part of the soul, which required no bodily organ to do its work.[22] It could think in abstract terms, infer universals from singulars, and contemplate other immaterial intelligences, all without any help from matter.[23] For Aquinas, this offered persuasive evidence that the human soul would survive the death of the body. The operations of its organ-dependent faculties would simply be suspended until the general Resurrection.[24]

Aquinas's soul–body composite soon gained the status of orthodoxy in Christendom.[25] But it had never gone undisputed, and dissent grew louder at the turn of the sixteenth century. The northern Italian universities of Padua and Bologna had, by this time, gained a reputation for fostering heterodox strains of Aristotelianism. Some of their faculty members were known to follow Aristotle's twelfth-century Arabic commentator Averroës, whose teachings had been determinedly scored off academic curricula by the church over the course of the two preceding centuries.[26] Averroës, like Aquinas, believed that humans partook of an immortal intellect. Unlike Aquinas, he thought that this was *one* universal intellect, shared among all of its partakers. The survival of the individual after death was therefore impossible, for individuality arose only from the interaction of the universal intellect with the particularity of a single, perishable organic soul.[27] Even worse, other northern Italian scholars were persuaded by the third-century Greek Aristotelian Alexander of Aphrodisias (newly available in

[22] Thomas Aquinas, *Summa theologiae* (hereafter *ST*), Ia, qq. 75–89, in Franciscus de Nerito et al. (eds.), *Summa theologiae: Pars prima* (Venice, 1477), pp. 391–495.

[23] Aquinas, *ST*, Ia, q. 89.

[24] Ibid., Ia, q. 75, a. 6. On the resurrection of the body, see *ST*, Suppl. IIIae, q. 69, a. 1. See also Lorenzo Casini, 'The Renaissance Debate on the Immortality of the Soul', in Paul J. J. M. Bakker and Johannes M. M. H. Thijssen (eds.), *Mind, Cognition, and Representation: The Tradition of Commentaries on Aristotle's* De anima (London: Routledge, 2016), pp. 129–130; Robert Pasnau, *Thomas Aquinas on Human Nature: A Philosophical Study of the* Summa Theologiae *1a, 75–89* (Cambridge: Cambridge University Press), ch. 5.

[25] Serjeantson, 'The Soul', p. 123.

[26] Michael, 'Renaissance Theories', pp. 150–152.

[27] Ibid., pp. 149–152.

Latin translation from 1495), who had argued that the human intellect was unqualifiedly mortal.[28]

And Alexander was not even the worst of the ancient leviathans that these well-meaning Renaissance humanists had managed to dredge up from the depths of Europe's monastic libraries. In 1417, one of them had unearthed a complete manuscript of *De rerum natura* ('On the nature of things'), the long-lost masterpiece of the Roman poet Titus Lucretius Carus (c. 99–55 BCE).[29] A follower of the ancient Greek atomist Epicurus (341–270 BCE), Lucretius had helpfully summed up the tenets of Epicurean philosophy in 7,400 lines of beautifully crafted Latin verse. Unfortunately, unlike Aristotle, Epicurus had not minced his words about the nature of the human *psychē*: it was mortal. And Lucretius could offer proof:

> in bodily diseases the mind [*animus*] often wanders astray; for it is demented and talks deliriously ... Therefore you must confess that the mind also is dissolved, since the contagion of disease penetrates it; ... But that which is immortal does not permit its parts to be transposed, or anything to be added, or one jot to ebb away; for whatever by being changed passes outside its own boundaries, at once that is death for that which was before. Therefore, if the mind is sick, it gives indications of mortality, as I have shown.[30]

The list of equivalent proofs continues: the fragility and frangibility of the mind can also be seen in infancy, old age, and drunkenness. It was this passage that Davies and Bryskett had taken such pains to refute (and Bryskett's choice of a mouthpiece was probably not accidental; Spenser had been a little too enamoured by Lucretius's poem).[31] Yet, although this passage was evidently deeply shocking to its sixteenth-century readers, it could at least be dismissed wholesale. For no church father had ever attempted to redeem Lucretius, or to render any tenet of his philosophy compatible with Christianity.

Unfortunately, the second-century 'prince of physicians', Galen, had said something worryingly similar in a treatise known to Latin readers as

[28] Ibid., p. 152; Casini, 'The Renaissance Debate', pp. 130–132.

[29] Michael Reeve, 'Lucretius in the Middle Ages and Early Renaissance', in Stuart Gillespie and Stuart Hardy (eds.), *The Cambridge Companion to Lucretius* (Cambridge: Cambridge University Press, 2007), p. 206.

[30] Lucretius, *On the Nature of Things*, trans. W. H. D. Rouse, revised by Martin F. Smith, LCL 181 (Cambridge, MA: Harvard University Press, 1924), pp. 222–225.

[31] Stuart Gillespie, 'Lucretius in the English Renaissance', in Gillespie and Hardy (eds.), *The Cambridge Companion to Lucretius*, pp. 243–247.

Quod animi mores corporis temperamenta sequantur ('That the soul's traits depend on bodily temperament').[32] Experience had taught him that the soul was easily 'overcome by the evils of the body in melancholia, *phrenitis*, and mania'.[33] If Plato was right and it *was* incorporeal, Galen mused, then

> why does the soul completely leave the body which is severely cooled or overheated? I have not found out after much investigation, just as I have not found out why, when yellow bile abounds in the brain, we are drawn to delirium (*paraphrosynē*) ... For as far as forgetfulness, mindlessness, immobility, or numbness follow ... someone might say the soul is being impeded in functioning with the capacities it has naturally. However, when someone thinks he sees things that are not visible or hears things no one has uttered, or says something that is shameful, or unspeakable, or completely unthinkable, not only is this evidence of loss of the innate capacities which the soul has, but also of the entrance of the opposites. This, then, already carries a certain strong suspicion regarding the whole substance of the soul, that it is not incorporeal.[34]

Although Galen was opposed to most aspects of Epicurean philosophy, Lucretius's poem may nonetheless have informed his reflections on the metaphysical ramifications of brain disease. Christendom never quite forgave Galen for this lapse into crude physicalism, and his early modern successors were always vulnerable to being tarred with the same brush.[35] 'Physitions hold that [our souls] ... Complexions bee', Davies announced scathingly, sprung 'from the Bodies humors tempred right'.[36] Unfortunately, by the turn of the sixteenth century, Aristotle and Galen – unlike Lucretius – were already far too deeply embedded in the edifice of European natural knowledge for anyone to extract them. The only thing to do was to ignore their more unpalatable comments about the soul, and (of course) the ones added by their heathen commentators. This was the rationale behind the papal ban on teaching Averroës. Yet the fact that so many repetitions of the ban had been required suggests that the

[32] Galen, 'The Soul's Traits Depend on Bodily Temperament', in Ian Johnston (trans.), *On Temperaments. On Non-Uniform Distemperment. The Soul's Traits Depend on Bodily Temperament*, LCL 546 (Cambridge, MA: Harvard University Press, 2020). Hereafter, for brevity's sake, I will refer to this treatise as *Quod animi mores.*

[33] Galen, 'Quod animi mores', in Karl Gottlob Kühn (trans.), *Claudii Galeni Opera Omnia* (Leipzig: Cnobloch, 1821), vol. 4, p. 788; in Johnston (trans.), *On Temperaments*, pp. 366–367.

[34] Galen, 'Quod animi mores', pp. 777, 787–788, in Johnston (trans.), *On Temperaments*, pp. 346–347, 364–365.

[35] See Charles T. Wolfe, '*Tres medici, duae athei?* The Physician as Atheist and the Medicalization of the Soul', in Peter Distelzweig, Benjamin Goldberg, and Evan Ragland (eds.), *Early Modern Medicine and Natural Philosophy* (Dordrecht: Springer, 2015), pp. 343–366.

[36] Davies, *Nosce teipsum*, pp. 10, 13.

church's ability to keep the universities in check had always been limited. It was in this context that the independent northern city-states of the Italian peninsula had gained a reputation as shelters for non-compliant natural philosophers.

In 1513, Rome's patience with the universities wore thin. The eighth meeting of Pope Leo X's Fifth Lateran Council declared the non-negotiability of the doctrine of natural personal immortality, decrying certain 'extremely pernicious errors ... namely that the soul is mortal or one in all men'.[37] More radically, the Council demanded that Christian natural philosophers prove the soul's immortality by the light of natural reason. The Council's ambitions were thwarted three years later, when the leading Aristotelian at Padua, Pietro Pomponazzi (1462–1525), published his *Treatise on the Immortality of the Soul* (1516).[38] For Pomponazzi, Aquinas's arguments did not stand up to scrutiny. In truth, he declared, 'no natural reasons can be brought forth to prove that the soul is immortal'.[39] Aristotle had clearly indicated that all knowledge was ultimately derived from the senses; this held for abstractions and generalizations as much as it did for singulars. It was just about feasible that the human intellect needed no organic instrument to think *through* or *with*; but it at least needed a source base of sensory impressions – the *phantasmata* presented by the imagination – to think *upon*.[40] Thus reasoning always depended on the sense organs, albeit by one remove. It was impossible for a substance to be unqualifiedly material and immaterial at the same time; it made most sense to conclude that the intellect was substantively material, and therefore mortal. Pomponazzi did end the treatise with a fideistic caveat: despite all the evidence to the contrary, the soul *would* survive the death of the body. His point was that this knowledge could not be proven by the light of natural reason; it had to be revealed to the faithful by God.[41] This was precisely the opposite of what the Fifth Lateran Council had asked for. The thesis was roundly condemned, but this did not stop it from being read all over Europe.[42]

37 Giuseppe Alberigo et al. (eds.), *Conciliorum oecumenicorum decreta* (Basel: Herder, 1962), pp. 581–582; Michael, 'Renaissance Theories', p. 152.

38 Eckhard Kessler, 'Psychology: The Intellective Soul', in Schmitt et al. (eds.), *The Cambridge History of Renaissance Philosophy*, pp. 500–504.

39 Pietro Pomponazzi, *Tractatus de immortalitate animae* (Bologna, 1516), sig. Cviii.

40 Michael, 'Renaissance Theories', pp. 153–155.

41 Pomponazzi, *Tractatus*, sig. Cviii.

42 For a survey of these responses, see Étienne Gilson, 'L'affaire de l'immortalité de l'âme à Venise au debut du XVI e siècle', in Vittore Branca (ed.), *Umanesimo europeo e umanesimo veneziano* (Florence: Sansoni, 1964), pp. 31–61, esp. 58–59; Paul Richard Blum, 'The Immortality of the Soul', in James Hankins (ed.), *The Cambridge Companion to Renaissance Philosophy* (Cambridge:

The Pluralist Solution

The Council's efforts were not entirely in vain; Pomponazzi's treatise spurred many of its sixteenth-century readers to articulate theories of soul which would offer firmer support for personal immortality.[43] Leading the way in Northern Europe was Martin Luther's collaborator Philip Melanchthon (1497–1560), who had embarked on an ambitious programme of educational reform at Wittenberg in the 1540s.[44] Central to the syllabus was a new, distinctively Lutheran version of Aristotelian natural philosophy, and its capstone was a new treatise on the soul.[45] Melanchthon's *Commentarius de anima* (1540) deliberately sidestepped Aquinas's unified soul and its pitfalls. He argued that the individual human being contained a plurality of forms, whose organic and rational parts were ontologically and not just conceptually distinct. Organic souls were generated from parental seed; the rational soul was superadded by God.[46] The former dissolved and corrupted with matter; the latter lived on, indivisible and incorruptible. Melanchthon was not the first to adopt this approach. Pluralism had always been a branch of the Aristotelian *De anima* tradition, but it had been overshadowed by Aquinas and blighted by its proximity to Averroës. Melanchthon acknowledged the scholastic friar William of Ockham (c. 1287–1347) as his source, but whereas Ockham had bisected the human into one corporeal and one incorporeal soul, Melanchthon identified three: the 'vegetative, sensitive, and rational, as Plato, Aristotle and Galen say'.[47] Strictly speaking, neither the vegetative nor the sensitive soul was a soul, but rather a kind of breath of life, bestowed by God, described by Melanchthon as an 'agitation' or 'continuous motion'.[48] Only the rational soul truly merited the name 'soul' (*anima*).[49]

Cambridge University Press, 2007), pp. 223–229; Kessler, 'Psychology: The Intellective Soul', pp. 504–507.

43 Michael, 'Renaissance Theories', p. 160.

44 See Kusukawa, *Transformation of Natural Philosophy*, ch. 2.

45 Ibid., ch. 3.

46 'Inspirauit in faciem eius spiraculum uitae . . . Sed anima sentiens & uegetatiua sunt ex traduce, hoc est, propagantur & oriuntur ex natura seminum'. Philip Melanchthon, *Commentarius de anima* (Wittenberg, 1548), ff. 12r–v.

47 'An uero sint distinctae animae in homine, uegetatiua, sentiens, & rationalis, sicut Plato, Aristotle, & Galenus loquuntur'. Ibid., ff. 11r–v.

48 'continua quaedam agitatio. . . quaedam ἐνδελεχεια'. Ibid., f. 10v. There was a longstanding debate over whether Aristotle had intended to use the word *entelechy* ('actualization', 'realization') or *endelechy* ('activity', 'continuous motion', 'persistence'). Cicero thought the latter, and Melanchthon endorsed his reading. See Kusukawa, *Transformation of Natural Philosophy*, pp. 91, 108.

49 'Nunc addenda est communis sententia de Anima, quam Christiana doctrina probat'. Melanchthon, *Commentarius*, f. 10v.

The followers of Aquinas had been left with the unenviable task of explaining how one immaterial soul was responsible for such heterogeneous operations as divine contemplation and digestion. Melanchthon's pluralism did away with this problem, but it helped little with the question of how these apparently incommensurable entities – one material, the other immaterial – interacted with one another. Melanchthon thought that the key to the answer might be found in the bodily spirits.[50] As we saw in the last two chapters, after several rounds of rarefaction, the animal spirits ended up more like light or fire than liquid. As such, they were matter which hovered at the very edge of materiality, and this made them a plausible enough conductive medium between the organic and the rational soul.[51] In the 1550s, Melanchthon even considered the possibility that the spirits served as the material cause of the vegetative and sensitive souls.[52] This idea was taken even further by the Calabrian natural philosopher Bernardino Telesio (1509–1588), for whom the organic soul and the spirits were one and the same: a corporeal, extended, corruptible substance.[53]

Melanchthon and Telesio were both familiar figures to the learned elites of Protestant England, and their pluralism influenced several English treatments of the soul. In his *De dignitate et augmentis scientiarum* (first published in 1623), Francis Bacon advanced a theory of soul and spirit clearly based on Telesio's.[54] But Aquinas's unified soul had survived the century of Reformations, too, and it had proven much more compatible with the Protestant confession embraced by Elizabeth I and her heirs. It had its roots in Augustine's body/soul dualism, and it was this church father's doctrines which lay at the heart of Reformed Protestantism.[55] The

50 In Latin these 'spirits' were known as *spiritus* (plural), creating ample opportunities for confusion (or conscious conflation) with the immortal Christian *Spiritus*. See Daniel P. Walker, 'Medical Spirits and God and the Soul', in Marta Fattori and Massimo Bianchi (eds.), *Spiritus. IV° Colloquio internazionale del Lessico Intellectuale Europeo, Rome, 7–9 gennaio, 1983* (Rome: Edizioni dell'Ateneo, 1984), pp. 233–244; Kusukawa, *Transformation of Natural Philosophy*, p. 120; Cellamare, 'Anatomy and the Body', pp. 347–348, n. 17.

51 Elena Carrera, 'Anger and the Mind–Body Connection', in Carrera (ed.), *Emotions and Health 1200–1700*, p. 113. Aquinas had considered and rejected the possibility of a material intermediary. See *ST*, Ia q.76 a. 6.

52 Park, 'Psychology: The Organic Soul', p. 483.

53 Ibid., pp. 483–484. This corporeal rational soul came 'from the seed' (*e semine educta*); Telesio, like Melanchthon, also recognized another soul 'infused by God' (*a Deo immissa*). Fabrizio Bigotti has argued that, in Galenic terms, Telesio envisioned the former as the soul's substantive instrument (*instrumentum*), and the latter as its essence (*essentia*). See Bigotti, *Physiology of the Soul*, p. 156.

54 Francis Bacon, *De dignitate et augmentis scientarium* (London, 1638), lib. 4, cap. 3, pp. 127–133.

55 See Mark Taplin, 'Confessions of Faith (Reformed)', and Thomas Curran, 'Anglicanism', in Karla Pollmann and Willemien Otten (eds.), *The Oxford Guide to the Historical Reception of*

result was that while few inhabitants of sixteenth-century England would have denied that they had an immortal soul, many were unclear on the question of how exactly it differed from – and interfaced with – the mortal remainder. They might well have heard from their local parish priest that every person was a composite of one body and one soul, and that that soul was single, indivisible, and (of course) immortal. But anyone with a smattering of natural philosophy could have insisted afterwards that he was wrong – that his description in fact applied to only one of their two (or three) souls. For the majority who were not well-enough versed in the *De anima* commentary tradition to pick a side, the mixed messages must have been baffling.

Stress-Testing the Soul

The preachers of the Reformed Church of England were supposed to teach their flocks that the human soul was unified, immortal, and indivisible (following Augustine) *and* the substantial form and animating principle of the body (following Aquinas). But this meant that they had to tread very carefully in their discussions of soul–body relations. And they were not always careful. Thomas Adams (1583–1652) was a brilliant preacher, but he was also capable of stretching a good metaphor too far. In a series of sermons entitled *Mystical bedlam, or the world of mad-men* (1615), he developed an extended parallel between 'corporal' madness and the 'spirituall' madness of sin.[56] It was a neat conceit, as far as it went. His mistake was to try to nail down the precise differences between these two types of madness:

> To vnderstand the force of *madnesse,* we must conceiue in the *brayne* three ventricles; as houses assign'd by Physitians for three dwellers, *Imagination, Reason,* and *Memorie.* According to these three internal *senses* or *faculties,* there be three kinds of *Phrensies* or *Madnesses* . . . For spirituall relation, we may conceiue in the soule; *vnderstanding, reason, will.*[57]

'Reason' is counted twice in this passage: once as an embodied faculty, a 'dweller' of the brain's middle ventricle, and then again as a possession of the immortal 'soule'. Adams's listeners and readers could have been forgiven for wondering exactly how many faculties there were *per capita.*

Augustine (Oxford: Oxford University Press, 2013); Richard A. Muller, *Christ and the Decree: Christology and Predestination in Reformed Theology from Calvin to Perkins* (Durham, NC: Labyrinth Press, 1986), ch. 6.

[56] Thomas Adams, *Mystical bedlam, or the vvorld of mad-men* (London, 1615). [57] Ibid., p. 35.

Adams had brought them to the troubled boundary between the soul's most sophisticated sensitive faculties (imagination, estimation, and memory) and its truly rational ones (reason, understanding, and will).

Today, all of these faculties fall under the heading 'mind', but for Adams, they fell across a critical metaphysical border. No wonder that pinpointing the precise difference between corporal and spiritual frenzy was harder than it looked. Later in the same sermon, Adams tried again:

> Now whereas they distinguish Soule. 1. *in vegetabilem*, that giueth life. 2. *in sensibilem*, that giueth feeling. 3. *in rationalem*, that giueth reason: the first desiring *esse*, to be; the second, *benè*, to bee well; the third *optimè esse*, to be best; so not resting till it be with God: behold, this spiritual madnesse eneruates this last action of the soule, as corporall endeuors to extinguish the two former.[58]

As a statement of humanity's God-given place on the 'ladder of nature', this account was completely unobjectionable.[59] But as an account of 'corporall' madness, it was seriously wanting. Frenzy did not simply extinguish 'life' and 'feeling': anyone who had encountered the disease in any capacity knew that it also caused failures of 'reason'. There was no species of madness which did not. Having likened diseases of the immortal soul to diseases of the embodied mind, Adams found himself struggling to draw a precise line between the two.

If Adams backed himself into this corner unintentionally, others went there of their own accord. Sir John Davies and Lodowick Bryskett were not the only people in early modern England to wonder aloud (or to get straw men to wonder aloud) why a supposedly impassible soul was passible to organic disease. The best-known English theologian of their generation, William Perkins (1558–1602), even begged the question from the pulpit. There were several possible reasons why a Christian might suffer distress of mind, Perkins noted: earthly affliction, resistance to God's will, diabolic temptation, or a guilty conscience. But there was a 'Fifth and last kinde of Temptation or Trouble of mind', and it arose 'from a mans owne bodie'.[60]

58 Ibid., p. 36.

59 The better-read members of Adams's audience might have recognized this as a quotation from the Catalan theologian Raymond of Sabunde's *Theologia Naturalis* (c. 1434–1436), glossed by one seventeenth-century English reader as follows: 'Some only bee, some bee, & live wi*th*all/& some have Beeing, life, & sense beside/But Man, by Reasons light, transcends them all' (London, Middle Temple Library, BAY L530). For a full transcription and discussion, see John O'Brien, 'In Praise of the *Theologie Naturelle*', *Review of English Studies* 65(269) (2013), 236–251.

60 William Perkins, *The first part of The cases of conscience* (Cambridge, 1604), p. 173.

The mind was easily disturbed by 'strange alterations' in its parts. When, for example, 'a man beginnes to enter into a Phrensie, if the braine admit never so little alteration . . . presently the reason is corrupted'.[61] Perkins took pause:

> Before I enter to speake thereof, one Question, in the meane time, must be answered, namely, How the bodie should, or how it can trouble the minde, considering that the soule or mind, is not bodily, but spirituall: and it is against reason, that that which is bodily, should either alter or trouble a spirit.[62]

Perkins began his answer with a quick primer on the human soul: 'the actions of man, doe proceede from one onely fountaine, and common cause, the soule; and are done by the power thereof'.[63] If Perkins's soul was single, immortal, and indivisible, this was not for lack of awareness of the other options. His comment that 'the soule of man is a spirit or spirituall substance, wheras the soule of a beast is no substance, but a naturall vigour or qualitie' showed his familiarity with Melanchthon's *Commentarius.*[64] Yet where Melanchthon (following Ockham) had given human nature one immortal *anima* and two vegetative and sensitive *agitationes*, Perkins allowed for no such frivolous additions. Aware that pluralism was an option, he decided firmly against it. Like Adams, Perkins was a devoted follower of Augustine; in this rulebook, the phrase 'organic soul' was an oxymoron.[65]

Returning to the question with which he had begun, Perkins returned to the standard answer of the Thomist Aristotelian tradition: any apparent damage to the soul was only damage to its 'next instrument', the body.[66] 'The bodie of it self', Perkins declared, 'is not an agent in any work, but as it were a dead instrument, in & by which the soule produceth all actions and workes'.[67] Yet the body and the soul

[61] Ibid., p. 181. [62] Ibid., p. 174. [63] Ibid., p. 174.

[64] William Perkins, *A salve for a sicke man* (London, 1611), p. 11.

[65] On Perkins's Augustinianism, see Richard A. Muller, *Grace and Freedom: William Perkins and the Early Modern Reformed Understanding of Free Choice and Divine Grace* (Oxford: Oxford University Press, 2020); Muller, *Christ and the Decree*, ch. 6; Donald K. McKim, 'Perkins, William', in Pollman and Otten (eds.), *The Oxford Guide to the Historical Reception of Augustine.*

[66] This was barely a metaphor at all; Aristotle had named these body parts the '*órgana*' ('instruments') of the *psychē* for a reason. Medieval proponents of the 'body-as-instrument' argument included William of Auvergne, John Blund, and Nicholas of Amsterdam. For overviews, see R. C. Dales, *The Problem of the Rational Soul in the Thirteenth Century* (Leiden: Brill, 1995); S. W. de Boer, *The Science of the Soul: The Commentary Tradition on Aristotle's* De anima, *c. 1260–c. 1360* (Leuven: Leuven University Press, 2013).

[67] Perkins, *The first part*, p. 174.

> are so ioyned together, that they make one person, and thus, the bodie beeing troubled, the soule is also troubled: yet is not this done, by any diuiding of the soule. For it cannot be diuided. Neither by diminishing the parts of the soule, but onely by corrupting the action of the minde, or more properly, by corrupting the next instrument of the minde.[68]

It was not the 'minde' which was corrupted by disease, but only its 'next instrument', the brain:

> This may be conceiued by a comparison. A skilful artificer in any science, hath an vnfit toole, and a naughtie instrument to worke withall: his skill is good, and his abilitie is sufficient, but his instrument whereby he worketh is vnperfect: and therefore he brings forth an imperfect worke. Now his toole takes not away the skill of his workmanship, nor his power of working, but keepes him from doing that well, which otherwise he should and could doe well. In like manner, the body beeing corrupted, hinders the worke of the soule. It doth not take away the worke of the soule, nor the abilitie of working: but because it is a corrupt instrument, it makes the soule to bring forth a corrupt worke.[69]

An organ with warped pipes was bound to produce discord, but the powers of the organist remained perfectly intact. It might *look* very much like frenzy had deranged the mind, but in fact it had only warped its 'next instrument', the brain. A workman sometimes had good reason to blame his tools.

We have already encountered this explanation in Davies's 1599 poem *Nosce teipsum*. The same motif recurs throughout the poem: the soul is a craftsperson, the quality of whose work depends on the quality of the tools; a musician, the sweetness of whose music depends on the tuning of the harp.[70] It was central to the refutation of Galen's *Quod animi mores* offered by a young Cambridge divine named Andrew Willet in 1585: 'If a skilled craftsman were hired for a price, he would not lose his skill or his praise if he lacked the tools for his work ... thus, the soul is not robbed of its honour when the body is in a state of defect'.[71] Different tasks called for different tools, and the brain – and, even more importantly, the animal spirits – were the tools of the mind.[72] Everyone knew that a diseased brain impeded the soul's activities more profoundly than an injured hand or

[68] Ibid., p. 175. [69] Ibid., p. 174. [70] Davies, *Nosce teipsum*, pp. 15–17.

[71] 'se pretio peritus aliquis artifex conductus fuerit, nihil ille de peritia sua, aut laude amittet, si operi suo desit, cùm apta & utilia instrumenta non adeptus fuerit: sic anima nec honore suo spoliatur, cùm corpus in vitio est'. Andrew Willet, *De animae natura et viribus quaestiones quadam* (Cambridge, 1585), p. 85.

[72] Ibid., pp. 83, 85.

foot, but in none of these instances had it been harmed by the body's injury.[73]

Of course, Pomponazzi had been familiar with this same Thomist analogy; in fact, he had worked it into his argument. For the soul to be proven immortal, he had argued, it had to be shown to have some operation which relied on the body *neither* as instrument *nor* as a bank of sense data. Perkins was no philosopher, and he made no attempt to offer a fresh refutation of Pomponazzi's claim: for him, it was self-evident that 'some actions of the soule & mind, are done without the helpe of the bodie'.[74] He was backed up in this by the vast majority of English religious writers who had put pen to paper on the subject. Throughout *Nosce teipsum*, Davies had insisted that 'sense' and 'fancie' relied upon the brain, but 'wit' and 'will' did not.[75] Bryskett had advanced the same argument in his rebuttal of Spenser's ghost: intellection was an '*actus purus*, a pure vnderstanding, not needing the bodie either as an obiect, or as a subiect'.[76] This was not to say that the intellect was never led astray by its organ-bound inferiors. It did not *need* the body, but – sitting as it did at one remove from the coalface of the material world – it inevitably came to rely upon the senses for information. And its judgements were only as good as its servants' reports: just 'as a cunning Prince that vseth Spies, If they returne no newes, doth nothing know; But if they make aduertizement of Lyes; The Princes Counsell all awrie do go'.[77] The lies did not damage the sovereign prince's power of judgement, but his misplaced trust in his false informants could lead him into error all the same. 'The soul does not need its instruments', Willet explained in 1585, but 'performs its duty with greater alacrity, if the body presents itself as a faithful and diligent servant'.[78]

These arguments were staples of the scholastic tradition, and Perkins, Davies, Bryskett, and Willet were not alone in finding them both elegant and convincing.[79] The fact that they were sourced from the *De anima*

[73] 'Nam si pes condoluerit, nihi est, aut manus vulneretur, verum si caput affligatur, laedatur cerebrum . . . pertimescendum malum est'; 'Corpus animam non laedit'. Ibid., pp. 81–82, 85.

[74] Perkins, *The first part*, p. 174. [75] Davies, *Nosce teipsum*, pp. 14, 17, 29, 49, 93.

[76] Lodowick Bryskett, *A discourse of ciuill life containing the ethike part of morall philosophie* (London, 1606), p. 276.

[77] Davies, *Nosce teipsum*, p. 89.

[78] 'Nec aliquis tamen hoc ita nobis dictum putet, ac si animae instrumentorum subsidio opus aliquando sit . . . Illud igitur effectum est, animam non corpori morem gerere, sed maiori alacritate munum suum exequi, si fidelem se seruum corpus & sedulum praebeat.' Willet, *De animae natura*, p. 88.

[79] I have not managed to do justice to the variety and nuance of these arguments. For detailed analyses of the counterarguments to Galen's *Quod animi mores*, see Bigotti, *Physiology of the Soul*, pp. 190–224; Des Chene, *Life's Form*, pp. 69–76. For counterarguments to Pomponazzi's

commentaries did not mean that they were stale – it meant that, over the course of four centuries, they had been refined and elaborated by some of the sharpest minds in Christendom. Besides, it would be wrong to suggest that every early modern Christian was troubled by the spectres of Lucretius, Galen, and Pomponazzi. Many would never have even heard of them, and we should not imagine that all those who had were kept up at night by their heretical claims. Some even appreciated the opportunity to shoot them down. In 1609, for example, the Cistercian philosopher Eustachius à Sancto Paulo declared that, although for Christians the soul's immortality was beyond doubt, it could 'be proved by physical reasons' in order 'to defeat heretics and pagans'.[80]

But not every seventeenth-century defender of the faith was confident that these enemies had been routed once and for all. In the 'Dedicatory Letter to the Sorbonne' which prefaced his *Meditations on First Philosophy* (1641), the French philosopher René Descartes expressed concern that

> some have even had the audacity to assert that, as far as human reasoning goes, there are persuasive grounds for holding that the soul dies along with the body and that the opposite view is based on faith alone. But in its eighth session the Lateran Council held under Leo X condemned those who take this position, and expressly enjoined Christian philosophers to refute their arguments and use all their powers to establish the truth: so I have not hesitated to attempt this task as well.[81]

Evidently, in Descartes's view, the 'body-as-instrument' argument was not sufficiently robust. And, in its more simplified iterations – like the ones which Perkins and Adams presented in their sermons – it did seem to give rise to inconsistencies. Perkins had stated both that the soul reasoned 'without the helpe of the bodie' *and* that if 'the braine admit never so little alteration . . . presently the reason is corrupted'. But surely – a sharp sermon-goer might have objected – if the body contributed nothing to the act of reasoning, it was hardly fair to blame it when that act went wrong.[82] If the soul did *not* rely on the brain for the use of this faculty, a corrupted reason could not be blamed on the brain. If the soul *did* rely on the brain,

Tractatus, see Gilson, 'L'affaire de l'immortalité de l'âme', pp. 31–61; Blum, 'The Immortality of the Soul', pp. 223–229.

80 'Et si rationales animas spirituales esse ac immortales non liceat homini Christiano dubitare . . . ad revincendos haereticos & paganos, poterit hoc ipsum physicis rationibus comprobari.' Eustachius a Sancto Paulo, *Summa philosophiae quadripartita* (Cambridge, 1648), vol. 3, tract. 4, q. 2, p. 328.

81 René Descartes, 'Dedicatory Letter to the Sorbonne', in John Cottingham et al. (trans.), *The Philosophical Writings of Descartes* (Cambridge: Cambridge University Press, 1985), vol. 2, p. 4.

82 Perkins, *The first part*, p. 174.

then Aquinas's old proof of immortality could not stand. For how was the soul supposed to continue reasoning when its material instruments had dissolved into dust? To admit two different kinds of reason – one mortal and the other immortal – was to accept the existence of plural souls. For many early modern Christians – both Catholic and Protestant – this option was simply not on the table. Any viable defence of the soul's immortality also needed to preserve its oneness.

Mortalism Strikes Back

Blithely unaware of this cross-confessional consensus, frenzy continued to show itself perfectly capable of disrupting the operations of the rational soul. Two years after the publication of Descartes's *Meditations*, the breakdown of censorship during England's first civil war made it possible to make this point in print – and not, this time, in the voice of a straw man waiting to be shot down. In 1643, the Leveller Richard Overton stated it as a syllogism: 'Mans Faculties ... are Temperatures: *Ergo [therefore]*, Mortall ... yea those of *Reason, Consideration, Science,* &c. all that distinguish Man from a Beast, are augmented by Learning, Education, &c. lessened by Negligence, Idlenesse, &c. and quite nullified by Madnesse: *Ergo* [mortal].'[83] Overton willingly embraced the point which Adams had skirted around: it was precisely the noblest faculties of the mind – 'Reason, Consideration, Science, &c.' – which were 'nullified by Madnesse'. He went on:

> experience tels us, If the former *Brain-pan* be hurt, the *Senses* are hindred, but the *Cogitation* remaineth sound. If onely the *Middle-pan* be harmed, the *Cogitation* is maimed; but the *Seat of Sense* keeps all the *five Senses* whole: If any hurt befall both to the *Former* and *Middle-pan,* both *Sense* and *Cogitation* decay. If the *Hinder-pan* be disordered only, the *Memorie* alone, and neither *Sense* nor *Cogitation* receive harme.[84]

We have no reason to doubt Overton's claim to have come to this knowledge 'by experience', but his interpretation of those experiences had certainly been informed by Galenic medical theory. If this enumeration of the three 'Brain-pans' and their operations sounds familiar, it is because it was sourced from the textbook medical description of frenzy. It was the observed effects of this disease which had first prompted Galen to disaggregate the faculties of the rational soul (*hēgemonikon psychēs*), and

[83] Richard Overton, *Mans mortalitie* (London, 1643), p. 9. [84] Ibid., p. 10.

which had prompted his later readers to allocate each of those faculties its own seat in the brain. Frantic patients had always provided key data points for modelling brain–soul relations. No wonder, then, that the disease was so often invoked in early modern debates on the soul's materiality. For Overton, frenzy was proof enough that the soul was material, and what was material was doomed to die.

Overton was no Epicurean, although his enemies did not hesitate to brand him as one; it would be fairer to describe him as a God-fearing 'mortalist'.[85] Historians have used the term 'mortalism' to encompass several different strands of heterodox belief about the afterlife, but what all of them had in common was the belief that, after the death of the body, the individuated human soul would not continue to exist in a conscious state.[86] We have no reason to doubt the sincerity of Overton's faith; he professed sincere belief in the Bible's promise of a general resurrection, and, for the saved, of eternal life in heaven. What he rejected was the notion that the fulfilment of this promise was a foregone conclusion; that is, that immortality was a natural consequence of the indestructability of a disembodied, immaterial soul.[87] This amounted to taking God's grace for granted; when He fulfilled his promise, his immortalizing of his naturally mortal children would be nothing less than a miracle.

Overton opened his treatise with the promise that he would prove the soul's mortality 'both theologically and philosophically … both by Scripture and Reason'.[88] Although he was not consistent about citing his philosophical sources, for his university-educated readers, his arguments had a distinct savour of Galen, Lucretius, and Pomponazzi. One of his critics, the English Jesuit Guy Holland, commented archly that, 'during the night of Gentilisme', it was bound to be the case that 'an Epicurus … should stumble and fall into an errour: but now after the sun is up, it were a great shame for a Pomponatius … to fall into a ditch, and teach such doctrine as the wisest of the most early ages judged to be erroneus and

[85] B. J. Gibbons, 'Overton, Richard (*fl.* 1640–1663), Leveller and Pamphleteer', *ODNB*, 27 May 2010, https://doi.org/10.1093/ref:odnb/20974; Nigel Smith, 'The Charge of Atheism and the Language of Radical Speculation, 1640–1660', in Michael Hunter and David Wootton (eds.), *Atheism from the Reformation to the Enlightenment* (Oxford: Oxford University Press, 1992), pp. 139–141.

[86] See Ann Thomson, *Bodies of Thought: Science, Religion and the Soul in the Early Enlightenment* (Oxford: Oxford University Press, 2008), pp. 15, 42–44; Smith, 'The Charge of Atheism', pp. 139–141.

[87] Smith, 'The Charge of Atheism'.

[88] Overton, *Mans mortalitie*, title page.

absurd'.[89] If Overton was a second Pomponazzi, his critics had no lack of long-dead scholastics to summon to their aid. To say 'there is no *habit* or faculty of reason in a *mad man*, because the *act* of reasoning is hindered', exclaimed the Anglican minister Alexander Ross, was 'as if you should say, that a *Musician* hath lost his skill in Musick, when he ceaseth to play'.[90] The soul had suffered no damage to its rational faculties; it was simply temporarily prevented from using them by a defect in its 'next instrument', the brain.[91] And yet Overton's opponents also continued to insist on the old Thomist exception to the rule – that, in the words of Thomas Hooker, 'the power of reason and understanding . . . worketh of it selfe without the body'.[92] These three divines hardly presented a united front: Holland was a Jesuit, Hooker a Puritan, and Ross a high churchman.[93] But the unanimity of their attacks on Overton should not surprise us; faced with a fresh attempt to prove the soul's mortality 'philosophically', they had all sourced their material from the same place: the scholastic commentaries on Aristotle's *De anima*.

The irony was that the Aristotelian natural philosophical edifice on which these arguments rested was rapidly losing ground to new competitors.[94] In his *Discourse* (1637) and *Meditations* (1641), Descartes had scrapped one of its most fundamental principles: the need for a 'substantial form' to actuate the undifferentiated, boundless potentiality of matter. There were no such 'forms', Descartes had declared. Everything in the cosmos was one of two possible types of thing: matter, unthinking and extended (occupying space), or mind, thinking and unextended.[95] Descartes's intended objective – stated explicitly in his dedicatory letter to the Sorbonne– was to demonstrate the natural immortality of the

89 Guy Holland, *The grand prerogative of humane nature namely, the souls naturall or native immortality* (London, 1653), p. 26.

90 Alexander Ross, *The philosophicall touch-stone* (London, 1645), p. 125.

91 See Holland, *The grand prerogative*, pp. 29–30; Thomas Hooker, *The immortality of mans soule* (London, 1645), pp. 40–43; Ross, *The philosophicall touch-stone*, pp. 123–126.

92 Hooker, *The immortality of mans soule*, p. 40.

93 Thompson Cooper, 'Holland, Guy (1585/6–1660), Jesuit', *ODNB*, 23 September 2004, https://doi.org/10.1093/ref:odnb/13520; David Allan, 'Ross, Alexander (1591–1654), Church of England Clergyman and Writer on Philosophy', *ODNB*, 4 October 2007, https://doi.org/10.1093/ref:odnb/24110; Sargent Bush, Jr., 'Hooker, Thomas (1586?–1647), Minister in America', *ODNB*, 3 January 2008, https://doi.org/10.1093/ref:odnb/13697.

94 Serjeantson, 'The Soul', pp. 128–129.

95 René Descartes, 'Discourse on the Method', in John Cottingham et al. (trans.), *The Philosophical Writings of René Descartes* (Cambridge: Cambridge University Press, 1985), vol. 1, pp. 131–141; René Descartes, 'Second Meditation' and 'Sixth Meditation', in John Cottingham (trans.), *Meditations on First Philosophy, With Selections from the Objections and Replies*, 2nd ed. (Cambridge: Cambridge University Press, 2017), pp. 20–27, 57–72.

human soul.[96] And his rejection of Aristotle *did* make that task simpler. If all organic bodies were divinely wrought perpetual motion machines, they needed neither a form to give them shape, nor an animating principle to give them life. The Aristotelians had already moved as far as they could in this direction: recall Perkins's description of the body as a 'dead instrument'.[97] But the option of automating all the body's functions had not occurred to them, or – if it had – it had not seemed plausible. Thus, the unified rational soul described by Perkins had remained burdened with all its old, organ-bound Aristotelian duties.[98] It was Descartes's newly mechanized, hydraulic model of physiology which allowed him to release the soul from this contract to keep the body running.[99] All sensitive and vegetative functions could now be explained mechanically – that is, by reference to matter in motion. This made it far easier insulate the 'mind' or 'soul' (terms which, for Descartes, were synonymous) from diseases of the body (including the brain).[100]

At first, English theologians were delighted by this development; Descartes had offered a new and excitingly non-Aristotelian refutation of Pomponazzi. But, as the 1650s wore on, the dangers of his radical new philosophy became increasingly apparent. In removing the need for substantial forms, Descartes had undone the stitching which had guaranteed the close enmeshment of the material and immaterial worlds. Now, anyone who found themselves agreeing with the Epicurean vision of the cosmos was better equipped than ever to explain how it might work: they could simply take up the hydraulic, mechanistic half of Descartes's philosophy, and leave the other half on the shelf.[101] This, in a series of devastating works published over the course of that decade, was exactly what the English philosopher Thomas Hobbes (1588–1679) proceeded to do. 'Man', his *Leviathan* (1651) made clear, was naturally mortal; he did not possess a separable, immortal soul. It was the whole being – breath and body – which would be resurrected at the end of days. And there would be nothing natural about that resurrection; the fact that it was possible was thanks only to God's omnipotence.[102] The soul was not immaterial,

96 Descartes, 'Dedicatory Letter to the Sorbonne', p. 4.

97 Perkins, *The first part*, p. 174.

98 See Des Chene, *Life's Form*, pp. 6–9.

99 See Des Chene, *Spirits and Clocks*, esp. pp. 40–45, 53–69.

100 Descartes, 'Discourse on the Method', p. 127; Descartes, 'Second Meditation', pp. 22–23.

101 Margaret J. Osler, *Divine Will and the Mechanical Philosophy: Gassendi and Descartes on Contingency and Necessity in the Created World* (Cambridge: Cambridge University Press, 1994), p. 297.

102 Thomas Hobbes, *Leviathan, or, The matter, forme, and power of a common wealth, ecclesiasticall and civil* (London, 1651), ch. 38, esp. p. 241.

simply because the very notion of an immaterial substance was a fiction. The universe, he declared, 'is Body; and that which is not Body, is no part of the Universe'.[103] It was no mystery why frenzy deranged the reason, for it was just as Lucretius had said: the mind was of 'Body' just as much as was the brain. This was the worst case of 'Epicurism' seventeenth-century England had ever seen. It was so bad that the Cambridge Platonist Henry More was forced to come up with a new label for it: Hobbes was a '*Materialist*'.[104]

As Hobbes's ideas gained notoriety, the defenders of the immaterial soul increasingly distanced themselves from Cartesianism. The mechanical philosophy was useful to them only to the extent that it proved the total lifelessness of matter, and thus 'the necessity of the assistance of a substance distinct from matter, that is, of a spirit, or being incorporeal' to make sense of all the varied phenomena of life.[105] Descartes had gone too far in reducing 'soul' to 'mind', and in refusing it to all creatures but humans. As the full extent of the threat posed by his philosophy became apparent (thanks in no small part to Hobbes), England's Protestant theologians declared a state of spiritual emergency.[106] Disbelief in the immateriality of the human soul was the first step on a slippery slope to atheism, and the inhabitants of England seemed – to them – to be sliding down it in droves.[107]

For those who had fallen out of love with Descartes's dualism, the list of alternatives had changed little. One option was to endow *all* living beings with naturally immortal, immaterial souls, but this meant *either* admitting 'brute' beasts to heaven (and what kind of paradise had wasps in it?), *or* insisting that God destroyed each non-human soul at death (which, given that He had created it to be naturally indestructible, required a miracle). The latter's implications were less than ideal – redundancy was not the Creator's style – but to More it looked like the best option on the table. It allowed him to restore all the sensitive faculties which Descartes had stripped from the soul, and to insist on their manifest existence as proof of

103 Ibid., ch. 46, p. 371.

104 Henry More, *Divine dialogues containing sundry disquisitions & instructions concerning the attributes and providence of God* (London, 1668), p. 6.

105 Thomson, *Bodies of Thought*, pp. 45–46.

106 John Henry, 'The Matter of Souls: Medical Theory and Theology in Seventeenth-Century England', in French and Wear (eds.), *Medical Revolution*, pp. 87–88, 92–93.

107 Thomson, *Bodies of Thought*, pp. 47–48; Michael Hunter, *Science and the Shape of Orthodoxy: Intellectual Change in Late Seventeenth-Century Britain* (Woodbridge: Boydell, 1995), pp. 229–244.

the limits of materialism. Living, sensing, feeling, and imagining – just as much as thinking – were operations of which matter was patently incapable.

But this made it no easier than before to solve the old Lucretian riddle about madness. In a late reply to Overton, More declared: 'As to *Madness*, there are no Apprehensions so frantick but are arguments of the Souls Immortality, not as they are frantick, but as Apprehensions. For *Matter* cannot apprehend any thing, either wildly or soberly, as I have already sufficiently demonstrated.'[108] No matter how deranged the results, the act of apprehension *always* revealed the presence of an immaterial soul. Like his forebears, however, More still had to find a way of explaining the breach: if immateriality did not guarantee immunity to damage, then the whole case for natural immortality fell down. Some of the soul's faculties, he explained, being 'very fatally passive' and in too close 'commerce with matter', 'are not so absolutely in her own power, but that her levity and mindlesness of the divine light may bring her into subjection to them'.[109] This maddened soul had not been defeated by the material body (as Descartes would have had it). It had been defeated by its own faculties – the 'fatally passive' ones, corrupted by their 'commerce with matter'.

Thus far, More had followed the old argument: it was not the soul that received the damage, but its material instruments. But he was about to strike out in a very different direction. With all due respect to Aquinas, it was simply untrue that the soul could exercise some of its faculties without these instruments. *All* of the soul's operations were dependent on matter, and reasoning was no exception to the rule. If it was, then 'Distemper and Diseasedness, could not prejudice her in her *Inventive* and purely Intellectual Operations; but it is manifest that they do, and that a man's Mind is much more cloudy at one time than an other'.[110] This was as good as admitting that Lucretius had been right all along. But More was no crypto-Epicurean: he remained adamant both that the soul was naturally immortal *and* that it would always be dependent on matter. For many early modern natural philosophers this would have sounded like a contradiction in terms, but for More it did not; in his Neoplatonic cosmos, the material and the immaterial shared so many attributes that the division of

108 Henry More, *The immortality of the soul, so farre forth as it is demonstrable from the knowledge of nature and the light of reason* (London, 1659), p. 479.
109 Ibid., p. 479. 110 Ibid., p. 205.

labour between them was often far from clear.[111] Here, the individual human consciousness needed only two things to survive: an invisible, extended, immaterial soul and an invisible, extended, material body. This material body was not the 'gross', heavily appendaged bulk most familiar to the senses, but an intangible, invisible, spirituous substance. It had to be made of the finest, purest, most rarefied matter: surely, this was the substance which physicians called the 'animal spirits'.[112] Material though they were, the soul would not leave all of them behind at death, but would 'collect herself, and the small residue of spirits, (that may haply serve her in the inchoation of her new Vehicle), either into the heart, whence is an easy passage into the Lungs, and so out at the mouth; or else into the Head, out of which there are more doors open than I will stand to number'.[113] The soul would then use these spirits to knit itself a new 'aethereal' body, which would carry it through to the general resurrection.[114]

As we have seen in previous chapters, the animal spirits had always been considered vital to cognition. But More's decision to make them the *only* necessary instrument of the soul obliged him to show that the brain was superfluous to its needs. These spirits needed a receptacle, he conceded, and the brain was fit for that purpose. In its embodied state, the soul sat in its fourth ventricle, the wellspring of the animal spirits, in order to direct their flow. But one only had to handle a brain – to feel its 'clammy and sluggish' consistency under one's fingertips – to realize it had nothing to contribute to this process.[115] Whatever this wobbly 'mess of Curds' did, it was not thinking.[116] This rhetoric was evidently intended to counter crude materialism (although, paradoxically, More had ended up making matter more indispensable than ever).[117] Yet for a pious anatomist like Thomas Willis – for whom every inch of the human body testified to the ingenuity of its maker – the Cambridge theologian's derisiveness towards the brain must have come as a shock.

[111] See Walker, 'Medical Spirits and God and the Soul', pp. 235–240; John Henry, 'A Cambridge Platonist's Materialism: Henry More and the Concept of Soul', *Journal of the Warburg and Courtauld Institutes* 49 (1986), 172–195.

[112] More, *The immortality of the soul*, pp. 199–209. [113] Ibid., p. 129.

[114] This was More's reworking of the Neoplatonic doctrine of the 'astral body'. See Ilinca Tanaseanu-Döbler, 'Synesius and the Pneumatic Vehicle of the Soul in Early Neoplatonism', in Donald Russell et al. (eds.), *On Prophecy, Dreams and Human Imagination: Synesius, De insomniis* (Tübingen: Mohr Siebeck, 2014), pp. 125–156; D. P. Walker, 'The Astral Body in Renaissance Medicine', *Journal of the Warburg and Courtauld Institutes* 21 (1958), 119–133. I owe this point to Reader C.

[115] More, *The immortality of the soul*, p. 205. [116] Ibid., p. 174.

[117] Henry, 'A Cambridge Platonist's Materialism', pp. 177–195.

Dissecting the Soul (Again)

Hobbes had declared that there was nothing *but* the brain; More had compared it to a 'mess of Curds'. The natural theologians of seventeenth-century England would have been hard-pressed to say who had insulted the Creator more. More's comments may well have goaded Willis to commence work on the *Cerebri anatome*, a textual-visual panegyric to the organ's structural complexity, purposefulness, and beauty. Yet, as I suggested in the last chapter, Willis turned his attention to the brain for other reasons too. As a practising physician, he had seen what frenzy did to its sufferers. And if Galen's point about the metaphysical ramifications of those effects had ever needled at him, works like Overton's *Mans mortalitie* and Hobbes's *Leviathan* can only have rubbed salt into the wound. It is hard not to read the claims of Willis's *De anima brutorum* (1672) in the light of a passing comment in the preface: the task of completing the manuscript had seemed impossible, until 'after the Death of my Dear Wife, being lonely . . . that I might the less think on my Grief, I have at last finished [it]'.[118] The result was Willis's most fully articulated defence of the rational soul's separateness from the body. His anatomical project was – at least in part – an attempt to underwrite the Bible's promise of human immortality.

Unfortunately, mind–matter dualism was no help at all in immunizing the soul to brain disease (and More's Neoplatonist version was no more palatable to Willis than Descartes's had been). There was one remaining option available to him: the pluralist solution. First developed in the early fourteenth century, this theory of soul was hardly cutting edge, but fortunately it had just been given a makeover by one of the most respected 'new philosophers' of the day: the Catholic priest and polymath Pierre Gassendi (1592–1655).[119] 'The human soul', Gassendi had announced in his *Syntagma Philosophicum* (published posthumously in 1658), 'is composed of two parts . . . the irrational, encompassing the vegetative and sensitive, [which] is corporeal . . . and the rational, or intellective, which is incorporeal'.[120]

[118] Willis, *Two discourses*, sig. A3v.

[119] See Margaret J. Osler, 'Baptizing Epicurean Atomism: Pierre Gassendi on the Immortality of the Soul', in Margaret J. Osler and Paul Lawrence Farber (eds.), *Religion, Science, and Worldview: Essays in Honor of Richard S. Westfall* (Cambridge: Cambridge University Press, 1985), pp. 163–183.

[120] Pierre Gassendi, *Opera Omnia* (Lyon, 1658), vol. 2, p. 256. Osler suggests that Gassendi's distinction between *animus* ('that by which we reason') and *anima* ('that by which we are

It was Gassendi's pluralist account which seemed – to Willis – to offer the best solution to the problem posed by madness. Man, he declared in 1683, was a two-souled creature: the incorporeal soul resembled those of the angels; the corporeal soul he shared in common with the 'brutes'.[121] Following Melanchthon, Willis sub-divided it into two parts: 'one Vital Portion living in the Blood, to be a certain inkindling of it, and another Sensitive, to be only an heap of Animal Spirits every where diffused thorow the Brain and Nervous Stock'.[122] It was this sensitive portion that was prone to 'extend its Sicknesses, not only to the Body, but to the Mind or rational Soul, which is of an higher linage'.[123] In most brain diseases, the effects on the rational soul were relatively slight: the intellect, 'like the eye placed in an obscure place', 'beholds . . . either not at all, or a few objects only of a more rude appearance, but is not easily snatched into any great error or fury'.[124] But in 'Phrensie',

> the Imagination is so disturbed, or perverted, that it falsly conceives, or evilly composes or divides, the species and notions brought from the Sense or Memory; presently for that reason the intellect beholds or forms conceptions and thoughts only deformed, distracted one from another, and very confused: Which indeed are represented to it from the Brain evilly affected, and as it were monsters from a multiplying or distorted Glass . . . by which the Imagination, and by consequence the mind and will, and the other powers of the superior soul, are wont to be perverted or depraved.[125]

An abscess in the meninges would block the movement of the animal spirits, and as such it could be expected to cause 'stupidity', lethargy, or a coma. But it could not, for Willis, explain the continual welling up of 'confused', 'perverted', and 'depraved' thoughts in his frantic patients' minds. It was this metaphysical problem – as much as his post-mortem findings – which drove him to move frenzy from the solid structures of the brain to its spirits. For 'truly a Phrensie cannot be more aptly defined', he declared, 'than that it is a burning or inflammation of the whole sensitive soul . . . This burning always beginning from the spirits inhabiting the Brain, and wandring from thence into the other parts of the sensitive soul'.[126] The disease spread like wildfire through the 'whole sensitive soul' – that is, the total mass of animal spirits circulating through 'the Brain and Nervous Stock'. No wonder that the reason soon became

nourished and that by which we feel') was adopted 'directly from Lucretius'. But if the borrowing was direct, it was not wholesale: Gassendi's *animus* was incorporeal, where Lucretius's most emphatically was not. See Osler, 'Baptizing Epicurean Atomism', p. 63.

121 Willis, *Two discourses*, sigs. A3v–A4v. 122 Ibid., sig. A3v. 123 Ibid., sig. A4r.

124 Ibid., p. 179. 125 Ibid., p. 179. 126 Ibid., p. 183.

entangled in its 'failings and faults'.[127] The fact that the immortal soul could be led astray so easily by a diseased imagination was regrettable, but then many aspects of life on this mortal coil were. The important thing was that the disease had not reached the rational soul itself. This was the only good argument 'against Epicurism, and Atheism', that 'our Sensitive Soul ... as that of the Brutes, miscarrying, the other perpetually survives'.[128]

Willis was nervous about how his newly divided human soul would go down among his contemporaries; he was a faithful Anglican, and the established church still endorsed the Augustinian body/soul dyad.[129] He need not have worried. In truth, his rearrangement of the soul was about as influential as his redefinition of frenzy: it won him some support, but was never at risk of becoming mainstream. Nor did it quell the rising tide of 'Epicurism'. In fact, in working out such detailed and plausible corporeal accounts of psychic disturbances, Willis had only furnished the materialists with new material.[130] In the 1690s, Henry Layton – the most outspoken Christian mortalist to come forward since Overton – repeatedly summoned the late 'Dr Willis' to his side.[131] Had not this pious doctor described the soul as 'a Material Spirit extracted ... [from] the Particles of Blood, inflamed in the Lungs, and made lucid in the Brain'?[132] Willis had suffered the same fate as Descartes: his account of human nature had been stripped of what – for him – had been the most important thing about it.

Conclusion

The battle for the immortality of the soul was very far from over at the end of the seventeenth century. In the era known as the Enlightenment, the conflict between orthodox Anglicans and 'freethinking' mortalists only grew fiercer. And, despite the best efforts of preceding generations to show that brain disease did *not* spread to the rational soul, its effects could still sow doubts in pious hearts. In *The nature and immortality of the soul proved* (1682), the nonconformist minister Richard Baxter began by reproducing a letter which he claimed to have received from '*one who professed*

[127] Ibid., sig. A4r. [128] Ibid., sig. A4r. [129] Ibid., sigs. A2r–A4v.
[130] Thomson, *Bodies of Thought*, pp. 83–84; Porter, *Flesh in the Age of Reason*, p. 60.
[131] Henry Layton, *Observations upon a sermon intituled, A confutation of atheism from the faculties of the soul...* (London, 1692), pp. 4, 13–14.
[132] Henry Layton, *Observations upon a short treatise, written by Mr. Timothy Manlove: Intituled, The Immortality of the Soul Asserted* (London, 1697), p. 62.

perplexing doubtfulness' on the subject.[133] This anonymous doubter had no difficulty believing in God. But, if he had grave doubts about the immortality of the soul, it was because

> by several accidents happening to the body, the man is incapacited from acting rationally, ... there is not in some of them so much a sign of a reasonable Soul, as to distinguish them from Bruits: Whereas were the Soul such as represented, it would rather cease to act, than act at a rate below it self. Did it know its Excellencies, such as we make them, it would as soon desert its being, as degrade its self by such bruitish acts: ... Tho the Workman breaks his Tools, his hands do not lose their skill, but ceaseth to act, rather than to do ought irregularly: so likewise would the Soul then act contrary to its own nature.[134]

Baxter gave short shrift to most of the points raised by this unfortunate letter-writer, but this one, he admitted, was 'the hardest Objection'.[135] The question which had haunted the defenders of human immortality for so long had been metaphysical: how was it possible for a material body to plunge an immaterial one into madness? But this doubter's question was not *how* but *why*: why would the rational soul choose to live on in this reduced condition?

The question was troubling, and so was Baxter's answer. The reason why the workman decided to put down his broken tools rather than embarrass himself was that he had the power to exercise his free will. Mad persons had lost that power: their souls' acts were not '*free-acts,* but necessitated by God by the order of nature'.[136] Although frenzy could not erase the rational faculties (reason and will), it could prevent the sufferer from exercising them so completely that – in this life – the outcome was the same. And God was apparently willing to let that happen. In the next two chapters, we turn to consider how the belief that frantic persons had lost the use of these faculties influenced their treatment in the here and now. Chapter 4 focuses primarily on the perceived consequences of the loss of 'will', and Chapter 5 on the loss of 'reason'.

[133] Richard Baxter, *The nature and immortality of the soul proved in answer to one who professed perplexing doubtfulness* (London, 1682), title page.
[134] Ibid., p. 10. [135] Ibid., p. 36. [136] Ibid., pp. 37–38.

CHAPTER 4

Judging by Intentions

Introduction

The fact that the faculties of the rational soul could be disabled (if not destroyed) had this-worldly implications. The same faculties – reason, understanding, and will – were central to the English common law's concept of criminal responsibility. When in 1628 the common lawyer Edward Coke wrote that 'the act and wrong of a madman shall not be imputed to him, for . . . *Actus non facit reum, nisi mens sit rea* [the act is not culpable unless the mind is guilty]', he was reminding his fellow barristers of what they already knew.[1] If a defendant had not acted knowingly and voluntarily, the act was no crime, no matter how terrible the consequences. The proper verdict in such cases was non compos mentis ('unsound in mind'), and once granted, it nullified the indictment and acquitted the perpetrator.

This tenet of common law was to form the basis of what, in the Anglo-American legal tradition, would come to be known as the 'insanity defence'. The most high-profile and best-known instances of this plea (in early modern England as today) were made by the defendants of suspected murderers. And it was not uncommon for courts to hear that such persons had killed their loved ones while in a 'frenzy'.[2] This side of the story has received considerable attention from legal and social historians.[3] In this chapter, I focus not on homicide but on suicide, and not on trials, but on a distinct but closely related type of jurisprudential procedure: the coroner's

[1] Edward Coke, *The first part of the Institvtes of the laws of England, or, A commentarie upon Littleton* (London, 1656), lib. 3, cap. 6, section 405, f. 247v.

[2] For examples of 'frantic' homicide, see: Kew, TNA, ASSI/35/7/5, mm. 13, 15, 20 (Henry Pelling, 1565); ASSI 35/99/11 m. 96 (Frances Edwards, 1657); *Old Bailey Proceedings Online*, 'Trial of Francis Brereton' (25 April 1688), ref. t16880425–28.

[3] See Nigel Walker, *Crime and Insanity in England, Vol. 1: The Historical Perspective* (Edinburgh: Edinburgh University Press, 1968); Nigel Walker, 'The Insanity Defence before 1800', *Annals of the American Academy of Political and Social Science* 477 (1985), 25–30.

inquest. The English coroner's task was to investigate and make a record of every unexpected or suspicious death which occurred in his locality. A particular story about frenzy recurs in these inquests; this chapter asks what it can tell us about lay and legal understandings of the relationship between sickness, culpability, the body, and the mind.

Coroners' Inquests

Death could be a lucrative business for the English crown. Homicide and suicide were felonies in post-Conquest law, and all of the felon's worldly goods and chattels were forfeit to the king. Even in cases of death by misfortune, the instrument of death (known as the *deodand*) belonged to the king. Careful investigation of any unexpected death was needed to ensure that local communities rendered every penny of what was due.[4] The solution, at the end of the twelfth century, was the creation of the crown-appointed office of the county coroner. On the discovery of a body, the coroner summoned around twelve to fourteen propertied men from the local community to act as his jury. Having viewed the body together, they issued a joint statement on the cause of death.

A still-unrivalled authority on the early English coroners' records, Ralph F. Hunnisett, commented in 1961 that 'some verdicts of misadventure, especially by drowning, may conceal suicides'.[5] In 1987, erring on the side of caution, S. J. Stevenson included *all* cases of ambiguous drowning in his attempt to calculate a suicide rate for sixteenth-century England. Producing three estimated rates, ranging from minimal to maximal gloom, he speculated that 'approximately 65 per cent of verdicts of accidental death by drowning may have been suicides'.[6] Working with this degree of uncertainty, he admitted that few positive conclusions about the prevalence of early modern suicide could be drawn from a quantitative study.[7] Nonetheless, Stevenson observed, these two verdicts – *per infortunium* (by misfortune) and *felo de se* (self-murder) – were liable to bleed into one another. In focusing on cases of ambiguous drowning, this chapter explores the implications of Stevenson's observation. In cases involving

4 Sara M. Butler, *Forensic Medicine and Death Investigation in Medieval England* (London: Routledge, 2014), p. 3.

5 Ralph F. Hunnisett, *The Medieval Coroner* (Cambridge: Cambridge University Press, 1961), p. 21.

6 S. J. Stevenson, 'The Rise of Suicide Verdicts in South East England, 1530–1590: The Legal Process', *Continuity and Change* 2(1) (1987), 65.

7 Ibid., p. 38.

frenzy, I argue, coroners' jurors tended to swing between one of these two verdicts: suicide or misfortune. Where the phrase non compos mentis appears, it usually seems intended to supplement the verdict, rather than replace it.

This claim serves to complicate the central thesis of Michael MacDonald and Terence Murphy's landmark study, *Sleepless Souls: Suicide in Early Modern England* (1990). Despite a brief nod towards Stevenson's work, MacDonald and Murphy's study focused on cases in which the deceased was presented to the court as having died by his or her own hand. They concluded that Tudor juries chose between two rival verdicts 'to distinguish the guilty from the innocent. A self-killer whom they deemed sane was returned a *felo de se*, a felon of himself; one who was insane was proclaimed *non compos mentis*'.[8] The deceased could not be both, for '[t]o be a self-murderer, to be judged guilty of felonious suicide, one had to be sane. Men and women who slew themselves when they were mad or otherwise mentally incompetent were not convicted for their crime'.[9] MacDonald and Murphy found that Tudor juries had pardoned less than 2 per cent of self-killers as non compos mentis, and slotted their finding into a compelling narrative of epochal change. The early modern period had been an 'era of severity', in which suicides were universally condemned as sinners and criminals.[10] Attitudes only began to soften after 1660, as a newly secularized society began to reclassify suicide as a sign and consequence of mental pathology. This argument is still persuasive. Yet in distinguishing only between cases ruled *felo de se* or non compos mentis, it suffered from having left out accidents.

It was not that MacDonald and Murphy had failed to notice Stevenson's estimates. But where he had seen the glass of the milk of human kindness half full, they saw it half empty: 'up to one half of all the suicides by drowning could just as plausibly have been returned as accidents'.[11] In other words, what seemed significant to them was that coroners' juries did not conceal *more* suicides (given the opportunity). But since we cannot know how many suicides were successfully concealed as accidental drownings, it is difficult to put this claim in perspective. For in many cases in which the trial jury's ultimate verdict was 'by misfortune', this most clement of possible outcomes rested on a good story about an unsound mind.

8 Michael MacDonald and Terence R. Murphy, *Sleepless Souls: Suicide in Early Modern England* (Oxford: Clarendon Press, 1990), p. 16.

9 Ibid., pp. 15–16. 10 Ibid., p. 15. 11 Ibid., p. 57.

Death by Frenzy

Steering his barge through the Huntingdonshire fens in early December 1525, the waterman William Broke of Over spotted a body in the water. The drowned man – it turned out – was John Nicholas, a husbandman from the nearby village of Needingham. A coroner's jury was called to investigate, and eventually reached a consensus on how Nicholas had died. Prior to his death, the jurors declared, the husbandman had been 'oppressed by frenzy and diverse other infirmities'. He had 'languished' at home until 6 December, when

> by reason of his aforesaid illness . . . between the hours of ten and eleven p. m. . . . he went out from his house at Nedyngworth alone to a place unknown to him, and so wandering in this way, he came to a certain lake of water known as Austenslake . . . in which very same lake John Nicholas, vexed by the disease of frenzy, as said above, fell into the water and was drowned.[12]

In its basic elements, this is a narrative template which appears again and again in the English coroners' records. The story had been told since at least the thirteenth century, and it was still being told at the end of the seventeenth.[13] It was told, for example, on 23 March 1685, by a Sussex coroners' jury who had been summoned to conduct an inquest into the death of a weaver named John Attersole. On 22 March, they declared, Attersole had been walking 'alone near "Blackbrooke" stream in Lindfield', when, being 'not of sound mind but franticke and distracted in mind and senses . . . he suddenly threw himself into the stream and drowned under the water, dying immediately'.[14]

Only eleven days later, on 3 April 1685, the same Sussex coroner, Alexander Luxford, was obliged to perform an inquest into a second death. This time the village was Ditchling, a seven-mile ride from Linfield. Luxford and his seventeen jurors (none of whom had served at Attersole's inquest) declared that

[12] 'existens ex frenesi & alijs diuersis infirmitatibus aggravatur . . . diu & per magnum tempus ibidem languebat et postea racione infirmitatis predicte . . . inter horas decimae & vndecimae eiusdem diei post meridiem exivit solus domum suam apud Nedyngworth ad loca sibi ignota & incognita & sic vagans tandem venit ad quemdam lacum aquae voc. Austenslake . . . in quem quidem lacumi Iohannes Nicholas ex passione frenesis vt predicitur vexatus cecidit in aquam et submersus est'. KB 9/501/2/60.

[13] For pre-1500 examples, see Kew, TNA, KB 9/201/4, m. 58; PRO JUST 2/34, mm. 18–19; PRO JUST 2/106, m. 9.

[14] KB 11/11, unnumbered membrane, trans. Ralph Hunnisett, in *Sussex Coroners' Inquests, 1603–1688* (Kew: PRO Publications, 1998), no. 510, p. 132.

> About 4 a.m. on 1 Apr, when Thomas Browne late of Ditchling, 'wheelewright', who was then not of sound mind but 'franticke' and 'distracted' in mind and senses, was alone near a pit which was full of water in his close in Ditchling, he suddenly threw himself into the pit and drowned under the water, dying immediately.[15]

Why did coroners and their juries continue to tell the same story? One simple answer is that these events did sometimes occur. Feverish diseases were known killers in early modern England. In *Contours of Death and Disease in Early Modern England*, Mary Dobson noted thirty-seven types of fever among the causes of death listed in the parish registers of just one small town.[16] Contemporaries regularly christened the latest outbreak the 'new ague', 'grief', or 'sweat', while medical theorists spilled much ink over how far each was genuinely 'new'.[17]

It is possible, then, that the deaths of Attersole and Browne were not a coincidence: their villages may have been overtaken by a new wave of infectious disease. The coroners' inquests provide even more vivid lay nicknames for these 'new diseases'. In 1545, a coroner's jury swore that, at the time of her death, Helen Armerod of Kirkby had been 'suffering from an illness in her body called "the Wood Agoo" . . . for the space of a quarter of a year':

> by reason of which [she] was out of her mind, and being in her house in a great fury . . . suddenly got up and ran into a garden outside her house, to a place nearby where there was a well of water. By misfortune and by the vehemence of her senses, there and then against her will she fell into the said well and was drowned against her will, and so went to her death.[18]

'Wodeness' was one of the most common words for raging madness in sixteenth-century England.[19] That an ague could earn this epithet suggests something of the terrible effects which it must have wreaked on its sufferers. Twenty years later, Ralph Jackson of Wakefield was judged

[15] KB 11/11, unnumbered membrane, trans. Ralph Hunnisett, in *Sussex Coroners' Inquests, 1603–1688*, no. 511, p. 132.

[16] Dobson, *Contours of Death and Disease*, pp. 237–239.

[17] Lloyd G. Stevenson, '"New Diseases" in the Seventeenth Century', *Bulletin of the History of Medicine* 39 (1965), 1–21.

[18] 'predicta Elena Armerod . . . infirmibatur de una infirmitate existente in corpore suo vocatur "le Wood Agoo" & sic de infirmitate predicta laborabat per spacium quarterni unius anni pretextu cuius predicta Elena erat extra memoriam suam & eo in domo sua propria in magno furore adtunc & ibidem existens subito surgebat & in uno orto extra domum currebat iuxta unum puteum aque ibidem existentem & per infortunam ac per vehementatem cuiusdem sences ad tunc & ibidem contra voluntatem suam cecidit in puteum predictum & ibidem fuit submersa contra voluntatem suam & sic ad eius mortem devenit'. KB 9/563/138.

[19] See *Oxford English Dictionary*, s.v. 'wood (adv.)'.

to have died in much the same circumstances while suffering from 'the wode Agoo' :

> by reason of which sickness he was out of his mind. And from his bed where he was then and then lying in a great fury, he suddenly rose up and ran to the back of his own house, where close by there was a well without a lid. By misfortune then and there he climbed into the said well and was suddenly submerged, and so the said Ralph Jacson went to his death and not otherwise.[20]

Although the coroners' jurors described the madness suffered by the deceased only as an effect of the 'wode ague', to a learned physician, the condition would have been recognizable as frenzy. Frenzy could extinguish life all by itself, but the coroners' inquests suggest that the erratic behaviour provoked in its sufferers could be equally deadly. A great many of these stories unfolded in the hours of darkness and on the outskirts of the parish. For a frantic person – wandering alone, in the dark – uncovered bodies of water would have been a very real hazard.

The fact that coroners often took pains to plot out the precise route taken by the deceased suggests that this commonsense notion formed part of their general bid for plausibility. Roger Frankwell, for example, who had been 'mad and out of his mind and not of sound memory' for sixteen days before his death, had been

> travelling from the said parish of Isfeld to the parish of Barcombe, through a certain wood called 'Barcombe wood', there being nearby in the said wood a large water called 'Barcombe Rivere' . . . the said Roger, straying from the said footpath . . . came to the aforesaid brook, and there and then by unhappy misfortune fell in.[21]

Before the onset of his illness, Frankwell must have possessed a mental map of the route between these two parishes; without access to it, straying into dangerous territory was all too easy. The frantic husbandman John Nicholas, too, was described as 'wandering in a place unknown and unfamiliar to him'.[22] Whether his lack of recognition lay in the fact that

20 'infirmabatur de una infirmitate vocatur "le wode Agoo" . . . pretextu cuius predicte infirmitatis erat extra memoriam suam et eo a lecto suo in magna furore adtunc & ibidem iacente, subito Surgebat et in dorsum domum suam proprem currebat iuxta unam fontem ibidem existens sine tectu per infortunam suam. Ad tunc & ibidem cendit in dicta fonte & subito submersus fuit et sic predictus Radulphus Jacson ad eius mortem devenit & non aliter'. KB 9/605/2/204.

21 'in transcendum a predicta parochia de Isfeld vsque parochiam de Barcombe in quadam silva vocatur "Barcombe wood" magna aqua in dicta silva existente. . . aque ibidem essente vocatur "Barcombe Rivere" dictus Rogerius in dicta silva sic ambulante via pedestralis . . . predictus Rogerius Frankenwell in Rivulum predictum ad tunc & ibidem ex infelicia infortune Cecidit'. KB 9/517/98.

22 'Ad loca sibi ignota & incognita & sic vagrans'. KB 9/501/2/60.

he had never visited the place, or in his inability to remember, was unclear. It is probably not a coincidence that the metaphor of getting lost underpinned most common vernacular idioms for madness. In its most literal sense, the Latin word *delirium* described a plough slipping out of its furrow. The 'wits' could stick to the route, but they could also stray from it. They could abandon their owner, or their owner could go 'beside' or 'out of' them. Either way, the result was the same: the alienation of the person from his or her internal compass.

The language of frenzy also served to accelerate the story's tempo. In these inquests, the victim typically rises up from his or her bed, runs, falls, and drowns in a single sentence; 'suddenly' (*subito*) can recur twice or three times in one telling. William Marshall, for example, had been 'lying in his bed in a great fury', when 'suddenly he got up and ran into the fields of the same town near a water called "Swaille", and by his misfortune there and then fell in the said water and suddenly was drowned'.[23] The hearer is swept headlong through the fields and into the river. According to the jurors who had investigated Dorothea Cawthorn's death, she

> got up from her bed went to the kitchen of the said Marie Elers, and broke a hole in the wall of the said kitchen, and passing through the wall and wandering as one mad came to a certain 'Crofte' or 'hop garth' of the said Marie Elers, in which there was a certain well of water five foot deep, into which well the said Dorothea accidentally fell with the result that she was immediately submerged in said well.[24]

The story is driven forward by these sudden, unexpected surges of movement. There had been – it suggests – no time for pause. Even had such victims been capable of reflection (which they had not), the disease had moved too fast for them. Premeditation was an impossibility.

Frenzy was not, of course, the only inciting cause of accidental drowning. The basic narrative was adaptable to any condition which might bring the sufferer to this end, whether through lapses of consciousness or unbearable pain. If the drowned individual was discovered to have a

[23] 'eo in lectu [sic] suo in magna furore ad tunc & ibidem Iacente subito surgebat & currebat in campos eiusdem villa iuxta unam aquam vocatur Swaille et per infortunam suam ad tunc & ibidem cecidit in dictam aquam & subito submersus fuit'. KB 9/560/109.

[24] 'surrexit e lecto suo et usque coquinam predicte Marie Elers adivit et foramen in muro eiusdem coquine fregit et perstravit et sic per foramen illud pertransiens ac vagrans ut demens venit in quodam "Crofte" vocatur "a hop garth" predicte marie Elers in quo erat quidam puteum aque profunditatis quinque pedum in quoquidem puteo predicta Dorothea ad tunc et ibidem casualiter cecedit occasione cuius predicta Dorothea Cawthorn in puteo predicto submersa'. KB 9/599/1/91.

history of 'the falling sickness' (epilepsy), this became the default cause.[25] When Elizabeth Richardson was found drowned near her home on 9 May 1534, the local jurors deposed that she had been sick for half a year 'with a certain disease or illness in the right part of her breast called "a Rotten brest"'. The pain had 'so gravely vexed and disturbed [her] that she was not only weak from it, but by reason of the said infirmity had lost her mind or her reason'.[26] She had drowned herself 'as much due to the debility of her body as of her mind'.[27] Thomas Page, meanwhile, had been suffering from a sickness called 'le stone', when

> by the vehemence and acuteness of the said disease [he] became demented, and continued mad and without remission or constant memory until the fifteenth day of the said month of December in the said year, on which day . . . the said Thomas Page, being thus mad, ran out of his house, and wandering and running unadvisedly and as one mad, by misfortune fell into a certain ditch or well.[28]

These stories did not differ substantially from the standard template of 'death by frenzy'; they were simply less common.

Were the stories told in these inquests true? The disappointing yet predictable answer is that – barring a one-in-a-million archaeological find – we will never know. It seems improbable that every one of them offers a faithful reconstruction of events; none of the jurors even claimed to have been eyewitnesses of the deaths of which they told. What we *can* say with certainty, however, is that the stories which the coroners were willing to undersign were plausible.[29] The court of King's Bench regularly called upon local officeholders to amend defective or irregular paperwork; few county coroners can have relished the prospect of restarting an inquest from scratch.[30] It was simply not in their interest to spin tall tales. The

[25] See, e.g., KB 9/686/2/206; KB 9/558/51; KB 9/594/119; KB 9/1065/24; KB 9/683/262.

[26] 'infirma fuit de quadam morbo sive infirmitate in dextra parte pectoris sue vocatur "a Rotten brest" qua quidem infirmitas tam graviter vexabat et perturbabat predictam Elizabeth quod . . . racione eiusdem non solum debilis fuit set eorum mentem siue racionem suam racione infirmitate predicte amiset'. KB 9/529/93.

[27] 'racione infirmitate & debilitate tam corporis quam mentis predict' ad tunc et ibidem in puteo predicto submersa fuit'. Ibid.

[28] 'per Vigorem & aegrotatem predicto morbi sui demenscia devenit & demens continuit absque illa perfect' sine constante memoria usque xv° diem eiusdem mensis decembris . . . eiusdem diei . . . predictus Thomas Page sic demens existente domum suum excurrit ac vagrans & currens inadviso ac quasi demens per infortunam in quodam fossulo' sive puteo perijt'. KB 9/1110/ unnumbered membrane.

[29] Tim Stretton, *Women Waging Law in Elizabethan England* (Cambridge: Cambridge University Press, 2005), p. 179.

[30] MacDonald and Murphy, *Sleepless Souls*, p. 26.

notion that pain or fever could literally send a person mad was apparently entirely believable.

The typical story of 'death by frenzy' balanced a stress on excess (of suffering, sickness, or fury), with one on deprivation (of mind). Excess and absence go hand-in-hand: the disease has swept through the body with such violence that it has stripped the person of his or her faculties. Thus far, we have encountered 'alienation of mind' as a diagnostic sign of frenzy, but alienation – of mental and material possessions – was also a central concern of the English common law. Looking at these records, it is worth attending to what is being alienated, and from whom. In these inquests, it is usually the invalid who has been taken *away from* his or her mental possessions. The formulae align the individual's sudden, violent exit from bed (*extra lectulum suum*), home (*extra domum*), and mind (*extra mentem suam*). The unlit fields through which the sufferer stumbles mirror this second, less tangible exile.

It was also possible for the coroner to describe the deceased as having lost – rather than left – his or her mind. Elizabeth Richardson, tormented by her 'Rotten brest', 'had lost her mind or reason'.[31] But this formula is rare among the inquests returned as *per infortunium*. Situating the deceased as the subject and her mind as the lost object, the active construction of this formula implies that Elizabeth was still present at the time of death – still in some sense *herself* – albeit with some of her faculties 'lost'. To judge by its usage, this was the less compelling of the two idioms. Asking why this was this case brings us to the crossroads between tragic accident and suicide.

Self-Murder

Someone had left his or her home in the middle of the night, and had later been found drowned. For early modern hearers, these bare plot points were enough to warrant suspicion of suicide. At least one third of deaths ruled self-murder (*felo de se*) in early modern England were drownings; as Hunnisett and Stevenson suggested, the real incidence rate was almost certainly higher still.[32] Turning to the inquests suggests just how finely the line between *per infortunium* and *felo de se* could be drawn. In September 1538, for example, a man named John Hudson 'being

31 KB 9/529/93.

32 MacDonald and Murphy, *Sleepless Souls*, p. 57; Hunnisett, *The Medieval Coroner*, p. 21; Stevenson, 'The Rise of Suicide Verdicts', pp. 63–65.

neither of sound memory nor mind, went to the river Trent within a mile of Beeston, and then … jumped into the said water of Trent, and so drowned himself there'. The inquest insists, twice, that Hudson was not 'of sound mind' at the time of his death. The circumstances in which he died seem virtually identical to those described in the 'death by frenzy' story. And yet Hudson was ruled a self-murderer.[33]

What was it that set Hudson's case apart? It could have been an instance of malpractice, inconsistency, or clerical error. Or, just as likely, it could have been a tussle over the goods of deceased. As a felon, a suicide's goods, lands, and chattels were forfeit to the crown. They were supposed to go to the royal almoner, and – on paper – once he had received them, he was supposed to redistribute them as alms. In practice, however, the monarch often gave local grandees – whether mayors, manorial lords, corporations, or courtiers – the right to collect forfeitures in their area of jurisdiction. These local officials were supposed to wait until each case had been investigated, presented, and ruled a felony. Sometimes, however, they cut out the middleman and simply turned up at the door of the deceased.

This was the fate suffered by Simon Springold, the adult son of the 'frantic' yeoman Thomas Springold. In 1560, he complained to the Court of Requests that the mayor of King's Lynn had turned up outside the house mere hours after his father's death. The mayor and his men

> did enter and with great force and violence did breake upp the Chestes which [belonged] to the saide Thomas in his lief tyme. And … dyvers severall somes of money amounting to four score Poundes and more, that hadd and found, did take and carry awaye. And not so content did also take and dryve awaie … the goodes and chattells of the saide Thomas Springold at tyme of his deathe, clamyng and pretendyng to have and enjoy the same by reason of certeyne liberties graunted unto them of all felones goodes.[34]

A local vicar corroborated Springold's testimony; he had seen 'certayne Cattell that were brought into the street and the maior did theare sease them. and Cause them to be dryvene awaye'.[35] Having the household's goods and chattels ransacked, appraised, and driven away through the streets must have been deeply humiliating for still-living relatives. For many, it also meant instant bankruptcy. A family like the Springolds had

[33] 'Johannes Hudson … non sane memorie nec compos mentis existens ivit ad ripam aque de Trent in Com' predict' infra miliare de Beeston predict' et de ripa illa, predictus Johannes Hudson tunc saltavit in dictam aquam de Trent, et sic seipsum ibidem submersit. Et sic predictus Johannes Hudson non sane memorie nec compos mentis existens … ad mortem suam devenit et non aliter … felo de se'. KB 9/541/130.

[34] Kew, TNA, REQ 2/84/12/7. [35] Ibid., m. 1.

good reasons to make sure that the householder's death was *not* ruled a suicide. Men like the Mayor of King's Lynn – for whom the acquisition of 'all felones goodes' was a perk of the job – had their own reasons to make sure that it *was*.

In *Sleepless Souls*, MacDonald and Murphy argued that the only way in which the relatives of suicides could hope to hold onto their inheritance was by securing a verdict of non compos mentis – voiding one of *felo de se* – and that this was scarcely ever awarded.[36] It seems likely that coroners, jurors, and the relatives of the deceased would have been aware of this low success rate. If the circumstances permitted it, for them, a tragic accident was infinitely preferable to a pardonable suicide. It is possible, then, that the death of John Hudson was inscribed as a suicide simply because, ultimately, the crown-appointed franchise holder had won out.

The conflict over Thomas Springold's chattels had kicked off on his son's doorstep, but sometimes the trouble began only when the inquest reached the court of King's Bench. When, in June 1685, King's Bench received the inquests which the Sussex coroner Alexander Luxford had conducted into the deaths of John Attersole and Thomas Browne – both of whom had drowned in the same parish, in the same fortnight, while suffering from the same disease – the county sheriff was immediately ordered to conduct his own independent inquiry into the deaths.[37] The sheriff's reports are missing, but he and his jurors seem to have endorsed the verdict of misfortune in Attersole's case, and overturned it in Browne's. The new verdict must have been suicide, for the following autumn, a yeoman named Joseph Browne was summoned to King's Bench to answer for his deceased relative's goods and chattels (valued at just under £133).[38] Although the sheriff's detective methods must remain a mystery, the fact that Thomas had been the possessor of a small fortune was probably not irrelevant to the outcome.

These drownings were evidently borderline cases, ones in which the more clement interpretation of events had apparently been mooted and then dismissed. It is worth attending particularly closely to the 'madness words' which they invoked. For, *pace* MacDonald and Murphy, one did not have to be sane to be a judged a self-murderer in early modern England.[39] Hudson was one of many individuals whose disordered minds

[36] MacDonald and Murphy, *Sleepless Souls*, p. 57.
[37] KB 29/344/89, KB 29/344/119. See Hunnisett, *Sussex Coroners' Inquests, 1603–1688*, p. 132.
[38] KB 29/344/142d. [39] MacDonald and Murphy, *Sleepless Souls*, pp. 15–16.

did not acquit them.[40] In 1609, Richard Deering of Maidstone was declared a suicide despite being 'not at all sane' and 'not of sound memory nor mind but very insane'.[41] 'On 1 Oct [1603], when John Paige was of unsound mind, he wilfully drowned himself in the harbour of New Shoreham', declared one Sussex coroners' jury.[42] At the bottom of the inquest was written both *felo de se* and *lunaticus*. Twenty-three years later, another coroners' jury ruled that 'Mary wife of John Peeter of Washington, "husbandman", being non compos mentis, voluntarily threw herself into "Duckly Ponde" in Washington and so died'.[43] On 9 April 1645, a Wiltshire man named Henry James 'voluntarily' threw himself into the river Avon while 'non Compos Mentis'.[44] Despite the ruling of non compos mentis, the ultimate verdict in all of these cases was felonious suicide. As I have suggested, these cases may have involved the kind of behind-the-scenes wrangling between rival stakeholders described above, procedural error, or both. Taking a closer look at contemporary legal theory, however, suggests another possible line of interpretation.

Legal Categories of Madness

English legal theorists had their own centuries-old hermeneutic framework for use in cases of suspected madness. Many of this framework's diagnostic categories had been borrowed straight from ancient Roman legal theory; others were loans from Hippocratic-Galenic medicine. *Phrenitis* (in medieval Latin, *phrenesis*) was in the latter camp, and – by the thirteenth century – it had become one of the commonest diseases of mind to be invoked in cases of suspected homicide and suicide.[45] In fact, the 'linguistic limitations' of the thirteenth-century coroners' records have prompted historians to wonder whether 'not enough "madness words" were available

40 KB 9 728/3, m. 204.

41 'mentis suis nullo modo compos sed lunaticus existens . . . non fuit sane memorie nec compos mentis sed valde insanus'. KB 9 728/3/204. For other similar verdicts, see KB 9/514/78 (John Prout, 1530); KB 9/567/105 (Johanna Mallome, 1546); KB 9/584/84 (Margaret Hobby, 1553).

42 KB 9/714/6, trans. Hunnisett, in *Sussex Coroners' Inquests, 1603–1688*, no. 8, p. 2.

43 KB 9/1094/105, ibid., no. 280, p. 70.

44 'predictus Henricus James decimo Nono die Aprilis Anno supradicto apud dauntesey predict' existens adtunc & ibidem non Compos Mentis seipsum in unam flumen vocatur Avon voluntarie proiecit'. KB 9/845/2/246.

45 See Walker, *Crime and Insanity in England*, vol. 1, pp. 19–24; Butler, *Forensic Medicine*, pp. 199–201.

to clerks for them to make an accurate, concise translation of the words of the jurors'.[46]

By the sixteenth century – while these time-honoured diagnostic categories were still in use – a veritable smorgasbord of new alternatives had sprung up alongside them. A Tudor coroner's clerk might have chosen to characterize a dead man as *expers mentis* ('out of his mind'), *de non saine memoire* ('of unsound memory'), *carens ratione* ('lacking reason'), *sine discretionem* ('without discretion'), *extra sensum* ('out of his senses'), *demens, amens, furiosus, freneticus, insanus, lunaticus, mente fracta et distracta* ('crazed and distracted in mind'), or just plain 'madd'. In 1628, Coke praised his fifteenth-century predecessor, the common lawyer Sir Thomas Littleton, for avoiding '*Amens, demons, furiosus, lunaticus, fatuus, stultus*, or the like, for *Non compos mentis* is most sure and legall'.[47] Glossing Littleton, Coke added that to speak of 'a man of non sane memory', was the same as 'to say in Latin, *Qui non est compos mentis*'.[48] In other words, the phrase *non sanae memoriae* ('unsound in memory') was to be understood as a synonym of non compos mentis ('unsound in mind), rather than as a specific reference to an impaired memory.[49] This makes it harder for us to pick out instances in which clerks and coroners *were* referring to that specific faculty (and where the record invokes the full phrase, I will assume that they were not). Yet the fact that the common lawyers' terminology had developed in this way is in itself suggestive: when it came to establishing legal personhood (or its absence), 'memory' was apparently important enough to serve as a synecdoche for 'mind'.

Despite Coke's best attempts at standardization, the same confusing medley of Latin, Law French and English was still current at the end of the seventeenth century. In his layperson's guide, *Non compos mentis, or, The law relating to natural fools, mad-folks, and lunatick persons* (1700), the barrister John Brydall echoed Coke: 'A Man of Non sane Memorie, is termed among the Latines Insanus, Fatuus, Amens, Demens, Mente Captus, Maniacus, Furiosus, Stultus, Errore Mentis Affectus, a Rationis usu Destitutus, Lunaticus; and Non Compos Mentis.'[50] If medieval clerks

46 Gwen Seabourne and Alice Seabourne, 'The Law on Suicide in Medieval England', *Journal of Legal History* 21(1) (2000), 31.
47 Coke, *The first part of the Institvtes*, lib. 3, cap. 6, section 405, f. 246v.
48 Thomas Littleton, in Eugene Wambaugh (ed.), *Littleton's Tenures* (Washington, DC: John Byrne, 1903), p. 193; Coke, *The first part of the Institvtes*, lib. 3, cap. 6, section 405, f. 246v. For later paraphrases, see *The Compleat justice* (London, 1661), p. 194; John Brydall, *Non compos mentis* (London, 1700), p. 5 (quotation on the next page).
49 I would like to thank Reader C for setting me right on this point.
50 Brydall, *Non compos mentis*, p. 5.

had too few 'madness words' at their disposal, it is tempting to conclude that their early modern successors had rather too many. No wonder Coke thought it necessary to insist on non compos mentis as the 'most sure and legal' choice. Behind this messy melange of 'madness words', however, lay a reasonably coherent set of principles. The common law, Coke explained, counted 'four sorts' of persons non compos mentis:

> 1. Idiota which from his nativity, by a perpetuall infirmity, is Non compos mentis. 2. He that by sickness, griefe, or other accident, wholly loseth his memorie and understanding. 3. A Lunatique that hath sometimes his understanding and sometimes not ... and therefore he is called Non compos mentis, so long as he has not understanding. Lastly, he that by his own vicious act for a time depriveth himself of his memory and understanding, as he that is drunken.[51]

This list remained more or less unchanged throughout the seventeenth century, although not everybody deigned to include drunkards. In his handbook for local justices of the peace, *The countrey justice* (1618), the barrister Michael Dalton counted only the first three types of persons non compos mentis: '1. A foole naturall, ... 2. Hee who was once of good and sound memorie, and after (by sicknesse, hurt, or other accident, or visitation of God) looseth his memorie. 3. A lunatike.'[52] In fact, it is unclear why Coke decided to add the fourth category, for he was adamant that 'that kinde of Non compos mentis shall give no privilege to him or to his Heires'.[53] If heavy drinkers ended up in the same sort of state as 'Mad-folks', Brydall concurred, this did not diminish their responsibility for their actions, for they 'were made so by their own Default'.[54]

It was at least reasonably easy for a coroner's jury to identify a 'Drunkard' (it cannot have been easy to keep a drink problem a secret in a rural parish). Establishing the status of an 'Idiota' or 'foole naturall' was a fairly straightforward process too: friends and neighbours were asked whether the individual had been that way since birth, whether they had known the value of 20 pence, and so on.[55] But establishing whether the deceased had belonged to either the second or third category on the list was

[51] Coke, *The first part of the Institvtes*, lib. 3, cap. 6, section 405, ff. 246v–247r.
[52] Michael Dalton, *The countrey justice* (London, 1619), p. 223.
[53] Coke, *The first part of the Institvtes*, lib. 3, cap. 6, section 405, f. 247r.
[54] Brydall, *Non compos mentis*, sig. A2r.
[55] Margaret McGlynn, 'Idiots, Lunatics and the Royal Prerogative in Early Tudor England', *Journal of Legal History* 26(1) (2005), 9–10.

a more complex matter. For, as blanket terms, neither non compos mentis nor lunacy covered all possible manifestations of madness.

On suicide, for example, Dalton wrote that 'If a man kil himself (either with a meditate hatred against his own life, or out of distraction, or other humor) he is called Felo de se; and he shall forfeit to the King his goods and chattels real & personal'. 'Distraction' was a loose synonym for 'madness' in early modern England; etymologically, it derived from the Latin verb *distrahere*, meaning literally 'to draw apart'. Like 'delirium', the word expressed the notion that the 'wits' had somehow become distanced from their owner.[56] But, for Dalton, it did not automatically earn the afflicted individual the status of non compos mentis. Nor did any 'other humor' (and here Dalton might have been speaking of a troublesome bout of bile, its effects on the soul, or both at once). The fact that the suicide had been swayed by their humours was not enough to grant them a non compos mentis verdict. Only a person who lacked all trace of 'discretion', Dalton insisted, would qualify.[57]

This distinction between two degrees of madness – imperfect 'distraction' and complete and utter unreason – was not new.[58] Its earliest articulation was to be found in a thirteenth-century legal treatise entitled *De legibus et consuetidinibus angliae*, traditionally attributed to the English jurist Henry de Bracton (c. 1210–1268). According to Bracton, only the severest cases of mental alienation merited a non compos mentis verdict. These were raging madmen, or *furiosi*:

> But if a madman, one out of his mind, phrenetic, or suffering from an acute illness has drowned himself or killed himself, does such a person commit a felony on his own account? It would seem that they do not, nor do they forfeit their goods or inheritance, because they lack sense and reason, and can no more commit a crime or a felony than a brute, since they are not far removed from the brutes.[59]

This passage from Bracton's *De legibus* became the definitive guide for anyone in early modern England angling for a non compos mentis

[56] For a fuller exploration of the meanings of 'distraction', see Neely, *Distracted Subjects*, pp. 1–26.

[57] Dalton, *The countrey justice*, pp. 216–217.

[58] For the later history of 'partial' versus 'total insanity', see Joel P. Eigen, 'Intentionality and Insanity: What the Eighteenth-Century Juror Heard', in William F. Bynum, Roy Porter, and Michael Shepherd (eds.), *The Anatomy of Madness, Vol. 2, Institutions and Society* (London: Tavistock, 1985), pp. 34–51; Joel P. Eigen, 'Delusion in the Courtroom: The Role of Partial Insanity in Early Forensic Testimony', *Medical History* 35 (1991), 25–49.

[59] Henry de Bracton, *Henrici de Bracton de Legibus & consuetudinibus Angliae* (London, 1569), lib. 3, tract. 2, f. 150r.

verdict. Brydall quoted Bracton extensively in his 1700 guide to the subject:

> No Felony, or Murder, can be committed without a Felonious Intent, or Purpose: But *Furiosus non intelligit quid agit & animo, & Ratione caret, & non multum distat a Brutis* [but the madman does not know what he is doing, and lacks mind and reason, and is not far removed from the brutes], as *Bracton* saith, and therefore he cannot have a Felonious Intent.[60]

Thus, concluded Coke, '[i]f a man lose his memory by the rage of sickness or infirmity, or otherwise, & kill himself while he is not *compos mentis*, he is not *Felo de se*'.[61]

Bracton's law was merciful – in its way – but the criteria for eligibility were extremely stringent. It was not enough to be subject to fits of violent passion or to see things which nobody else saw. What was required was nothing less than a total alienation of 'mind' and 'reason'. Elsewhere, Coke insisted that the sufferer's condition was to be no less than 'absolute madness and deprivation of memorie'.[62] At the end of the century, Coke's successor as Chief Justice of the Common Pleas, Sir Matthew Hale (1609–1676) set the bar at the same height as his predecessor:

> It is not every melancholy or hypochondriacal distemper, that denominates a man *non compos*, for there are few, who commit this offense, but are under such infirmities, but it must be such an alienation of mind, that renders them to be madmen or frantic, or destitute of the use of reason.[63]

No matter how disturbed their mind, if an individual had the wherewithal to 'doe the common offices of this life', they were also capable of crime.

In sum, the legal theorists of early modern England recognized three degrees of madness. Persons who had become fully alienated from their own minds – whether through sickness, injury, or misfortune – were judged incapable of forming intent (criminal or otherwise). They were grouped with other innocents (infants, 'idiots', and 'brutes'), and were instantly pardoned. More ambiguous forms of madness (described variously as 'melancholy', 'inconstancy', 'distemper', or 'distraction') did not necessarily disable all their sufferers' faculties, and thus could not be relied upon to earn them the status of non compos mentis. Lunacy, on the other hand, *did* guarantee it, but it was – in its strictest definition – episodic: its

60 Brydall, *Non compos mentis*, p. 75.

61 Edward Coke, *The third part of the Institutes of the laws of England concerning high treason, and other pleas of the crown, and criminall causes* (London, 1644), cap. 8, p. 54.

62 Ibid., p. 6.

63 Matthew Hale, *Historia placitorum coronae*, vol. 1 (London, 1736), p. 412.

sufferers euphemistically 'enjoyed lucid intervals'. If a lunatic had killed himself while non compos mentis, he was innocent; if he was in one of his 'lucid intervals', then he was guilty.

This was a framework with which county coroners would have been at least somewhat familiar (at least, the ones who had read their Dalton). And although their jurors would have been less likely to be able to read, they might have heard a version of the same framework preached from the pulpit.[64] For, if human law was always supposed to be patterned on divine law, this was one corner of the tapestry which Protestant divines felt confident that the lawyers had right. Thus, in *Lifes preservative against self-killing* (1637), the Reformed preacher John Sym assured his readers that, although suicide was a mortal sin, there were 'certaine exempt cases', such as when 'a man, destitute of *understanding,* or of the *use* of *reason,* kills himselfe, as . . . a mad man in his mad fits, . . . *or* in such fits or sicknesse as is accompanied with a *delirium* or phrensey, as, in a *calenture* [fever]', for

> the same is not in them properly *self-murder: because,* understanding in them is *deficient,* or *passively* depraved, and not *actively* and wilfully done by themselves: *so* that they cannot judge *morally,* nor sometimes naturally, of their owne actions; *neither* are able rightly to direct them, in a *state* of that impotency of understanding: *neither* is such an *act* in such persons to be deemed willing, or an *act* of the *will,* so long as reason is wanting, without which it is not possible for a mans *will rationally* to move. *And therefore,* in such prancks, and mad acts, the *will* whereby they are done, is but *brutus impetus, a brute motion or violence,* which motion is not from the understanding so much, as from accidents, making a man not to be himselfe.[65]

This was why, Sym concluded, in 'neither in the *Courts* of earth, nor heaven, are such persons condemned as *self murderers,* for killing themselves, because, they are not properly so much *agents,* as *sufferers*; both in the *act* doing; and also in the *effect,* or death thereupon ensuing'.[66] As a divine, Sym was more interested than his legal colleagues in how exactly 'depravation' cascaded from one cognitive faculty to the next: it was an 'impotency of understanding' and want of 'reason' which made 'an act of will' impossible. What was left was a mere 'brute motion or violence'. Although Sym did not quote Bracton, his choice of the word 'brute' was no coincidence; this was a notion which spanned legal, philosophical, and theological constructions of madness. Although this '*brutus impetus*' compelled the sufferer to move, it did not merit the name of 'will', for it did

[64] MacDonald and Murphy, *Sleepless Souls*, pp. 112–113.
[65] John Sym, *Lifes preservative against self-killing* (London, 1637), p. 172. [66] Ibid.

not stem 'from the understanding'. In Sym's eyes, the 'will' was a faculty of the rational soul; if it could not move rationally, then it could not move at all. And without it, a man was not 'himselfe' at all.

In *Self-homicide-murther* (1674), the Cambridge divinity graduate Thomas Philipot echoed Sym: all of the incremental steps towards self-murder were 'the results of deliberation and debate, or of consent and choice', acts which 'a will distorted with a Phrensy cannot be capable of'.[67] This was why if a fatal act was 'performed by persons that are assaulted by violent Fevers, as Calentures, and the like, which are usually accompanied with a Phrensy, and to such persons as these, upon just and evident proof of their distemper, they do not deny the Obsequies of Christian Funeral'.[68] Of course, the only 'just and evident proof' available in such cases was the testimony of other parishioners – the same group from whom the coroners' jury was drawn.

Circumstances of Death

Reading the coroners' inquests in the light of these prescriptive texts is illuminating. Even at a grammatical level, the crafting of these stories shows a sustained effort to cast the deceased in exactly the role described by Sym and Philipot: not as an 'agent', but as a 'passively depraved' sufferer. One interesting consequence of reading the inquests in dialogue with the theory is that the manner of death starts to look like a more significant indicator of outcome than the individual's purported mental state. If a person had strangled or stabbed themselves, angling for a non compos mentis verdict was not likely to be worth the effort. After all, even the most haphazard of such deaths required sourcing and wielding the appropriate instruments. This was proof of forethought and intent; it fatally weakened the plot of 'death by frenzy'. Parish communities must have spread the word that cases of hanging and self-wounding were lost causes. The physical signs of 'malice aforethought' were indelibly marked on the body.

Despite the odds, there was still the occasional valiant effort to frame a death of this sort as an accident. In 1538, the jurors of Standley witnessed that the chapman Thomas Paterdayll had been 'visited with a certain illness called "A Wode agoo", and there and then by misfortune fell on a certain knife against his will'. The trial jury seems to have accepted this

[67] Thomas Philipot, *Self-homicide-murther* (London, 1674), p. 8. [68] Ibid., p. 7.

assessment, and affirmed the verdict of 'by misfortune'.[69] More than a century later, on 21 June 1658, a coroners' jury swore that William Morley, who for the previous seventeen years 'was divers times taken and laboured of and with certaine fitts and turnes of the frenzey . . . was again seized with such a fit at Halnaker and at 4 p.m., while still labouring with it, struck himself in the middle of the throat with a knife of iron and steel . . . and then died'.[70] This inquest, too, seems to have been waved through. But successes of this kind were few and far between; many more were rejected by the King's Bench jury. In the case of the Kentish husbandman Thomas Gyles, the coroner's jury was willing to swear that he had been non compos mentis on the day of his death, and 'in his madness [had] cut his throat with a knife worth 1d'.[71] By the time the case was copied onto the controlment roll at Westminster, however, the verdict was *felo de se*. Coroners and their jurors could not have remained ignorant of the low success rate of the 'accidental self-stabbing' story, or not for long. They risked, at best, the time and expense of cross-examination at Westminster; at worst, a conviction for perjury. They would have needed very good reasons to swear to the truth of a story which ran against the grain of the material evidence.

A drowned body, on the other hand, presupposed nothing. It was a blank page, one which would bear a range of stories. One told of a sane man losing his footing and drowning by accident, but this risked questions as to what he had been doing leaving his house alone and at night. A second told of a chronic lunatic doing the same. This version resisted the suicide verdict twice over (the death was an accident *and* the victim had been non compos mentis), but it obliged its tellers to argue hard.[72] Where lunacy was claimed, it was up to the claimants to prove that death had not occurred during a 'lucid interval'.[73] Any other type of mental disturbance, meanwhile, had to be shown to have caused total 'deprivation of memorie'. It is hard to see how either point could have been proven beyond all doubt. Both left weak points in the story, easy for a suspicious trial jury or an eagle-eyed almoner to detect and exploit.

69 'non existens compos mentis & tunc & ibidem visitatus cum quadam infirmitate vocatur "A Wode agoo" & ad tunc & ibidem per infortunam Cecidit super unum Cultellum contra voluntatem suam . . . ex infortuna'. KB 9/539/96.

70 KB 9/879/426, trans. Hunnisett, in *Sussex Coroners' Inquests, 1603–1688*, no. 448, p. 115.

71 KB 9/517/97, trans. Hunnisett, in *Sussex Coroners' Inquests, 1485–1558* (Lewes: Sussex Record Society, 1985), no. 83, p. 22.

72 For just a few examples, see KB 9/517/61 (William Wale, 1530); KB 9/519/97 (William Dymmok, 1531); KB 9/979/197 (William Wyrall, 1541); KB 9/556/92 (Thomas Aston, 1543).

73 Dalton, *The countrey justice*, p. 217; Hale, *Historia Placitorum coronae*, vol. 1, p. 412.

The third story is the one with which this chapter began: the story of the 'wode ague'. Rereading this last narrative in the light of the legal framework sketched out above is illuminating. It suggests that this particular plotline – in which a feverish disease leads to a complete alienation of the mind – possessed a power to persuade which other claims to madness did not. It seems to have reliably convinced its hearers that the victim had been non compos mentis. Dalton and Hale both privileged mental alienation caused by 'sicknesse, infirmity, or accident' as a valid case of exemption from blame.[74] The theorists' certainty on this point must have informed the development of the clerical formulae used in the inquests, and the formulae, in turn, must have steered jurors' interpretation of new deaths.

These formulae are repetitive, but they merit attention. In cases ruled suicide, the movements of the deceased are always recounted in the active voice. Despite his unsoundness of mind, John Hudson leapt into the Thames and drowned himself (*saltavit ... et sic seipsum ibidem submersit*). Echoing the foregone conclusion of *felo de se*, the reflexive construction of this formula drives home its message: murderer and victim are one and the same. In the story of the 'wode ague', conversely, near-identical events are reframed in the passive. The victim *was* drowned (*submersus est*; *demersus est*; *mersus fuit*). Thing happened *to* him or her. Dorothy Cawthorn, who was 'sick with a certain quotidian fever ... was often so tortured by this sickness that she became as one mad, so much so that she did not know what she was doing or saying'.[75] Likewise, on 5 May 1534, 'Jane Barkeworth lay in her bed much vexed by illness and in agony, so that she did not have the reason to govern herself. Suddenly she leapt up from her bed, deprived [of reason] by her fury and agony, and then and there ran to a certain pool and was accidentally submerged'.[76]

The most common formula of all was the one we have encountered already: the one in which the sufferer has simply gone 'out' of his or her mind. This formula leaves no room for speculating as to whether there had been some residue of 'reason' or 'will' left. It was the possessor of these faculties – the subject capable of conscious intent – who had gone missing. With the human subject displaced, other actors moved to the fore. In the

74 Hale, *Historia Placitorum coronae*, vol. 1, p. 412; Dalton, *The countrey justice*, p. 223.

75 'fuit egrota de quadam febre quotidiana et de eadem egritudine plerumque adeo cruciebatur Ita ut se velut demens gerebat in tantum ut nesciabat quod faciebat aut loquebat'. KB 9/599/1/91.

76 'Johanna Barkeworth iacuit in lecto suo mult' vexabat cum infirmitate et agonia eo quod non habens Racionem se gubinari subbito [sic] surrexit a lecto suo in furiositatem agonie sue distracione sua deficiente & adtunc & ibidem concurrit in quadem stagnum et aqua ibidem ea casualiter submersit'. KB 9/529/106.

'wode ague' narrative, it was typically the disease itself which took on the leading role. When, in 1548, Thomas Halom was 'visited and tormented by a certain illness called An Agewe', his journey 'out of his bed . . . to a certain font called "a Well"' happened only 'through the great fury of the said sickness'.[77] In these inquests, the 'furious' behaviour seen in those suffering from frenzy transfers to the disease. Given affect, will, and motive power, it assumes the mantle of subjecthood, and thereby also of liability for the death. It was *its* fury – and not that of the human sufferer – which plunged the body into the water.

Given the need to present the deceased as a helpless victim – pushed around by agents they were too weak to control – it might seem surprising that none of these stories of 'death by frenzy' ever featured the Devil. If a person could not be blamed for the disabling effects of disease, surely – one might think – the double onslaught of disease *and* the Devil would make the victim doubly passive, and thereby doubly innocent. But this is not how early modern Christians saw it. Satan could stir up the humours, kindle the passions, abuse the imagination, and so on, but he could not – under any circumstances – hijack the rational soul. This was because sin *always* required the voluntary consent of the sinner. Even Reformed Protestants like Sym, who followed Augustine in insisting that the will was not 'free' in the sense of having the ability to choose between alternatives, believed in 'free will' in an attenuated sense. Human beings were never *forced* to sin, by Satan, God, or anyone else.[78] Even the staunchest believers in predestination agreed with Aquinas that the Devil could not 'cause sin in the way that the [Holy] Spirit causes grace'.[79] Christian theology fundamentally depended on the freedom of the human will to embrace evil.[80] If an act was done against the actor's will, it was no sin.

[77] 'visitatus et vexatus fuit de quadam infirmitate vocatur "an Agewe" . . . per magnam furiositatem dicti egritudinis exivit fforas extra lectulum suum vsque ad quandem fontem voc "a Well" . . . ad tunc & ibidem predictus Thomas Halom per furiositatem morbi predicti saltabat in fontem predictam et statim demersus fuit. Et sic . . . per furiositatem morbi predicti ad mortem suam devenit'. KB 9/570/93.

[78] John Calvin, *The institution of Christian religion* (London, 1561), book 2, chs. 1–2, 5, ff. 5r–17r, 27r–35v. Augustine's mature position has been described as 'non-free free will'. Human beings were never compelled to sin. See Kenneth M. Wilson, *Augustine's Conversion from Traditional Free Choice to 'Non-Free Free Will': A Comprehensive Methodology* (Tübingen: Mohr Siebeck, 2018). For the Reformed Protestant position, see Muller, *Christ and the Decree.*

[79] See Thomas Aquinas, *ST*, Ia IIae, q. 80, a. 3.

[80] To reject 'non-free free will' was to make God the author of sin. See John Calvin, *The institution of Christian religion, vvrytten in Latine by maister Ihon Caluin, and translated into Englysh*. . . trans. Thomas Norton (London, 1561), ff. 5r–v.

What stood in the courts of heaven also (on this occasion) stood in the courts of earth. Self-killing at the instigation of the Devil was *always* self-murder, for – no matter how distracted the individual had become – he or she had still *chosen* to listen to and act on the tempter's urgings. Even 'lunatic', 'distracted', or 'melancholy' persons could have enough use left of their rational faculties to follow this path. The husbandman Richard Hartley had been mad 'abowte xij [12] yeres paste before his deathe', but when he stabbed himself in April 1554, it was 'by the instigation of the Devil and by his [own] willfull means'.[81] This was where the means came to matter: mad persons who had hanged, stabbed, or suffocated themselves had always done so 'feloniously', 'voluntarily', and 'wickedly'. Their methods showed forethought – sometimes even ingenuity – and this suggested a measure of diabolic prompting. Victims of frenzy, on the other hand, were supposed to be altogether incapable of acts of will and understanding. It was thus safer to leave Satan out of the equation, for – if he had whispered words of persuasion in their ears – they were not supposed to have had the presence of mind to comprehend them.

The Devil stood at the centre of MacDonald and Murphy's argument about the 'secularization' of suicide. It was the looming presence of Satan in English Protestantism which ushered in the 'age of severity', they argued, and his declining presence in the so-called age of Enlightenment which brought about 'the revival of leniency'. It is certainly true that the phrase 'the instigation of the Devil' drops out of the late seventeenth-century coroners' inquests. And there is plenty of evidence to suggest that he was starting to play a less active role in goading on the suicidal (at least, in the minds of learned elites). Yet the diminishing immanence of the Devil did not necessarily make people either more or less compassionate towards those who had taken their own lives. In his 1674 *Self-Murther Suicide*, Philipot did not mention Satan once, but (as the title of his treatise suggests) he was not soft on 'Self-murderers'. He wrote approvingly of the ancient custom of dragging 'through the execrable Gates of Cities . . . and in other places to disgrace this Fact [deed], and make it more exemplary Criminal'.[82] Meanwhile, the list of exemptions was the same as it had always been, and – circumstances permitting – sympathetic jurors probably still preferred to angle for a verdict of *per infortunium* rather than the question-begging non compos mentis.

[81] KB 9/587/208. [82] Philipot, *Self-homicide-murther*, p. 6.

Disputed Verdicts

For those whose sympathies lay with the survivors of the deceased, the story of 'death by frenzy' was the surest means of getting an inquest past the clerks of King's Bench without attracting attention. When this did not happen (whether out of lack of sympathy or fear of perjury), the result was a verdict of *felo de se*. It was not uncommon, however, for locals to continue to resist this verdict. In their attempts to reclaim or to hold onto the forfeited goods of the deceased, heirs took counsel, and carefully moulded their stories to pass through the same framework. The equity courts in which these cases were pursued were generally recorded in the vernacular. These records are typically much fuller and less formulaic than the coroners' records, and can therefore give a richer sense of how ordinary people expected – or thought that magistrates would expect – a frantic person to act.

After the 'frantic' yeoman Thomas Springold's house had been pillaged in May 1560, his son and brother-in-law joined forces to sue the men responsible in the Court of Requests. The mayor of Lynn had wronged the family, they insisted, for he had had no right

> to take or sease any of the goodes cattelles or other moveables or any other thing belonging to the saide Thomas at tyme of his deathe, for that the saide Thomas was not then of whole mynd but madd and franticke and knew not what he did. And therefore by order of the lawe ought not to lose or forfett all his goodes and cattell (beyng *Felo de se*) which thing is most untrue, as your saide Subiectes are well able to prove.[83]

The bill requested that local commissioners be appointed to interrogate as 'many honest parsones as your said Subiectes shalbe able to produce, and to here and receyve such proofe and Testimonye they are able to make for and towching the premysses'. The fourteen 'parsones' whom Spryngold and Lemyng managed to assemble were – by the standards of the day – ideal witnesses: all were men between thirty and fifty; most were respectable tradesmen, two were gentlemen, and four were in fact parsons. In number and social standing, this was a panel intended to rival the coroner's 'twelve good men and true'.[84] Interestingly, although these witnesses were handpicked, their written testimonies were not identical. Several admitted ignorance or guesswork on the question of Thomas's wealth, and some even as to the number of his children. The only answer

[83] REQ 2/84/12/7r. [84] Thomas Smith, *De republica Anglorum* (London, 1583), p. 79.

which was consistently the same *and* always recorded in full was the third: its corresponding interrogatory (now missing) must have inquired as to the deportment of the deceased. To this question, a witness named William Peerse replied that he had been 'with the sayd Thomas divers and sondry tymes betwene the 27 of March and the 14 of Maye & at all tymes he fownd him mad and franticke and was with him abowt three of the Clocke in the afternoone the daye before he dyed and fownd him still in one Case and so died'.[85] These timings matched up perfectly with the timeline set out by Simon Springfield in his account of his father's death. It had been on 27 March that Thomas had first 'lost his wittes and understanding and became madd and frantycke and so contynued in his saide madnesse and francye until the 14 daie of Maye then next following at which daie the saide Thomas then beyng in his said francye and madnes at Seche aforesaid did hang hym self'.[86] Springold's repeated insistence that his father was 'in his said madness and francye' up to and including the moment of his death served to stop up any possible gaps in the story. Peerse's claim to have seen Thomas on several occasions during the last six weeks of his life – and to have found him 'in one Case' throughout – further bolstered its continuity. In fact, all fourteen witnesses stuck to the original timeline set out by Springold. Each encountered Thomas within the same six-week period; each swore that Thomas had 'continued in the case he was in when he was with him last & so continuell til the daye of his deathe'. All but one stated that Thomas had seemed both 'mad' and 'frantycke'. These testimonies were evidently engineered to block two of the diagnostic pathways outlined above: this was not an intermittent lunacy, for Thomas had been 'in one case' throughout. It was not a mere 'distraction' of mind, but a total 'madnesse and francye'. This was the sort of differential diagnosis which would have made a learned physician weep. But diagnostic accuracy was not the goal; the goal was to get a non compos mentis verdict. For non-specialists like Springold – men who had a working knowledge of the legal system, but limited exposure to the small print – it made sense to hedge one's bets.

Simon Springold was far from being the only bereaved heir to sue a crown official over a suicide verdict. But the reverse scenario was more common: if heirs resisted the verdict by simply refusing to hand over the forfeited goods, the king's almoner could prosecute them in Star Chamber at half the normal fee. Most almoners were vigilant about doing so, even over seemingly insignificant sums.[87] This was certainly true of George

85 REQ 2/84/12/1r. 86 REQ 2/84/12/7r. 87 MacDonald and Murphy, *Sleepless Souls*, p. 27.

Montaigne, who served as the king's almoner from 1619 to 1626. In November 1624, Montaigne sued a Staffordshire man named Thomas Crompton, whose brother-in-law George Copwood had stabbed himself to death in May that year. The coroner's inquest had given a verdict of *felo de se*, but Crompton had 'Denyed to Deliver or pay to the said Lord Bishopp or to any [of] his deputy or servant' Copwood's forfeited goods.[88] Crompton defended himself fiercely and at length. He insisted that he was

> able to prove by good & sufficient testimony that the said George Copwood by reason of great want of sleep and other Distemperature of body wherewith he was possessed for a good space before he became *felo de se* was at the time of such his act committed become *non compos mentis*, and overcome with a frensie or Lunacy, and that by his weakness caused thereby he soe made away himself, and not by malice forethought as by the said Bill or Informacion alledged.[89]

Crompton's retelling of his brother-in-law's death has much in common with Simon Springold's bill. He described how, in the last week of March,

> George Copwood being then of good and perfect memory and well and godlie disposed but finding his sleepe at that tyme to goe from him & fearing that he was falling into a fever or into some other Infirmity of body . . . resolved to settle and Dispose of his estate Whilest he continued able and fitt for to doe.[90]

Crompton's defence suggests one final advantage to the 'death by frenzy' story: the clean-cut nature of its beginning and ending. The disease's lifespan was familiar. Some agues could linger, but frenzy developed suddenly, dramatically, and without warning. It reached a crisis within days or weeks, after which the patient would recover or die. There was no middle ground; there was no such thing as a mild case. It divided time into clear-cut segments, eliminating all traces of ambiguity. The sufferer had been 'of good and perfect memory'; the disease had struck; thereafter he had been non compos mentis.

This was useful to Crompton, for his defence stood on shaky ground. Copwood had left him everything in his will, but he had made that will on 26 March, seven weeks before his death. It was a universally accepted tenet of English common law that 'Mad-folks, during the time of their furor, or Insanitie of Mind, cannot make a testament, nor dispose anie thing by

88 Kew, TNA, STAC 8/3/14/1. 89 Ibid., m. 2. 90 Ibid., m. 2.

will'.[91] If, however, 'a man that is of good and perfect memory, makes his will, and Afterwards . . . he becomes of unsound memory, this Act of God shall not be a Revocation of his Will'.[92] Crompton's story corresponds to this rubric even in its exact wording. Copwood had had the prescience to make over all of his goods and lands to his brother-in-law while still 'of good and perfect memory'; it was only afterwards that he had fallen into the alienation of mind in which he died. Few other diseases of mind were quite so pliable on this score, for most of any severity were believed to be chronic and treatment-resistant. Once a man had lost his mind, the law assumed him to remain in this condition unless proven to the contrary.[93]

This placed families seeking a ruling of non compos mentis in a difficult position. If the mind of the deceased had been unsound at any time before or at the moment of writing the will, the bequest was invalid and its named heirs suspect; if it had not been utterly unsound at the time of the death, then it was the non compos mentis verdict which was invalid. Crompton managed to steer a path between these two pitfalls. His carefully backdated story assured both that Copwood's deed of gift to him in March was valid *and* that the coroners' suicide verdict was invalid. Simon Springold's account was similarly tidy in its periodization, confining his father's illness to the six weeks before his father's death. The prognostic timeline for frenzy possessed its own narrative (rapid onset, deterioration, crisis, death). Its momentum could be harnessed to persuade.

Conclusion

Crompton stressed at every opportunity that his brother-in-law's condition had begun as an 'Infirmity of body'. It was on 'finding his sleepe at that tyme to goe from him' that Copwood knew to make his will, and ultimately it was 'great want of sleep and other Distemperature of body' which rendered him non compos mentis. Before this fever, Crompton insisted, Copwood had been 'well and godlie disposed'.[94] What precisely he meant by this – whether that his brother-in-law had enjoyed good health, a good disposition, godliness, or all three – was left unclear. And that served Crompton's purposes: the fever, it implied, was one tragic

[91] Henry Swinburne, *A briefe treatise of testaments and last willes* (London, 1591), p. 36.
[92] Brydall, *Non compos mentis*, p. 85.
[93] There were a few exceptions to this rule. If the testator had fallen 'into some frenzie upon some accidentall cause, which cause is afterwardes taken away . . . in these cases the testator is not presumed to continue in his former furor or frensie'. Swinburne, *A briefe treatise*, pp. 37–38.
[94] STAC 8/3/14/2.

episode in an otherwise healthy, happy, blessed, and blameless life. This was exactly the character arc plotted out in the coroners' inquests.

So far, we have seen frenzy prompt multiple attempts to articulate the enmeshment (and separability) of 'body' and 'soul'. Learned physicians treated psychic and physical symptoms as two sides of the same coin. Pluralist divines counted multiple souls; Reformed Protestant divines saw only one. Legal theorists put metaphysics to one side, and focused on the demonstrable signs of 'wit' and 'will'. It is harder to trace the outlines of the soul–body ontology to which lay defendants, witnesses, and jurors referred, and to gauge how it informed their judgements of guilt and innocence. What does seem apparent, however, is that those who were sick principally in 'mind' were more likely to have their record of personal conduct probed than whose frenzy had arisen as a direct consequence of a bodily disease.

All of these factors combined to lend the story of 'death by frenzy' a unique robustness. It erased the culpability of the deceased at every stage. He or she had fallen ill unwittingly; God and the disease itself had been the only players in the game. Once the latter had gained a foothold, it had ravaged the victim's body and alienated his or her mind. The transition from tormented invalid to person non compos mentis to corpse was near seamless. The story risked none of the difficult questions to which other madness words (like 'lunacy') were vulnerable. Frenzy, like other febrile diseases, was a known quantity. Its actions were so rapid and violent that premeditation was an impossibility, and death was almost inexorable. It emptied its sufferers (of will, wit, and memory), and filled them with its own uncontrollable fury.

This chapter thus adds to a growing body of scholarship which has resisted and complicated MacDonald and Murphy's account of this period as an 'era of severity'.[95] If there was a change, it was not in the hearts and minds of coroners' jurors, but in their confidence in their ability to navigate the system differently. The umbrella term of non compos mentis does seem to have gradually expanded to cover states of 'partial' or 'imperfect' madness (such as 'melancholy'); this may have been a response to the mounting protests at forfeiture, which had long been seen as an

[95] See Donna T. Andrew, 'The Secularisation of Suicide in England, 1660–1800', *Past & Present* 119 (1988), 158–165; Rab A. Houston, *Punishing the Dead? Suicide, Lordship, and Community in Britain, 1500–1830* (Oxford: Oxford University Press, 1998); Róisín Healy, 'Suicide in Early Modern and Modern Europe', *The Historical Journal* 49(3) (2006), 903–919; Elizabeth K. Hunter, '"Between the Bridge and the Brook": Suicide and Salvation in England, c. 1500–1650', *Reformation & Renaissance Review* 15(3) (2013), 237–257.

unjust punishment of the suicide's survivors.[96] And the more that non compos mentis verdicts passed through the king's almoner's hands without comment, the more confident coroners and the jurors would have felt about returning the same verdict. There was no need to craft a watertight story about fevers and unfenced bodies of water if mere madness would do.

Although of course the willingness to interpret non compos mentis more loosely does suggest a change of values at some level of the crown's legal apparatus, this was not the end of an era of 'severity' and the beginning of one of 'leniency'. Rather, it was a continuation of a centuries-old conflict between – on the one hand – suicide survivors and their supporters, and – on the other – the franchise-holders with a right to the forfeited goods. In her study of fourteenth-century Norfolk, Barbara Hanawalt found that most suicides in the region were concealed as accidents. 'Community feeling would [have been] with the surviving family', she concluded.[97] This general observation applies equally well to the communities of sixteenth- and seventeenth-century England.

A frenzy diagnosis could salvage the reputation of the accused, and restore the inheritance of his or her heirs. Yet innocence was bought at the price of rationality, and, as we have seen, this was a high cost. Bracton's adage that *furiosi* 'differed little from brutes' was intended to absolve them, but it also served to disempower and dehumanize them. The coroners' records examined in this chapter give little sense of this effect, but it becomes very clear in records documenting the treatment of still-living sufferers. It is to these records which we now turn.

96 MacDonald and Murphy, *Sleepless Souls*, pp. 78–86.

97 Barbara Hanawalt, *Crime and Conflict in English Communities, 1300–1348* (Cambridge, MA: Harvard University Press, 1979), p. 102.

CHAPTER 5

Ruling by Reason

Introduction

Medical theorists had explained how frenzy materially disordered the brain and animal spirits. Theologians had explained how it disabled (but did not damage) the rational faculties. Legal theorists had explained how it absolved sufferers from blame. Yet none of these explanations answered the question of *why* God allowed frenzy to occur. Why – as Heywood asked – would He choose to give its victims 'grace and then deprive them of the use of Reason'? And what was to be done with them while they remained in this state? This chapter seeks to deepen our understanding of what the loss of reason meant to contemporaries, by exploring how it informed decisions about still-living frantic persons' treatment. The hopes expressed for these treatments reveal varying degrees of optimism about the likelihood of recovery. Yet the justification of the methods reveals a strikingly consistent set of principles: rationality bestowed the right to rule, and reasserting rule was the best way restore reason.

It was these mutual relations – between the irrational and the rational, the rulers and the ruled – which formed the links in the 'chain of being' to which all God's creatures belonged. The conduct of frantic persons was a clear sign that they needed to be reinserted into that divinely ordained hierarchy – ideally by regaining the capacity for self-rule but, failing that, by submitting to be ruled by others. Yet the mere existence of frenzy was an unpleasant reminder of the instability of that order. For one thing, these diseases were no respecter of rank; formerly 'reasonable' men succumbed just as easily as anyone, prompting sudden reshuffles of the hierarchies of household and state. For another, frantic persons often proved immune to the sorts of corrective measures which could be relied upon to bring sane malefactors into line.

This chapter begins by examining the rhetoric of 'reason' and 'rule', showing how the descriptions of frenzy offered by medical theorists and moralists drew on a common vision of the ideal socio-political order.[1] It then turns to consider how this vision was used to justify a range of corrective interventions in the lives of sufferers, ranging from beating to blood transfusion. In the end, I argue, despite the solicitous rhetoric, restoring these persons to 'ruliness' was a more pressing imperative than restoring their rationality.

Empires of Reason

Divinity

Among all the descriptions of frenzy we have encountered in this book, a common motif has emerged: what the disease disturbed was the 'ruling' part of the soul: the 'soul-in-chief', the 'soueraigne' queen, the 'supream and principal form of the whole Man'.[2] To early modern thinkers, the political connotations of this language were not a coincidence. It was from '*the* Contemplation *of* our selves, in *the* Faculties *of* our Souls, and *the* Subservience *of* our Bodies', declared the Tory physician Nathaniel Johnston in 1686, that 'wise Men' had first 'fram'd *the Idaeas of* Government'.[3] The naturalness of the socio-political order was shown by the fact that it ran (in miniature) through every human heart.

Within that little principality, frenzy was a *coup d'état*, a violent deposition of the ruling soul by its inferiors. And although England's physicians subscribed to a broadly naturalistic account of brain disease, they were not blind to the moral implications of that defeat. Anxious to show that his two-soul theory was 'altogether Orthodox', 'agreeable to a good Life, and Pious Institution', Thomas Willis pointed out that it permitted 'the Wars and Strivings between our two Appetites, or between the Flesh and Spirit, both Morally and Theologically inculcated to us', to be 'also Physically understood', for

1 See Michael J. Braddick and John Walter, 'Grids of Power: Order, Hierarchy and Subordination in Early Modern Society', in Michael J. Braddick and John Walter (eds.), *Negotiating Power in Early Modern Society: Order, Hierarchy and Subordination in Britain and Ireland* (Cambridge: Cambridge University Press, 2001), pp. 1–42; Ethan Shagan, *The Rule of Moderation: Violence, Religion, and the Politics of Restraint in Early Modern England* (Cambridge: Cambridge University Press, 2011), esp. ch. 1.

2 Andreas Vesalius, *De humani corporis fabrica libri septem* (Basel, 1543), 7.6, p. 636, in Richardson and Carman (trans.), *On the Fabric of the Human Body*, vol. 5, p. 165; Davies, *Nosce teipsum*, p. 15; Willis, *Two discourses*, sig. A4r.

3 Nathaniel Johnston, *The excellency of monarchical government, especially of the English monarchy* (London, 1686), p. 1.

> *The Flesh lusts against the Spirit, and the Spirit against the Flesh.* So generally comes to pass in us, for as much as the Corporeal Soul adhering to the Flesh, inclines Man to Sensual Pleasures, whil'st in the mean time, the Rational Soul, being help'd by Ethical Rules, or Divine favours, invites it to good Manners, and the works of Piety.[4]

By 'Spirit', Willis inferred, what the Apostle Paul meant was the 'Rational Soul'. In fact, although he was bound to give priority to scripture as proof of his theory's orthodoxy, the three-way psychic struggle which he described had more in common with Plato's vision of human nature than with Paul's. In the *Phaedrus,* Plato had famously compared the rational soul to a charioteer, holding the reins of two horses: a 'good', obedient one representing the rational will, and a bad, disobedient one representing the sensitive appetites.[5]

This Platonic allegory enjoyed a long afterlife in early modern England. It was a particularly good fit with a verse from the Psalms: 'Be yee not as the horse and mule, which haue no vnderstanding: whose mouth must bee helde in with bit and bridle'.[6] Repeating the Psalmist's admonition, Thomas Adams added, 'Men haue vnderstanding, not beasts: yet when the frenzy of lust ouerwhelmeth their senses, wee may take vp the word of the Prophet, and powre [pour] it on them'.[7] By 'frenzy of lust', Adams meant the urges of the concupiscible appetite (the sensitive soul's equivalent of a 'will'). The rational will, Robert Burton explained, 'commaunds the other two in men, and is a curbe vnto them, or at least should be: but for the most part is captiuated and overruled by them, and men are led like beasts by sense, giving raines to their concupiscence and severall lusts'.[8] A war of this sort was recognizable to the learned as a '*psychomachia* . . . a war betwixt the soul and body'.[9] Madness was a sign that the reason had surrendered, and this complicated the question of how far the ensouled person was to blame. Materially, the loss of the rational faculties was explicable as a disruption in the animal spirits, but morally, it looked more like a failure of internal security. How had it been allowed it to happen?

England's divines were very capable of pointing the finger at the sufferers themselves. The 'more a man follows his lust', warned Thomas

[4] Willis, *Two discourses*, sig. A4r.

[5] See Plato, 'Phaedrus', in Christopher Emlyn-Jones and William Preddy (trans.), *Lysis. Symposium. Phaedrus*, LCL 166 (Cambridge, MA: Harvard University Press, 2022), pp. 436–441.

[6] KJV, Psalms 32:9. [7] Adams, *Mystical bedlam*, p. 45. [8] Burton, *The anatomy*, p. 37.

[9] Thomas Blount, 'Psychomachy', in *Glossographia* (London, 1659), sig. Ii5v. *Psychomachia* could also refer to a conflict between two distinct parts of the soul (as in Plato's 'Phaedrus'), or between different souls.

Hooker, 'the lesse is he led by his will . . . & the more he standeth upon pleasing of his sences, the lesse reason ordinarily useth he'.[10] It was the strength of the rational soul's resolve, the Anglican prelate Edward Stillingfleet preached in 1666, which made the difference

> between those who maintain the Empire of reason, assisted by the motives of Religion, over all the inferiour faculties, and such who dethrone their souls and make them slaves to every lust that will command them. And if men willingly subject themselves to that which they were born to rule, they have none to blame but themselves for it.[11]

Henry More agreed: it was only 'levity and mindlesness of the divine light' which could bring the rational soul 'into subjection' to the passions, and it was this which led to madness.[12]

For those who were inclined to see madness as self-inflicted (and not everybody did), the Bible offered some compelling templates. There was Deuteronomy 28:28, with which the English friar Bartholomeus Anglicus had opened his chapter 'of the Phrensie': 'Our lord shall smite thee with woodness [madness], and losse of wit and mind'.[13] The most memorable example of the Lord making good on this promise was to be found in Daniel 4, in which – the preacher Henry Smith reminded his readers – was 'laid down the pride, fall, and restitution of Nabuchadnezzar'.[14] The Babylonian king had been warned by the prophet Daniel that – if he did not repent of his sins within a year – his heart would 'be changed from man's, and . . . a beast's heart be given unto him'. But Nebuchadnezzar did not listen to Daniel; in fact, he ended his year-long grace period by boasting of his own majesty. The fulfilment of the prophecy was instant: he 'was driven from men, and did eat grass as oxen . . . till his hairs were grown like eagles' feathers, and his nails like birds' claws'.[15] The chapter ends with the recovered king's extraordinary first-person testimony:

> [A]t the end of the days I Nebuchadnezzar lifted up mine eyes unto heaven, and mine understanding returned unto me, . . . At the same time my reason returned unto me; . . . Now I Nebuchadnezzar praise and extol and honour

[10] Hooker, *The immortality of mans soule*, p. 37.
[11] Edward Stillingfleet, *A sermon preached before the King, March 13, 1666/7 by Edward Stillingfleet* (London, 1667), p. 18.
[12] More, *The immortality of the soul*, p. 479.
[13] Henry Smith, *The Fall of King Nabuchadnezzar* (London, 1591), p. 2.
[14] Bartholomaeus Anglicus, *De proprietatibus rerum*, in Stephen Bateman (trans.), *Batman vppon Bartholome, his booke De propiertatibus rerum, newly corrected, enlarged and amended* (London, 1582), f. 88r.
[15] KJV, Daniel 4: 24–37.

> the King of heaven, all whose works are truth, and his ways judgment: and those that walk in pride he is able to abase.[16]

This was the urtext for the proverb 'pride comes before a fall', and it never failed to fascinate and unsettle its early modern readers.[17] Sermons like Smith's *The Fall of Nebuchadnezzar* (published in 1591) reveal with particular clarity what a loss of reason meant to the divines of early modern England, and what they expected it would mean to their congregants. Nebuchadnezzar's fate was proof that – if sufficiently provoked – God really might take away His 'image' from a person, leaving a 'beast's heart' in a human body. For 'sinne and pleasure make men lyke beasts', Smith concluded, and 'when they haue abused their wits often, and peuerted their reason, at last God takes their vnderstanding from them, and they become like beastes'.[18]

And to be made 'degenerate like a beast' was not the end of it. Nebuchadnezzar would 'be driuen out of his palace', Smith continued, 'vntill his subiectes, and seruants, and pages, make their sport, and gaze and wonder at him . . . What a downfal was this to be brought vnder all his subiects, which spake euen now as though there were none but he: and now his seruants seruant would not be like vnto him?'[19] The king's reduction in soul had entailed an immediate reduction in rank; Smith did not have to waste time spelling out why. In a matter of moments, Nebuchadnezzar had slipped down several rungs on the 'great chain of being', from just below the angels to just above the grass. God had made him a 'wilde' creature in order to teach him his place on that ladder; He had placed 'a bitte' in Nebuchadnezzar's mouth, and 'checkt the king as boldly, as ever the king checkt his subiectes'.[20] Note the continuity of the Psalmist's motif: a loss of understanding called for the immediate application of 'bit and bridle'.[21] A 'brutish' soul merited the sort of measures used to control 'brutes'.

Medicine

We might expect that Hippocratic-Galenic medicine – with its penchant for naturalistic explanation – would be less likely than scripture to prompt sermonizing of this kind. Yet on the question of self-management there was a surprising accord between these ancient traditions of knowledge.

[16] Daniel 4: 34–37. [17] See Smith, *King Nabuchadnezzar*, p. 27. [18] Ibid., p. 32.
[19] Ibid., pp. 16, 26. [20] Ibid., pp. 17–18, 31. [21] Psalms 32:9.

Plato had claimed that the rational soul's capacity to curb the passions and appetites was vital to the health of the body, and this precept had become central to Galen's preventative medicine.[22] His advice about moderating one's habits had become codified under the heading of the 'six non-naturals', and the passions and the appetites were not the least among them.[23]

There was nothing especially novel, then, about Willis's blending of medicine, divinity, and moral philosophy. Similar cautionary amalgams had appeared in many earlier treatises on health management (known as *regimina*). In *The touchstone of complexions* (1576), for example, the Catholic priest and physician Levinus Lemnius (1505–1568) had warned that once the vital spirits 'haue attayned strength and power: they reiect and cast away the brydle of reason, & draw the spirit animal also (for they be al deryued out of one fountayne) into their faction & disordered rebellion'.[24] It was 'vntemperate dealing', 'gurmandyze, surphet, and dronkennesse' which fed the 'lewd affections, and vnbrydled motions' of the inferior soul. And once this soul had recruited the animal spirits to its cause, the reason was no longer able 'easely to subdue' them.[25] 'Hence it is', warned Willis a century later, 'that Drinking of Wine, Banquetting, and every Kind of Dissolute Life, because they render the Blood lawless, and not able to be restrain'd or bridl'd ... [that] Men become not only unable for Exercising the Acts of Judgment and Reason; but are found very prone to all manner of Wickedness and most filthy desires'.[26]

The difference between divinity and medicine was that, in medicine, the individual was not *always* to blame for a lapse of reason. Frenzy could be caused by immoderation, but – as we saw in Chapter 1 – it could also be caused by a range of factors over which the individual had much less control. It could be brought on by 'Strong Drinks' or 'Anger', the anonymous author of *The sick-mans rare jewel* (1674) warned his readers, but also by 'hot Air, the rise of the Sun' or 'a Contusion or a Wound'.[27]

[22] See Plato, 'Charmides', in W. R. M. Lamb (trans.), *Charmides. Alcibiades I and II. Hipparchus. The Lovers. Theages. Minos. Epinomis* (Cambridge, MA: Harvard University Press, 1927), esp. pp. 20–33. I owe this reference to Reader C.

[23] Saul Jarcho, 'Galen's Six Non-Naturals: A Bibliographic Note and Translation', *Bulletin of the History of Medicine* 44(4) (1970), 372–377.

[24] Lemnius had studied both divinity and medicine at Leuven. He spent most of his career as a practising physician, but took holy orders after the death of his wife. Quotation from Thomas Newton (trans.), *The touchstone of complexions* (London, 1576), f. 14r. Original text in Lemnius, *De habitu et constitutione corporis* (Antwerp, 1561), ff. 13r–14r.

[25] Lemnius, *The touchstone*, f. 10v.

[26] Willis, *Two discourses*, p. 47.

[27] B. A., *The sick-mans rare jewel* (London, 1674), pp. 165–166.

Sometimes it was 'through inward or outward distemperatures, defect of organs, which are vnapt or hindered, or otherwise contaminated', that the imagination was rendered 'vnapt, or hindered, and hurt', and then – misled by its sensitive informant – the rational soul could not help but lose its way.[28]

Early modern physicians found the prospect of the rational soul's defeat no less horrifying than had the divines. It was like 'a ciuill tumulte and sedicious vprore among the common people', Lemnius blanched, in which 'the Magistrate hath much ado to appease and mollifye the wilfull peoples rage and headinesse'.[29] In the 1660s, Willis tailored this time-honoured political-somatic analogy to fit his new anatomical-physiological account. The corporeal soul furnished both the 'Oeconomy' and 'Government' of the body, one in which the spirits were 'disposed, as it were an Army spread abroad thorow the whole Field'.[30] Each troop of this 'Animal regiment' had its distinct 'Orders and Offices, one thing in this part, and something different in that'.[31] The spirits had their different ranks (vital and animal), but they were also kept in line by the carefully planned layout of their barracks – the organs, ducts, and vessels of the body. And no site on this anatomical map was more carefully ordered than the brain. As we saw in Chapter 2, Willis had allocated each of the three orders of the Galenic-Aristotelian *psychē* its own floor on this building: the vegetative powers at the base (the cerebellum), the instinctive ones in the middle layers (the *corpus striatum* and *corpus callosum*) and the higher-level ones at the top (the cerebral cortex). The pecking order of the 'Animal Government' was given visible form in the spatial organization of its headquarters. In fact, Willis's preoccupation with the hierarchical order of this organ was so pronounced that it has led some historians to argue that it was intended – consciously or unconsciously – to shore up the newly reinstated ecclesiastical or religio-political order.[32]

Willis's hierarchically ordered brain may indeed have been a tacit religio-political manifesto; in the early 1660s, the solidity of the new regime was not to be taken for granted. Thus far, I have argued that Willis was driven to anatomize the brain not simply in order to admire its orderliness, but because he had been baffled by its capacity to produce *dis*order. Perhaps painful memories of the world 'turned upside down' *did*

[28] Burton, *The anatomy*, p. 123. [29] Lemnius, *The touchstone*, f. 10v.
[30] Willis, *Two discourses*, sig. A4r, pp. 2, 24. [31] Ibid., p. 24.
[32] Martensen, '"Habit of Reason"'; Caron, 'Thomas Willis'.

haunt his decades-long inquiry into disorders of 'the little world'.[33] Certainly, the language of 'overthrow', 'confusion', and 'tumult' is everywhere in his descriptions of 'Cephalick Diseases'.[34] Frenzy was an infiltration 'into the Pores and passages of the Brain' of 'either fierce and untameable particles, or such as are malignant and deadly to the Animal regiment'. These malignant particles stirred up rebellion among the animal spirits, compelling them 'into very confused troops . . . [so] that the Reins of the mind being shaken off, they turn thus all things upside down in their government'.[35] Yet, as the quotation from Lemnius suggests, the comparison of a properly ordered psyche to a hierarchical government – and its disorder to a 'sedicious vprore among the common people' – was centuries old. Willis may simply have been trying to gain acceptance of his new theories (and they were, after all, unverifiable) by grounding them in an analogy familiar to his readers.

Unruliness

Whether or not Willis's cerebral microcosm was intended to bolster the newly reordered macrocosm – and it is worth saying that he never explicitly connected the two – there is no question that what he wanted was a cure for disorder. And, in cases of frenzy, the real risk of disorder was usually closer to home: in the individual, the household, and the parish. For frantic persons did not keep the news of their inner regime change to themselves; their behaviour immediately spread the disruption to the social order in which they were embedded.[36] This is evident not merely in the rhetoric of sermons, but in the language of those who diagnosed and dealt with them as patients, wards, and neighbours. Updating his notes in 1617, a tired-sounding Richard Napier summed up his patient George Norris's condition in five words: 'he will not be ruled'.[37] The young man 'would not kepe his bed but rise and strike' and, shouting and hollering, 'runne into the pond'.[38] Of another young man named Richard Straker, the rector noted with consternation that he 'threatneth to mischiefe [harm] his father & some of the neighbours . . . stubborne. will not be ruled'.

[33] Christopher Love, *The naturall mans case stated, or, An exact map of the little world man* (London, 1658).

[34] Ibid., pp. 179–185, 201–206. [35] Willis, *Two discourses*, p. 180.

[36] Jonathan Andrews, 'The Politics of Committal to Early Modern Bedlam', in Jonathan Andrews et al. (eds.), *The History of Bethlem* (London: Routledge, 1997), p. 23.

[37] Kassell et al., *Casebooks*, case 46216. [38] Ibid., cases 45582, 46216.

Straker had recently set fire to a neighbour's house and been 'cast into prison for it'.[39]

At best, frantic persons were breakers of the peace; at worst, they threatened to cause serious harm to people and property. But most unsettling of all was the fact that they did not respond to 'correction' as ordinary miscreants did. Napier described his 'distracted' patient Elizabeth Piddington as 'testy & cholerik. she will fling [hit out] at her husband because he hath beaten her in her fits . . . [she] remembers when she has done evil & yet does not mend it & the more they strive with her the worse she is'.[40] Napier was perfectly capable of calling wife-beating 'abuse'; it is telling that on this occasion he reserved judgement.[41] In early modern England, the household was supposed to be every bit as orderly a body as its natural and political equivalents; the husband, as its head, was accounted both its most rational member and the one responsible for keeping the others under rule. Elizabeth Piddington's failure to 'mend' reflected badly not only on her, but on her husband.

For the great chain of being did not merely show 'Man' his place (above the 'brutes' and below the angels); it also showed the relations which God had ordained to obtain among members of his species. Kings had rule over subjects, husbands over wives, parents over children, and masters over servants. Everyone (barring God) was subordinate to someone, and they were expected to be ready to show it on request. In reality, this vision of order seems to have been honoured as often in the breach as in the observance.[42] But those guilty of such breaches were at least expected to respond to 'correction' with appropriate meekness. Frantic persons were unable to find their place in this script: sometimes rebuke prompted excessive grovelling, but – far more commonly – it prompted flagrant shows of defiance. The frantic housewife Mercy Fish 'loves not her husband but doth sckorne him', Napier wrote, and 'doth so strugle that 3 or 4 can scarce rule her'.[43] In his 'furious' fits, George Baker would rail 'agaynst his father because he is not maryed'.[44]

Mercy Fish and George Baker had been diagnosed with frenzy, and as such, they were not held to blame for their actions in the same way as they would have been had they been sane. Nevertheless, this sort of behaviour was an unwelcome reminder of what a 'world turned upside downward'

[39] Ibid., cases 27133, 27241. [40] Ibid., case 41459. [41] Ibid., cases 29865, 48944.
[42] See Laura Gowing, *Gender Relations in Early Modern England* (London: Routledge, 2014).
[43] Kassell et al., *Casebooks*, cases 66283, 66401, 66415. [44] Ibid., cases 70048, 22207.

would look like. Horses would 'ride in a Coach, men drawe it', Burton brooded darkly in 1621, 'Children rule ... women weare the breeches; sheepe demolish towns, devoure men, &c.'[45] This upended chain of being was patently unnatural because, if it came to pass, souls which God had endowed with a lesser degree of 'reason' would rule over their better-endowed superiors.

Women and children sat higher up on this scale than 'brutes' because they possessed rational souls; every human being bore the imprint of the image of God. And the fact that Burton baulked at the notion of women wearing 'the breeches' did not mean that he believed them altogether incapable of rule (he had after all grown up in the reign of Elizabeth I). The recently appointed Dean of St Paul's, John Donne (1572–1631), freely acknowledged women's capacity for some forms of governance. The female soul was a government, and all 'governments may justly represent God ... who is the God of Order, and fountain of all government'. And yet, he continued, while

> Wee are sure that women have *Soules* as well as men, but yet it is not so expressed, that God breathed a Soule into woman, as hee did into Man; All formes of government have this Soule, but yet God infuseth it more manifestly, and more effectually, in that forme, in a *Kingdome* ... a *Kingdome* is a more lively and more *masculin Organe*, and Instrument of this Soule of Soveraigntie, than the other forms are.[46]

This vision of male superiority drew its justification not only from scripture, but also from natural philosophy and medicine.[47] According to both Aristotle and Galen, women were physically and psychologically inferior to men because they possessed less 'vital heat', making their bodies slower and less effective at distilling animal spirits from the blood. The different humoral complexions of men and women underwrote this temperamental difference: men had more blood and choler, making them hotter and drier (more 'choleric') than women. It was a woman's underpowered 'phlegmatic' temperament – leading to a less impressive unfurling of her organs – which supposedly prevented her from exercising her rational

45 Burton, *The anatomy*, p. 35.

46 John Donne, 'A Sermon upon the fifth of November 1622', in George R. Potter and Evelyn M. Simpson (eds.), *The Sermons of John Donne* (Oakland: University of California Press, 1959), vol. 4, no. 9, p. 7.

47 See Ian Maclean, *The Renaissance Notion of Woman: A Study in the Fortunes of Scholasticism and Medical Science in European Intellectual Life* (Cambridge: Cambridge University Press, 1980); Joan Cadden, *The Meanings of Sex Difference in the Middle Ages: Medicine, Science, and Culture* (Cambridge: Cambridge University Press, 1995).

soul's powers to their fullest extent.[48] Willis managed to preserve this doctrine even in his reduced-choler version of human physiology.[49]

This temperamental ranking system extended not only across genders and life stages but also across species. The fox's subtlety was due to the fact that 'his temperament and constitution is hot', explained the cleric Edward Topsell in 1607, while the sheep, 'the moistest and coldest creature among all four-footed Beasts', was slow-witted and meek.[50] A castrated adult ram (a 'wether') was hotter and drier than a male lamb, but in comparison to an uncastrated one he was still accounted 'blockish' and 'dotish', 'the most foolish of all other, a coward and without courage'. Of all members of the species, female lambs were the most 'fearful', 'dumb', 'tame, humble, and tender'.[51] When the eponymous protagonist of William Shakespeare's *Hamlet* declared 'I am pidgion liuerd, and lacke gall [choler]', he was framing a deficiency of manhood as a demotion in species.[52] And (although we should not take Hamlet too literally here), these temperamental qualities *could* be transferred between species. Burton had read that if one were to switch 'a Kid and Lamb', and let 'either of them sucke of the others milke, the Lamb of the Goats, or the Kid of the Ewes, the wooll of the one will bee hard, the haire of the other soft'.[53] Attenuating the goat's drier, 'greaser, and hotter nature' with ewe's milk would soften its hair, and vice versa.[54]

Within this deterministic grid, frenzy presented something of a paradox. It was supposed to be their hotter, drier temperaments that made some creatures more quick-witted than others.[55] And yet it was also the hot humours – blood and choler – which caused the worst diseases of mind. 'The reason why Dogs and Wolves are more subject to madnesse then any other beast, is because their bodies are cholerick', Topsell explained.[56] What was true of canines was true of humans: 'adust choler' sending 'vp fumosities vnto the heade' was a danger 'specially to yonge men or colericke'.[57] If frenzy befell patients of 'a hot and dry Habit of Body',

[48] See Gowing, *Gender Relations*, pp. 6–8. [49] See Willis, *Oxford Lectures*, pp. 75, 89.
[50] Edward Topsell, *The history of four-footed beasts and serpents* (London, 1658), pp. 174, 495.
[51] Ibid., p. 495.
[52] William Shakespeare, *The tragedy of Hamlet Prince of Denmarke* (London, 1611), sig. F4v.
[53] Burton, *The anatomy*, p. 190.
[54] William Bullein, *A newe booke entituled the gouernement of healthe* (London, 1558), p. lxxxix.
[55] For a particularly deterministic account, see Juan Huarte de San Juan, *Examen de ingenios: The examination of mens vvits* (London, 1594).
[56] Topsell, *The history The history of four-footed beasts*, p. 580.
[57] Henry Wingfield, *A compendious or short treatise, gathered out of the chyefe and principall authors of phisycke* (London, 1551), sig. B4r.

Salmon noted gravely, it was 'rarely cured'.[58] By default, this made frenzy a disease to which men were more vulnerable than women. Most medical authors seem to have assumed that this was the case (although this is hard to say with certainty, given that the generic patient to whom they referred was always male). What *can* be said with certainty is that frenzy did not appear on their list of 'women's diseases' (except in the childbirth-specific context of a retained afterbirth).[59] This assumption about gender was borne out by Napier's diagnostic experience: of the sixty-six frantic patients I have identified in his casebooks, twenty-seven (41 per cent) were women and thirty-nine (59 per cent) men. When we consider that 60 per cent of all Napier's mentally ill patients were female, this skew in the gender ratio starts to look even more marked.

The frantic patients in Napier's casebooks also bear out the medical authors' assumptions about age. During a man's youth, the surgeon Peter Lowe had written,

> which is hot and drie, more hot than drie, and lasteth till 35. yeares, [he is] subiect to hot feuers, frenzies, and diuers other diseases, and is gouuerned by Venus, which ingendreth greate cupiditie of lust. Mans estate is most temperate of all, and lasteth vntill 50. yeares, ... in this time men are subiect to hot feuers, flux of blod ... frenzie, and such like, and is gouerned by the Sonne, who is author of wisdome and grauity.[60]

Twenty-nine of the thirty-three male patients whose ages Napier recorded (88 per cent) were under the age of fifty; twenty-three (70 per cent) were under the age of thirty-five. To contemporaries, the latter statistic would have been the least surprising of the two; as Lowe's remark suggests, youth was seen as a time when passions and appetites ran high. Young, single men were given much greater license to indulge those urges (in the hope that they would 'run [themselves] out of breath') than their female counterparts.[61] But apparently reaching 'Mans estate' – a 'temperate' age, a time of 'wisdome and grauity' – did not eliminate a man's risk of succumbing to frenzy.

The hot, 'lively' physiology which was supposed to make men the most rational of all God's creatures also predisposed them to 'frenzie ... the

58 Salmon, *Praxis medica*, p. 176.

59 See, e.g., James Primerose, *Popular errours* (London, 1651), pp. 311–313; James McMath, *The expert mid-wife a treatise of the diseases of women with child, and in child-bed* (Edinburgh, 1694), p. 261.

60 Lowe, *The whole course of chirurgerie*, sig. D3v.

61 Trosse, *The Life*, sig. A2r. The classic study of early modern masculinity remains Alexandra Shepard, *Meanings of Manhood in Early Modern England* (Oxford: Oxford University Press, 2003).

chiefest and greatest mischeif which can come to the brain'.[62] The same vital heat which was supposed to produce the fastest and purest animal spirits could also burn them up. The choler which was supposed to nourish manly courage could nourish senseless rage; the blood which was supposed to raise the spirits could raise them too high. A night's hard drinking or a romantic disappointment was all that it took to tip the scale from vigour into madness. Of his twenty-nine-year-old patient Roger Lawrence, Napier noted that, before the onset of the disease, he had been 'a witty & a chollerick fellowe'.[63] There was a curious irony to the fact that the same physiological factors which were supposed to equip adult males to rule made them uniquely vulnerable to a total loss of reason.

It is probably not a coincidence that – though all of Napier's frantic patients talked 'idly' – young men were uniquely prone to fall into delusions of grandeur. Lawrence, a manservant, was 'frentick with a vision that he should goe teach all nations'; a month later he was talking 'of kings'.[64] An 'overstudyed' 'scholer of Cambridge' named Mr Richardson was 'boasting' and 'vainglorious'.[65] Thomas Stiles said of the Devil 'that he is a fyne serving man'; George Baker that he could 'master god & Doe as mutch as god'.[66] Baker blamed his parents for the fact that he was not yet married, enjoined 'his father to marry him & to have his land made over to him', and threatened 'to kill his frends . . . [so] that he mayst have ther land'.[67] The oldest of these four bachelors was thirty-three; the youngest was twenty-five. This was precisely the age in which they were supposed to be coming into 'Mans estate' by becoming householders, husbands, fathers, masters – in short, by being anointed kings of their own little principalities.

If young men were disappointed in these hopes, they were also socialized to deal with those disappointments in gender-specific ways: by redoubling their efforts to attain what they had been denied, by fighting their opponents, or by drowning their sorrows. None of these methods was conducive to better mental health. The sort of downward spiral which dashed hopes could precipitate can be seen particularly clearly in the case of the thirty-two-year-old clerk Robert Matthews. Between late December and early February 1602/3, Matthews's relatives came to see Napier five times. At first, Napier was unsympathetic: the young man was 'very pleasant in his frensy with latyne & pedlers french', he noted sardonically, but his 'brayne [was] idle & ill as if the wits were perished & wasted.

[62] Blount, 'Phrenetick', in *Glossographia*, sig. Gg5v. [63] Kassell et al., *Casebooks*, case 49372.
[64] Ibid., cases 49372, 49608. [65] Ibid., case 62015. [66] Ibid., cases 55170, 66981.
[67] Ibid., cases 70048, 22207.

laugheth madly with it. took it with surfeting & drinkinge amis this 12 month'.[68] The clerk was clearly capable of reading a medical self-help guide or listening to a sermon; Napier was evidently inclined to think that he only he had himself to blame. But it was not until almost a month later that the rector heard the full story. Matthews had indeed taken 'a surfett and . . . [been] dronken at London', but it was not until afterwards that

> he tooke such a Conceit that he was never well after, but his maisters maides made him beleeve sometymes that one of them loved him and sometimes another so that at length his mynd came altogither upon their love and he became sottish and now speaks he Cannot tell what and talks idly never ceassing as long as he hath any Company.[69]

'[T]his fellow loved 2 wenches one after another & was defrauded of them boathe', Napier wrote indignantly a week later.[70] Matthews was from a little village in rural Northamptonshire; his time in London must have been disorienting, exhilarating, and lonely in equal measure. No wonder that he had taken the maids' flirting too seriously.

We saw in Chapter 1 that young men were likelier than their female counterparts to become frantic after receiving a head wound. Matthews's story suggests that the expectation that they would prove themselves as suitors and drinking companions could be just as damaging to their health. And the failure of these men to prove their 'manhood' in these all-important arenas manifested in their madness. Matthews had styled himself as a lover and a wit; in his frenzy, he would talk incessantly, laugh, quip in Latin and French, and make 'rimes'.[71] Thomas Stiles had been assaulted by two men who 'fought with him & cut his head with a long staffe & feld him'; ever since he had been 'furious', 'very choleric & quarlesom', 'wonderfull stubborne', and 'very wild'. He would 'walke all the night . . . with a staffe & sayeth that he would beate him if he could find him'.[72] Matthews had responded to romantic, heterosexual humiliation by becoming a caricature of the sanguine man; Stiles had responded to physical, homosocial humiliation by becoming the choleric equivalent.

Correction

For a Christian moralist, the plight of men like Matthews and Stiles was clear. By failing to curb his longings, Matthews had let his 'concupiscible

[68] Ibid., case 18460. [69] Ibid., case 18546. [70] Ibid., case 18571. [71] Ibid., case 18517.
[72] Ibid., cases 53649, 55170, 58292.

appetite' overwhelm his rational soul. By letting his wounded pride rankle into rage, Stiles had handed the reins to his 'irascible appetite'. Yet the fact that these men had 'none to blame but themselves for it' was also cause for hope: a disease brought on by poor self-rule might prove amenable to correction. The solution was simple: repent, pray for God's mercy, and forswear the excesses which had caused the disease.

For a learned physician – intimately familiar with the diagnostic small print – deciding on a course of treatment was less straightforward. Frenzy was virtually indistinguishable from mania, but there were two crucial differences: first, it was accompanied by a fever, and second, the patient might die within days. For some physicians, this meant treating it like any other deadly ague (of which there were many). For others – notwithstanding the fever – it was to be treated exactly like mania, its closest sibling on the family tree of madness. How far this made a difference to treatment depended a good deal on the background and outlook of the practitioner. Andrew Boorde was happy to take a one-size-fits-all approach. The chapter on 'Phrenesy' in his *Breuiarie of health* (first ed. 1547) ended on a particularly brief note: 'keepe him as it is specified in the Chapter named *Mania*'.[73] In the sixteenth century, this interchangeability of treatments made sense: the two diseases still shared near-identical lines of causation (blood and choler), and their sufferers behaved in near-identical ways. By the late seventeenth century, however, the models of causation had diversified, and so too had the treatment options.

At this point, it is worth reminding ourselves that – in early modern England – the people who adhered closely to this ancient medical framework were always outnumbered by those who did not. For the vast majority of the English population who did not have a medical degree – and for whom 'frenzy' and 'madness' were basically synonyms for the same condition – sufferers merited the same treatment as they always had. Yet, although the people who we will encounter 'correcting' frenzy came from very different walks of life, and although they justified what they were doing differently, there was also plenty of common ground. Rather than presupposing a hard distinction between medical cures and non-medical correctives, this section focuses on the similarities of rationale offered by physicians, experimental philosophers, crown officials, relatives, and – very occasionally – by sufferers themselves.

[73] Boorde, *The breuiarie*, f. 92v.

Reminders of Rule

Much ink has been spilt over the question of whether pre-Enlightenment individuals were less humane towards the mentally ill than their post-Enlightenment successors. I cannot hope to provide an aggregate score for early modern England in this transhistorical ethics test. But if we attend to what contemporaries thought they were doing, one thing becomes clear: the only thing that made the treatment of the mentally ill crueller than the treatment of anyone else was their failure to respond appropriately to 'correction'. Frantic persons were 'wilfully . . . froward', 'untoward', 'unruly'.[74] By responding to heads of households' chastisement with recalcitrance, they had let the revolt in their souls spread to the domestic realm. For a wife, child, or servant, this came perilously close to *lèse-majesté*: an act of treason, an insult to the ruler's sovereignty. The fact that the offender was not technically guilty was neither here nor there; the husband, father, or master who did not respond by reasserting his authority had failed in his duty. Elizabeth Piddington's husband may well have believed that he was fulfilling that duty by beating her 'in her fits'.

There is no doubt that most of those who were physically violent towards the frantic believed that what they were doing was for the sufferer's own good. This was certainly true of Sir Thomas More, who, during his time as Lord Chancellor, had been called upon to deal with a man who had fallen into a 'playne open fransye'. The man had previously 'ben put vppe in bedelem', More recalled, 'and afterwarde by betyng and correcyon gathered hys remembraunce to him, and begann to come agayne to hym selfe'. But after his release 'hys old fansyes beganne to fall agayne in his hed', and he began to misbehave as he had before. Having been requested 'to take some other order wyth him', More declared,

> I . . . caused him as he came wanderyng by my dore, to be taken by the constables and bounded to a tre in the streete byfore the whole towne, and there they stryped him with roddys therfore til he waxed wery and somwhat longer. And it appered well that hys remembraunce was good inough, saue that it wente about in grasynge [grazing] tyl it was beten home.[75]

Note the recurrence of the same animalizing language we encountered earlier: if a man's wits had gone about grazing, then so too had the man.

[74] Kassell et al., *Casebooks*, cases 73340, 68959, 65331.

[75] Sir Thomas More, *The apologye of syr Thomas More knyghte* (London, 1533), ff. 197r–198v.

And if his superiors could not appeal to his 'reason', the use of the rod was every bit as justified as the use of 'bit and bridle'.

There is evidence to suggest that the same order was given by crown officials across the land throughout these two centuries. In 1690/91, for example, the constable of the Huntingdonshire parish of Great Staunton recorded a payment to a contractor for 'taking up a distracted woman watching her and wipping her the next day'.[76] Shocking as this order is, it is important to keep it in context. Corporeal punishment was ubiquitous in early modern England. At the turn of the sixteenth century, for example, the mayor of Norwich was making regular payments to a man who went by the name of 'Barnabye the whipper'. In a typical three-month quarter, Barnaby would be ordered to whip between ten and twenty persons.[77] By contrast, when a 'madd woman' arrived in the city in the winter of 1601, the mayor ordered him simply to carry her 'to heverlond [Haveringland]'.[78] This was probably not an act of compassion: the likelihood was that this woman was not a native of Norwich, and the mayor was taking care to make sure that she was not treated as one. 'Correction' might be taken to imply belonging, and belonging implied a duty of care. Carrying 'a madd woman' across the county border and leaving her there sent a much clearer message: whoever she was, she was not the city's problem.

In the eyes of contemporaries, then, the refusal to provide 'correction' was likelier to signal neglect than mercy. For how could a person who had shown themselves no longer capable of self-correction hope to mend, if not by the correction of others? Physicians too embraced this principle of 'tough love'. In a letter endorsing 'the use of whipping in medicine', the Danish anatomist Thomas Bartholin (1616–1680) quoted with approval a passage from Augustine: 'A physician is uneasy [harsh] to a patient in a frenzy, and so is a father to an disobedient son – the one by tying him down, and the other by whipping, but both by loving them . . . if they should neglect them, and suffer them to perish, that false clemency is rather a cruelty.'[79] 'This cure by whipping, altho' it may seem rough, yet

[76] Huntingdon, Huntingdonshire Archives, HP82/9/1, f. 52v.

[77] Norwich, Norfolk Record Office, NCR 18d/13, ff. 101v–144v. See Krista Kesselring, 'Law, Status, and the Lash: Judicial Whipping in Early Modern England', *Journal of British Studies* 60(3) (2021), 511–533.

[78] NCR 18d/13, f. 139r.

[79] Thomas Bartholin and Johann Heinrich Meibom, *De usu flagrorum in re medica & veneria* (Frankfurt, 1669), pp. 16–17. This and further quotations from *De usu flagrorum* are taken from an anonymous 1761 English translation: 'A letter from Thomas Bartholin on the Medicinal Use of

ought not a physician to abstain from it, if it has good effect', Bartholin concluded.[80] It was especially useful in cases of madness; Bartholin himself 'knew a very honest man, who was often mad, forced by the threatenings and blows of a stronger person to lye quiet as a lamb'.[81]

The Danish anatomist offered several suggestions as to why it was that this cure worked; whipping recalled the 'mind from wandering thoughts', and induced 'the fear of pain', both of which served to keep 'the patient within the bounds of reason'.[82] Physiologically, it served to increase the pulse and 'raise the temperature'.[83] In Bartholin's experience, this effect was generally well-tolerated; in cold diseases (like epilepsy) it was downright beneficial.[84] Even in mania, the physician did not need to be 'afraid of raising the heat, because it is without fever or a small pulse, which distinguishes it from *phrenitis*'.[85] Evidently, frenzy was to be treated as an exception to the rule.

Not all early modern medical authors observed this distinction between frenzy and mania, and the divergence of treatment recommendations became more marked in the seventeenth century than it had been in the sixteenth. Back in the 1540s, physical 'correction' was one of the treatments for mania which Boorde had been happy to extend to frenzy: the patient was to be 'keept in feare of one man or an other, & if neede require he muste be punished and beaten'.[86] For Willis, this catch-all approach was unacceptable. It was only mania, in his book, that called for 'threatnings, bonds, or strokes, as well as Physick':

> indeed for the curing of Mad people, there is nothing more effectual or necessary than their reverence or standing in awe of such as they think their Tormentors. For by this means, the Corporeal Soul being in some measure depressed and restrained, is compell'd to remit its pride and fierceness; and so afterwards by degrees grows more mild, and returns in order: Wherefore, Furious Mad-men are sooner, and more certainly cured by punishments, and hard usage, in a strait room, than by Physick or Medicines.[87]

Rods', in *A treatise of the use of flogging in venerial affairs . . . made English from the Latin original by a physician* (London, 1801), p. 19.

80 Bartholin, *De usu flagrorum*, p. 16; 'A letter', p. 19.

81 Bartholin, *De usu flagrorum*, p. 13; 'A letter', p. 17.

82 'A letter' p. 17; Thomas Bartholin, *De morbis biblicis miscellanea medica* (Frankfurt, 1672), p. 85. Translation from Johan Schioldann-Nielsen and Kurt Sørensen (eds.) and James Willis (trans.), *On Diseases of the Bible: A Medical Miscellany. Acta historica scientiarum naturalium et medicinalium*, vol. 41 (Copenhagen: Danish National Library of Science and Medicine, 1994), p. 75.

83 Bartholin, *De morbis biblicis*, p. 85.

84 Bartholin, *De usu flagrorum*, pp. 9–10; 'A letter', p. 15.

85 Bartholin, *De usu flagrorum*, p. 13; 'A letter', p. 17.

86 Boorde, *The breuiarie*, f. 75v.

87 Willis, *Two discourses*, p. 206.

It is possible that Willis was simply following Bartholin's advice; the sufferers of mania were not acutely feverish, and therefore 'hard usage' did not threaten their health in the same way. Yet there is also a distinctly censorious ring to this passage; it sounds much more like the moralizing censures with which this chapter began than does any of his guidance on frenzy.

This difference in tone reflected Willis's belief that these two diseases did not typically share a common cause. In his Oxford lectures, Willis had contrasted 'disorders of the animal spirits from external causes such as phrenzy', with 'conditions caused by the bad *diathesis* [constitution] of the patients themselves, as in mania'.[88] This *diathesis* could be hereditary, but it could also be caused by 'A bad mode of life, which imposes a taint on the blood of the brain'.[89] Mania, in other words, was likelier to be self-inflicted than frenzy. This moral distinction had sometimes been drawn in the sixteenth century, and not just by physicians: as we saw in the last chapter, laypersons were perfectly capable of situating a madness on a sliding scale of personal accountability. A person who fell frantic while desperately sick with an ague was not in the same camp as a person who did so after a week of hard drinking. Nonetheless, the Restoration physicians' reconfiguration of pathology – especially conceptions of 'external' and 'internal' causes – does seem to have sharpened the divide.

Of course, the belief that frantic persons did not deserve punishment did not rule out the therapeutic use of physical shocks. Of 'the Cure of the *Phrensie*', Willis recalled one 'rare instance':

> I was one time sent for to Cure a Maid, that was strong, and having a Feavour, was highly raging, being continually bound in her Bed ... I therefore bid them (for that it was Summer time) that in the middle of the Night she should be carried by Women forth of doors, and put into a Boat, and her Cloths being pull'd off, and she tyed fast with a Cord, should be drenched into the depth of a River, the Rope being tyed only about her middle, that she might not be stifled in the Water.[90]

Willis had probably gleaned this idea from the writings of Jan Baptist van Helmont, the chemical physician whose writings on physiology had so much influenced his own. The cure worked, Helmont's son explained in 1694, because 'Water puts a stop to the too violent and exorbitant Operation of the fiery life, or doth mortifie the same'.[91] Willis would have

[88] Willis, *Oxford Lectures*, p. 122. [89] Ibid., p. 131. [90] Willis, *Two discourses*, p. 187.
[91] Franciscus Mercurius Van Helmont, *The Spirit of Diseases; or, Diseases from the Spirit* (London, 1694), p. 45.

agreed. Of the frantic 'Maid', he reported with satisfaction that '[t]his Cure succeeded so happily and so suddenly, forasmuch as the excess both of the Vital and the Animal flame, being together immensly increased, was taken away by a proper Remedy for the more intense Fire; to wit, by the moistning, and cooling of the Water'.[92] A ducking was the cold, wet equivalent of a beating: it mortified the corporeal soul.

Of course, corporeal 'correction' was only one way of bringing a frantic person 'back to hym selfe', and it was not the subtlest. Many early modern medical practitioners preferred milder methods, and they had at least one ancient medical authority on their side. The Byzantine Galenist Alexander of Tralles (525–605 CE), whose *Therapeutics* circulated in early modern Europe as the *Practica Alexandri*, had permitted 'some familiar friends ... [to] stay with him, so that their mild rebukes influence him in his actions. On the other hand, no servant or relative, whom he once angered or was angered with, may be allowed to come to him. For this sight would irritate and distress the patient and, of course, cause great excitement'.[93] Alexander's advice was often redacted and adjusted by his early modern medical readers.[94] 'Let his dearest frindes come to him', Barrough instructed, 'and let them sometime speake gently and softely unto him, & sometime rebuke him sharply'.[95] Alternating between mild and strong drugs was a common practice among early modern physicians, and the principle was easily extended to psychological therapies. Sharp words could be salutary, but only the patient's 'dearest frindes' could be trusted to deliver them with care. In general, however, the recommendation was to reduce rather than increase stimulation. 'All great Perturbations of the Mind, as Anger, Grief, Love, &c. are to be avoided', Salmon advised, 'for they excite the Animal Spirits with great violence'.[96] As Alexander had warned, if chastisement was helpful, 'excitement' was to be avoided at all costs. Their diet was to be 'slender and not delicate, their cloathing course

[92] Willis, *Two discourses*, p. 187.

[93] 'Einige vertraute Freunde mögen bei ihm bleiben, damit deren milde Zurechtweisungen ihn in seinem Thun beeinflussen. Dagegen darf kein Diener oder Verwandter, über welchen er sich einmal geärgert oder erzürnt hat, zu ihm gelassen werden. Denn (sein Anblick) würde den Kranken reizen und beunruhigen und selbstverständlich in gewaltige Aufregung versetzun'. German translation by Theodor Puschmann, in Puschmann (trans.), *Alexander von Tralles, Original-Text und Übersetzung* (Vienna: Braumüller, 1878–1879), p. 518.

[94] See, e.g., *Practica Alexandri yatros greci* (Lyons, 1504), lib. 1, cap. 57, f. 8v: 'Neither should friends come to him frequently, nor a multitude of people ... nor should sadness or anger be stirred up in or expressed to him'. 'nec amici frequenter aut multitudo hominum ingrediat ad ipsum ... neque tristicia neque iracundia ei movenda est aut indicenda'.

[95] Barrough, *The methode*, p. 17. [96] Salmon, *Praxis medica*, p. 176.

[sic], their beds hard, and their handling severe and rigid'.[97] No images were to be allowed in their rooms, 'to take away the imagination that commeth by the sight'.[98] Although the express intent of these measures was to calm the sensitive soul, it was also exactly the sort of 'keeping' which a sane offender could expect in gaol.

Some reminders of rule were even subtler (if no less symbolically charged). In his *Touchstone of Complexions*, Lemnius reported that 'for the redress of certeyne diseases of the head, losse of right wittes, feeblenes of Brayne, dottry, phrensie . . . fury and franticke fittes, Phisitions deemed it the best way to have the hayre cleane shaven of'.[99] This made good sense, the Dutch physician continued, for 'every man after his beard hath been trimmed or cleane shaven of, feeleth himself a greate deale meryer, and lesse wayward and overthwart than he did before'.[100] Having unkempt hair made a man look 'wayward', and a man who looked 'wayward' *felt* 'wayward'. He was on a slippery slope to becoming Nebuchadnezzar, who had 'liued with beastes in the wilderness till his hairs were grown like Eagles feathers'.[101] Shaving was beneficial because it made a man feel differently about 'himself'. It was a therapy which was simultaneously interoceptive and relational: being groomed and restored to a neat, orderly outward appearance reminded the sufferer of his social identity (as an orderly person), and thus prompted him to feel and act less like an unruly one.

What Lemnius neglected to mention, of course, was that – while beard-trimming was no doubt a routine request in the barbershops of early modern Europe – head-shaving was not. There were plenty of classical and biblical precedents for seeing it as a ritual of humiliation.[102] And if it was humiliating for men, it was doubly so for women. The Apostle Paul had written that it was a shameful 'for a woman to be shorn or shaven', and later generations of bible-readers had taken him at his word.[103] In early modern England, it was a punishment reserved for witchcraft suspects and sexual offenders.[104] The same was true of being stripped naked. Yet whether they were understood as means of bringing low or raising up,

97 Willis, *Two discourses*, p. 206. 98 Boorde, *The breuiarie*, f. 75v.
99 Lemnius, *The touchstone*, p. 124. 100 Ibid., p. 124.
101 Smith, *The Fall of King Nabuchadnezzar*, p. 10.
102 For scripture, see Leviticus 21:5, Deuteronomy 21:12–14, Judges 16: 17–21; 1 Corinthians 11. For legal precedents, see Vern L. Bullough, 'Medieval Concepts of Adultery', *Arthuriana* 7(4) (1997), 5–15.
103 1 Corinthians 11: 5–6, 15.
104 Martin Ingram, *Carnal Knowledge: Regulating Sex in England, 1470–1600* (Cambridge: Cambridge University Press, 2017), pp. 288, 297, 339.

there was a consistent logic underpinning all of these corrective measures. The idea was to remind sufferers – whether by kind words, rebukes, personal care, or humiliation – of the social order to which they belonged, and which they had apparently forgotten.

The evidence of what the recipients of these treatments thought and felt about them is scarce, but some do seem to have grasped the underlying logic. Although George Trosse never applied a medical diagnosis to his 'miserable distracted Condition' – and I have no wish to do it for him – his account does offer a rare glimpse of what it was like to be on the receiving end of this sort of treatment.[105] At the first onset of his illness, he recalled, 'A Brother-in-Law of mine, standing by, demanded of me whether I would be rul'd . . . assuring me, that, in case I would, all might be well again. To whom I instantly reply'd I would do so'.[106] Yet Trosse's best intentions were scotched by the return of the 'terrifying and disquieting Visions and Voices'. Seeing no improvement, his relatives had him removed to a private madhouse. Eventually, Trosse recounted,

> thro' the Goodness of God, and by His *Blessing* upon *Physick*, a *low Diet*, and *hard Keeping*, I began to be somewhat *quiet* and *compos'd* in my Spirits; to be *orderly* and *civil* in my *Carriage* and *Converse*, and *gradually* to regain the Use of my *Reason*, and to be a fit *Companion* for my *Fellow Creatures*.[107]

If Trosse's refusal to be ruled was a sign that he had lost his 'Reason', he saw his renewed acceptance of 'hard' rule as the first sign of its restoration.

Cooling Agents

From a medical perspective, all of these treatments had a temperamental rationale. If whipping was to be eschewed in cases of frenzy, it was because it risked raising the patient's temperature; ducking was safe for the same reason. 'Perturbations of the Mind' and provocations of the imagination were banned because they altered the body's temperature and agitated the animal spirits. Shaving, conversely, cooled the body. Body hair was understood to consist of excreted humoral remains; if especially thick or coarse, it was liable to block up the pores, decreasing the efficacy of the body's natural ventilation system. Shaving the head unblocked the pores and thus

[105] Most first-person accounts of madness which survive from this period belong to the genre of spiritual self-writing. While their authors were fully willing to admit that they had been distracted, few were willing to label what they had experienced as 'frenzy' (or indeed 'mania').

[106] Trosse, *The Life*, p. 50. [107] Ibid., p. 63.

helped to cool and ventilate the brain. 'For thereby [the] grosse vapours . . . have more scope to evaporate and fume oute', Lemnius explained.[108]

Of course, the precise rationale for these therapeutic interventions varied according to one's definition of frenzy. Most medical authors sought to 'resolve' the abscess in the brain or meninges, and thus applied to the head the same sorts of warm compress which were used to draw out and drain external abscesses. For, as the learned physician James Primerose put it: 'These hot things in the height, and also in the declination of the disease, doe not heat, but resolve . . . for as *Galen* teaches, *Digesting remedies do by accident refrigerate and coole an inflammation*'.[109] Despite the fact that Willis had rejected this traditional definition of frenzy, he continued to recommend the use of warm compresses. They were not, he insisted, 'for the taking away the inflammation of the *Meninges*', but simply for helping the patient sleep.[110]

Despite the many edits made to frenzy in the late seventeenth century, the therapeutic principles tended to remain the same. Obstructions had to be cleared, passageways opened, and 'gross' fumes and other waste products evacuated.[111] Above all, the patient had to be returned to their natural temperament. In cases of frenzy, this always meant removing or attenuating the hot humours, and the quickest and most efficient way of doing it was to let blood. Although bloodletting was ubiquitous in early modern medicine, it seems to have been performed especially liberally on frantic patients.[112] It was not uncommon for a male patient to be let blood in multiple places at once. Napier's prescription for the thirty-eight-year-old Francis White was typical: 'Let blood under the tongue. Cephalic [vein] eight ounces . . . horse leaches a heten in his necke'.[113] The cephalic and jugular veins carried blood away from the head, and thus were obvious choices of release valves. The same was true of the frontal vein in the forehead. The thirty-year-old Richard Cockman was let blood 'in the heade', the 'median vayne of the right arm', and 'in the neck & shoulders'. He too had leeches applied 'to his browe & on to his neck'.[114]

This sort of regime was not for everyone; the learned physician was supposed to tailor the course of treatment according to the age and strength of the patient. Skipping the lancet in favour of leeches was recommended for weaker patients. Female patients (assumed to be in the

108 Lemnius, *The touchstone*, sig. C3v, p. 143. 109 Primerose, *Popular errours*, p. 398.
110 Willis, *Two discourses*, p. 186.
111 The mainstays were 'purges' (laxatives), 'vomits', and 'clysters' (enemas).
112 Barrough, *The methode*, p. 18. 113 Kassell et al., *Casebooks*, case 70795.
114 Ibid., cases 75729, 76748.

latter camp) were often let blood in the *saphena* vein in the ankle rather than the *cephalica*.[115] Opening this vein was believed to encourage the blood to return to its 'natural' female route; it was also smaller and more delicate, making it easier to staunch the blood.

How far such precautions mattered depended on how much blood was supposed to be drawn. Whereas some medieval physicians had positively encouraged bleeding frantic patients until they fainted, their early modern successors tended to be more conservative.[116] Bleed as much as 'the strength of the patient will suffer', Barrough advised, 'but take heed you let him not bleed vntill he sound [swoon], as many rashely do'.[117] Yet if bleeding till they dropped was not to be recommended, the subduing effects of blood loss were not unwelcome. It was by 'opening a vein . . . sometimes in the Arm, sometimes in the Neck Vein, Forehead, or Foot', Willis explained, that 'both the raging of the Spirits and the lifting up of the Soul, are best of all suppressed'.[118] And frantic patients' spirits were often too high for their doctors' liking. Cockman 'is exceding talking' – Napier wrote with gritted teeth – 'if he still continue talking idlely then let him blood in the ceph. of the arme'.[119]

Alongside these subtractive therapies were the additive ones: cold, moist substances, which – once absorbed by the body – would temper the patient's hot, dry complexion. The staple modes of delivery were topical poultices, medicated baths, drinks, and edible syrups or conserves. All were made up of different combinations of the same roster of ingredients: substances which had 'vertue to coole and moisten'.[120] The most common edibles were lettuce, endives, radishes, cucumbers, leeks, melons, apples, and lemons. Chief among the herbs and spices were cowslip, violets, roses, mallows, water lilies, bugloss, borage, fumitory, nutmeg, and saffron. By means of these medications, Willis declared, 'the rage of the Blood, and the burning of the Animal Spirits may be allayed'.[121]

These cooling, moistening substances did not simply serve to lower the patient's temperature; many of them were also gentle sedatives (learned physicians variously called them 'somniferents', 'stupefactives', 'hypnotics', and 'narcotics'). A cold, moist temperament was strongly associated not only

[115] See Boorde, *The breuiarie*, f. 92v; Bateman (trans.), *Batman vppon Bartholome*, f. 88v; Barrough, *The methode*, p. 18.

[116] See, e.g., Bernard de Gordon, *Opus lilium medicinae* (Lyon, 1559), p. 216: 'In primis . . . fiat phlebotomia de cephalica, usque ad syncopim, uel quasi syncopim'.

[117] Barrough, *The methode*, p. 18.

[118] Willis, *Two discourses*, p. 206.

[119] Kassell et al., *Casebooks*, cases 75729, 76748.

[120] Barrough, *The methode*, p. 18.

[121] Willis, *Two discourses*, p. 185.

with docility and slow-wittedness, but also with sleepiness. If the brain became oversaturated with phlegm, the result was lethargy (a disease in which the sufferer could scarcely be roused from sleep). Frenzy sat on the opposite end of this spectrum: a hot, dry, choleric brain would not permit sleep. Insomnia was understood to be both a symptom of frenzy *and* an aggravator of the mental alienation which accompanied it. 'Do we not find raveries, and frenzies the ordinary attendents of sleeplessness?', asked the divine Joseph Hall in 1646. What else was to be expected, given that nothing cooled and refreshed the body like sleep, and the soul followed 'the temper of the body'?[122]

The most powerful narcotics were those derived from the poppy, which 'in respect of their temperament and elementary qualitie' were 'colde in the fourth and higheste degree'.[123] Yet, although opiates had long been recommended as a treatment for frenzy, the recommendation was usually accompanied by a strongly worded safety warning.[124] At the end of a list of narcotic preparations, for example, Barrough added a few lines of small print: 'note that you must eschew continuall vse of stupefactiue medicines aswell inwardly as outwardly also. For in this disease, by ouermuch cooling you may turne the frenesy into a litargy [lethargy], wherby you may cause him to sleepe so, that you can awake him noe more'.[125] '*Hypnoticks* or Medicines causing rest, are often very necessary in this Disease', Willis wrote a century later, 'but yet . . . let them [not] be frequently used; because sleep caused by Opiates, carries more morbific matter to the Brain, and fixes it more deeply there'.[126] And the same caveat which obtained in bloodletting obtained here: 'if the patient be weake beware how you minister stupefactiue things to prouoke slepe, for in such as be weak . . . somnoriferous potions [sic] doe noe small hurte, and sometime they kill'.[127]

Despite these warnings, frenzy seems to have regularly driven early modern medical practitioners to this last resort. Napier's prescription for his thirty-year-old patient John Quarell, whom he described as 'frentick & distemperd . . . in his brayne', was typical: 'to procure sleepe at night. conserve of roses [and] cowslip: one and a half ounces each . . . extract of opium: eight grains'.[128] And it was not just the amateurs who often resorted to opiates to get their patients to sleep. Napier's better-qualified

122 Joseph Hall, *The balm of Gilead* (London, 1646), p. 278.
123 Lemnius, *The touchstone*, p. 62.
124 See, e.g., Avicenna [Ibn Sīnā], *al Qānūn*, in Giovanni Costeo Giovanni Costeo and Giovanni Paulo Mongio (eds.), *Avicennae arabum medicorum principis. . .* [*Canon Medicinae*] (Venice, 1595), p. 473; Gilbertus Anglicus, *Compendium medicinae* (Lyon, 1510), f. 102v; Johan van Heurne, *De morbis humani capitis* (Leiden, 1594), p. 118.
125 Barrough, *The methode*, p. 19.
126 Willis, *Two discourses*, p. 186.
127 Barrough, *The methode*, p. 19.
128 Kassell et al., *Casebooks*, case 70899.

contemporary, the physician Daniel Oxenbridge (1576–1642), was equally ready to give 'Sleepers' to his distracted patients.[129] One twenty-year-old patient who had fallen 'into a *Paraphrenitis*' was given two grains of laudanum dissolved in lettuce water, which – Oxenbridge noted with satisfaction – 'caused him to sleep'.[130]

The same qualitative grid which served to differentiate and rank living bodies in terms of gender, age, and species also extended to medicinal substances. The seeds of the plant known as *agnus castus* ('chaste lamb') – traditionally eaten to cool the 'desire of lechery' – were also 'good for the frensie'.[131] The 'flesh of lambs', being 'flegmaticke, watery, and moiste' was safe for frantic patients to consume, whereas the 'flesh of the old hee or male gotes' was not.[132] If the hot, dry flesh of a male goat would masculinize its eater, then cold, moist things would have the opposite effect. They would bring an excessively choleric woman back to her 'native' temperament. Thus, Willis reported, the frantic 'maid', once plunged into the river, 'fell to swimming, that scarce any Man could do it better ... After about a quarter of an hour, she came forth of the Water sound, and sober, and then being had to Bed, she slept'.[133] The young woman's unnatural heat had translated as manlike athleticism, aggression, and sleeplessness: her cold, wet immersion had cured all three.

This gendered logic is especially clear in the base prescribed for some of these remedies: woman's milk.[134] 'Great Housleek bruised with womans milk, and laid to the forehead, appeaseth a Phrensie', wrote Bayfield in 1663.[135] 'Housleek ... mixt with a Womans Milk, and applied to the hinder part of the Head being shaved, is wonderfully praised', echoed Willis.[136] The simplest remedy to procure sleep was known to 'euery good wife', Burton declared: 'Rosewater and Vineger, with a little womans milke ... applied to both temples'.[137] Medieval physicians had taken a more belt-and-braces approach: frenzy called for 'the milk of a woman

[129] Daniel Oxenbridge (attrib.), *General Observations and prescriptions in the practice of physick* (London, 1715), pp. 5–9, quotation on p. 9.

[130] Ibid., p. 5.

[131] William Langham, *The garden of health* (London, 1597), pp. 5–6. The plant is now commonly known as the 'chaste tree' (*Vitex agnus-castus*) or 'Abraham's balm'.

[132] Bullein, *Gouernement of healthe*, f. 89r.

[133] Willis, *Two discourses*, p. 187.

[134] Medieval physicians had probably borrowed this cure for frenzy from the first-century natural historian Pliny the Elder. See Pliny, 'Naturalis historia', in John Bostock and H. T. Riley (eds.), *The Natural History of Pliny* (London: Bohn, 1855), book 20, ch. 5. For an early modern version, see Heurne, *De morbis humani capitis*, p. 118.

[135] Robert Bayfield, *Tes iatrikes kartos* (London, 1663), p. 38.

[136] Willis, *Two discourses*, p. 186.

[137] Burton, *The anatomy*, p. 478.

nursing a girlchild'.[138] If no lactating women were available, 'asses milk' was the next best thing.[139] These stipulations show with particular clarity how the axes of humoral theory traversed age, species, and gender: the best milk would come from a young human mother nursing a female baby, but – at a pinch – a ruminant mother could produce an acceptable substitute.

If woman's milk could lull a squalling baby to sleep, it could be expected to have the same effect on a full-grown adult. If ewe's milk could soften a kid, it could also soften a man. After all, as Burton had written, 'Men and Beasts participate of her nature and conditions, by whose milke they are fed'.[140] The same belief still prevailed among the learned physicians of the Restoration. In November 1667, a certain 'Dr. Whistler' told the diarist Samuel Pepys a 'pretty story' about the Tudor physician John Caius, who

> being very old, and living only at that time upon woman's milk . . . while he fed upon the milk of an angry, fretful woman, was so himself; and then, being advised to take it of a good-natured, patient woman, he did become so, beyond the common temper of his age. Thus much nutriment, they observed, might do.[141]

The variously infantilizing, emasculating, and animalizing resonances of this therapy were not lost on mentally ill patients. In 1679, the poet and Bethlem inpatient James Carkesse complained bitterly that 'His *Diet* was most of it *Milk,*/To reduce him again to a *Child;*/And *Butter* as soft as *Silk,*/To smooth the *Fierce* and the *Wild*'.[142] Like Bartholin, Carkesse framed the reformation sought by his keepers as a change of species: 'The Roaring *Lyon* turns to *Lamb,*/Lies down and couches wondrous Tame'.[143]

In the 1650s, the experimental physiologists of Oxford, London, and Paris took this sort of temperament-altering therapy one step further: they began injecting 'nutriment' directly into the bloodstream.[144] Leading the way in England were Christopher Wren and Richard Lower, both of whom Willis would later recruit to work on the *Cerebri anatome*. They

[138] 'cum lacte mulieris puellam nutrientis'. Gordon, *Opus lilium*, 2.22, p. 217. See also Anglicus, *Compendium*, f. 102r; Otto Brunfels, *Iatrionices medicamentorum simplicium* (Strasbourg, 1533), book 3, f. 15v.

[139] Barrough, *The methode*, pp. 35, 72, 92.

[140] Burton, *The anatomy*, p. 190.

[141] Samuel Pepys, 21 November 1667, in Robert Latham and William Matthews (eds.), *The Diary of Samuel Pepys* (London: G. Bell, 1971), vol. 8, p. 543.

[142] James Carkesse, *Lucida intervalla* (London, 1679), p. 14.

[143] Ibid., p. 34.

[144] Simon Schaffer, 'Regeneration: The Body of Natural Philosophers in Restoration England', in Christopher Lawrence and Steven Shapin (eds.), *Science Incarnate: Historical Embodiments of Natural Knowledge* (Chicago: University of Chicago Press, 1998), pp. 94–105.

began by injecting dogs with the same substances which were typically given to patients orally: milk, opium, and salt of antimony (a common purge).[145] Many of these early test subjects died in agony. Yet the virtuosos' efforts were not in vain, scoffed a disillusioned ex-colleague: they had proven beyond a shadow of doubt that 'such things as are innocently taken into the *Stomach*, are mortal when *injected immediately into the blood*'.[146]

Undeterred by these unpromising results, Lower turned his sights from infusion to transfusion. By February 1665, he had developed a method for passing blood from the artery of one dog into the vein of another. On hearing the news, his fellow experimentalist Robert Boyle (1627–1691) helpfully issued him with a list of questions: 'Whether by this way of Transfusing Blood, the disposition of Individual Animals of the same kind, may not be much altered? (As whether a fierce Dog, by being often quite new stocked with the blood of a cowardly Dog, may not become more tame; & vice versa, &c?)'[147] Blood transfusion promised the sort of radical transformation of temperament of which previous generations of physicians had only been able to dream. Neither bathing human patients in milk nor forcing them to drink it had ever achieved the like. Perhaps, Boyle suggested, it might even produce 'a change in species' – if not from lion to lamb, then at least between 'Animals near of kin'.

Although Boyle's list of questions referred only to quadrupeds, his mind was already racing ahead. Witnessing the early infusion experiments, he had already suggested that 'if it could be done, without either too much danger or cruelty, tryal might be made upon some humane subjects, especially on Malefactors'.[148] Still, the death toll among dogs gave the English experimentalists pause. 'Brute' souls were one thing; human souls (even those of 'Malefactors') were another. Not least, experimental philosophers were not immune to charges of manslaughter.[149] The method needed perfecting, and this would come only through practice. Lower began by teaching his techniques to the London physicians Edmund King and Thomas Coxe, who proceeded to perform a successful transfusion between two dogs on 14 November 1666. King's subsequent trials reveal a

[145] Robert Boyle, *Some considerations touching the vsefulnesse of experimental naturall philosophy* (Oxford, 1663), pp. 62–63; Richard Lower, *Tractatus de corde* (London, 1669), pp. 126–128; Henry Stubbe, *Legends no histories* (London, 1670), pp. 121–126.

[146] Stubbe, *Legends no histories*, p. 126.

[147] [Robert Boyle], 'Tryals proposed by Mr. Boyle to Dr. Lower', *Philosophical Transactions* 1(22) (1666), 386–388.

[148] Boyle, *Some considerations*, p. 64.

[149] [Henry Oldenburg], 'An Account of more Tryals of Transfusion', *Philosophical Transactions* 2(28) (1667), 522.

now-familiar symbolic logic at work. In April 1667, he transfused the blood of a male heifer into that of a female sheep, and observed that it left her 'strong and lusty'. Let loose from the table, she immediately caught sight of 'a Dog near her (which was a Spaniel, that had formerly suffered the tranfusion of Sheeps-Blood into him) . . . [and] butted with great violence at him three or four times'.[150] A bullish sheep had attacked a sheepish dog; if this was not a 'change in species', it came close enough. On 9 June, he tried transfusing the blood of a lamb into a fox, but the recipient sickened and died before any change of his vulpine disposition could be observed.[151]

At the same time as they were conducting these interspecies experiments, Lower and King were also busy developing 'a method of transfusing bloud into men'.[152] Unfortunately, their hopes of performing the first ever human blood transfusion were dashed within the month. At the end of June, the Royal Society received a letter from the Parisian physician Jean-Baptiste Denis, offering a full account of his transfusion of lambs' blood into two human subjects. One of them, a youth suffering from 'a contumacious and violent fever', had previously been bled twenty times 'to asswage the excessive heat', yet 'his wit seem'd wholly sunk' and 'his memory perfectly lost'. The transfusion had been transformative: 'he executes nimbly whatever is appointed him . . . and, in brief, is a subject of amazement of all those that know him'.[153]

The learned doctor, of course, had expected no less. The blood of animals was less 'full of impurities, than that of men', he wrote, because extreme passions, 'debauchedness and irregularity in eating and drinking' were not so 'ordinary to them, as to us'. Besides, 'If Physicians so successfully employ the milk of certain Animals, to which they oblige certain Patients for some whole years together . . . Why may we not hope greater advantages from the mixture of their blood with ours[?]'. Denis evidently saw a direct through line from these traditional milk based therapies to his new blood-based, intravenous alternative. He anticipated

150 [Henry Oldenburg], 'An Account of an easier and safer Way of Transfusing Blood out of one Animal into another', *Philosophical Transactions* 2(25) (1667), 451.

151 Edmond King, 'A Further Account Of some Experiments of Transfusion made by Dr King at his house', 1667, London, Royal Society, RBO/3/58, pp. 195–196.

152 Edmond King, 'A method of transfusing bloud into men', London, Royal Society, CLP/12i/12, m. 1r.

153 Jean Denis, 'A Letter Concerning a new way of sundry diseases by Transfusion of Blood', 22 July 1667. This letter was printed in an unauthorized issue of the *Philosophical Transactions* (no. 17), and later suppressed. It is reproduced in A. D. Farr, 'The First Human Blood Transfusion', *Medical History* 24 (1980), 154–162, quotations on pp. 160–161.

therapeutic applications in a whole range of diseases, not least 'Madness, Dotage, and other Maladies arising from the Malignity of the blood'.[154]

The English pioneers of blood transfusion had been pipped to the post by a Frenchman, and they did not accept the news with good grace.[155] The truth was, the secretary of the Royal Society commented icily, 'that the Philosophers in England ... [would have] practised it long agoe upon Man, if they had not been so tender in hazarding the Life of Man (which they take so much pains for to preserve and relieve)'.[156] Yet Denis had done the English transfusionists a favour: he had suggested to them a new sort of trial subject. Perhaps he was right; perhaps transfusion *could* offer a cure for madness. And, more importantly, if the outcome was unhappy, the trial was less likely to cause a scandal. If 'the Life of Man' was infinitely precious, the lives of the mad were surely a little more expendable than others.

Thus, on the 24 October 1667, the physicians of the Royal Society decided that it was 'most adviseable to try it upon some mad person in the hospital of Bethlem'. Lower and King (among others) were tasked with arranging procurement of a candidate with the hospital's in-house physician, Thomas Allen. To his credit, Allen refused to comply.[157] But Lower was nothing if not resourceful, and – with the help of his fellow virtuoso John Wilkins – he soon identified a suitable candidate. On 21 November, Pepys reported that the evening's alehouse conversation had been on the matter of

> a man that is a little frantic, that hath been a kind of minister ... that the College have hired for 20s. to have some of the blood of a sheep let into his body ... some think it may have a good effect upon him as a frantic man by cooling his blood, others that it will not have any effect at all.[158]

The 'frantic man' in question was a thirty-two-year-old Cambridge divinity graduate named Arthur Coga, who had for a time served as a reader in Wilkins's church. He was generally 'lookt upon as a very freakish and extravagant man', the secretary of the Royal Society wrote to Boyle the next day.[159]

[154] Ibid., p. 159.

[155] Denis had added insult to injury by claiming that the French had come up with the idea of transfusion 'some ten years agoe', long before it had occurred to the English. See, in ibid., pp. 146–147.

[156] [Oldenburg], 'An Account of more Tryals', p. 522.

[157] Thomas Birch, *The History of the Royal Society of London* (London, 1756), vol. 2, pp. 202, 204.

[158] Pepys, 21 November 1667, *Diary*, vol. 8, p. 543.

[159] 'Oldenburg to Boyle, 25 November 1667', in A. Rupert Hall and Marie Boas Hall (trans.), *The Correspondence of Henry Oldenburg* (Madison: University of Wisconsin Press, 1966), vol. 3, p. 611.

None of the Society's members seem to have been sure exactly what ailed Coga, and it is not clear that they cared to know. It is possible that Allen, 'scrupling to try the experiment of transfusion upon any of the mad people' in his care, had pointed out that his worst afflicted patients would be unable to consent to the procedure.[160] Certainly, Coga's recruiters took pains to stress not only that was that he was 'willing', but that he was sound enough in mind for that expressed will to count. Coga was 'a healthy man', Wilkins told Pepys, and as such would 'be able to give an account what alteration, if any, he do find in himself'.[161] He 'speaks Latin well when he is in that company he likes', King reassured Boyle, even if 'his brain is sometimes a little too warm'.[162]

The experiment was conducted two days later, Saturday 23 November, in an overcrowded room at Arundel House. King and Lower tied up a lamb, opened its carotid artery, and proceeded to feed the blood into the human recipient's vein via a series of interlinked pipes and quills. One of the witnesses asking him 'why he had not some other creature's blood', Coga announced, in Latin, that 'sheep's blood has some symbolic power, like the blood of Christ, for Christ is the lamb of God'.[163] The nature of this 'symbolic power' was plain to all. Coga had a reputation for being 'a debauched man'; now, an innocent lamb had blotted out his corruption with its purity.[164] Furthermore, as one commentator put it, 'a Lamb is esteemed to be the meekest and most peaceable Animal Nature has brought forth, why then might not his blood . . . introduce such a pacation [pacification] into the tumultuous blood of the Patient as was sufficient for his cure?'[165]

The signs were promising. On his return to his lodgings, Coga was 'very sober and quiet, more than before, as the people in the house tell us'.[166] Two days after the procedure, he was still 'more composed' than they had ever seen him.[167] The following week, he was brought along to a meeting of the Royal Society, where he presented 'a Latin paper of his own, giving an account of what he had observed in himself since he underwent the said

[160] Birch, *The History*, vol. 2, p. 204. [161] Pepys, 21 November 1667, *Diary*, vol. 8, p. 543.

[162] 'King to Boyle, 25 November 1667', in Thomas Birch (ed.), *The Works of the Honourable Robert Boyle* (London, 1772), vol. 6, p. 647.

[163] 'sanguis ovis symbolicam quamdam facultatem habet cum sanguine Christi; quia Christus est agnus Dei'. Ibid., p. 647.

[164] Pepys, 21 November 1667, *Diary*, vol. 8, p. 543.

[165] George Acton, *Physical Reflections upon a Letter . . . Concerning a New way of Curing sundry Diseases by Transfusion of Blood* (London, 1668), pp. 9–10.

[166] 'King to Boyle, 25 November 1667', in *The Works*, p. 647.

[167] 'Oldenburg to Boyle, 25 November 1667', in Hall and Hall (trans.), *Correspondence*, vol. 3, p. 611.

experiment'.[168] That evening, Pepys bumped into him at the alehouse, and was treated to the abridged version: 'he finds himself much better since, and as a new man'. Pepys had his doubts: for all that he spoke 'very reasonably, and very well', Coga nonetheless struck him as 'cracked a little in his head'.[169] But the fellows of the Royal Society were too elated by their success to worry about a few leftover eccentricities. Oldenburg had already written to one learned colleague that the procedure promised to be 'most beneficial to humanity . . . in the treatment of frenzy and many other diseases'.[170] Interspecies blood transfusion held out the promise of a root-and-branch cure. There would be no more need for blows, threats, or restraints: with lamb's blood in his veins, a frantic man would 'lye quiet as a lamb' of his own accord.

Unfortunately, Pepys's intuitions were not misplaced. By the end of the year, it had become impossible to ignore the fact that – frantic or not – Coga had a serious drinking problem. On 23 December, Oldenburg admitted to Denis that 'the wildness of his mind remains unchanged – or perhaps we ought rather to consider that the improvement of his brain is prevented by the incurable intemperance of which he is guilty'.[171] Coga was chastened repeatedly 'for disordering himself by intemperate drinking of wine', but his all-too-public pub crawls continued.[172] By January, rumour had it that London's coffeehouse-goers had deliberately 'endeavoured to debauch the fellow, and so consequently discredit the Royal Society and make the experiment ridiculous'.[173] What had started out as a paean paean to experimental philosophy was rapidly turning into a farce.

The virtuosos' suspicions were not unjustified. Whatever the truth of the rumour about Coga's Machiavellian coffeehouse companions, there *was* a campaign to 'make the experiment ridiculous'. In 1670, the transfusionists' arch-enemy Henry Stubbe even printed a letter signed by one 'Agnus Coga' ('Coga the Lamb'), begging the Royal Society for a further cash infusion. The letter's author described himself as 'Your Creature (for he was his own man till your Experiment transform'd him into another *species*)'. If he had been forced by poverty to pawn his clothes, this was the experimentalists' fault: it was 'very miserable, that the want of natural heat should rob him of his

[168] Birch, *The History*, vol. 2, p. 216. [169] Pepys, 30 November 1667, *Diary*, vol. 8, p. 554.

[170] 'Oldenburg to Sluse, 25 November 1667', in Hall and Hall (trans.), *Correspondence*, vol. 3, pp. 615–617.

[171] 'Oldenburg to Denis, 23 December 1667', in Hall and Hall (trans.), *Correspondence*, vol. 4, p. 77.

[172] 'Oldenburg to Boyle, 17 December 1667', in ibid., p. 55; Birch, *The History*, vol. 2, p. 227.

[173] Philip Skippon to John Ray, January 1667/8, in Edwin Lankester (ed.), *The Correspondence of John Ray* (London: The Ray Society, 1848), p. 23.

artificial too'.[174] Whether it was Coga or a good impersonator, the letter's author clearly understood how to turn the 'symbolic power' of transfusion on its head. Coga's wildness had been tamed, but 'the want of natural heat' now barred him from living a life of self-sufficiency. He had been his 'own man'; now he was scarcely a man at all.

The Messy Reality

If Coga had not been 'transform'd . . . into another species', he was very far from cured. The '*Transactions* report an *Untruth,* in saying that *Coga* was ever the *better* for it', concluded the Society's bitter ex-correspondent. It was those who claimed to be able to cure 'Madmen' who deserved 'to be sent to Bedlam'.[175] And perhaps this pessimism was not unfounded. The rhetoric of 'restoration' remained as alluring as ever: it promised to restore not just an individual's wits, but also the social order in which they were embedded. Yet the evidence for how ordinary patients were treated suggests that – if this high hope had ever informed the choices made by their caregivers – it was soon crowded out by more pragmatic concerns. The final section of this chapter revisits some of the prescribed treatments discussed above, showing how, in practice, their application often undermined their rationale.

Reminders of Rule

If an ordinary householder fell frantic in early modern England, it was the head of household who was supposed to bring him or her back in line. Unfortunately, the fact that frenzy was a disease most often diagnosed in men aged between twenty-five and fifty – that is, exactly the people most likely to be heads of households – was a major flaw in this projection. When the housewife Margery Sagar came before the Lancashire justices of the peace in 1641, she reported that her husband, who had lately fallen into a 'frensie', was 'lyinge bound in Cheanes, & featers, & not lessed att all for theise Fifteene weekes last past'. Everyone in the parish was 'fearfull, to come neare unto him, in his fittes, often befallinge upon him bothe night & day, in most fearfull & terrible skrikes [shrieks], & shouttinges'. The only person who dared approach her husband was

> his owne naturall father being an old, & aged man, of Threescore, & three yeares of age, whoe often adventures himself with him, to keepe him in

[174] Stubbe, *Legends no histories*, p. 179. [175] Ibid., pp. 133–144.

> some awe, & subjection, with if it should happen my saide father in lawe, to come to any great hurt, I myself my twoe poore children, and my mother in law, should be lefte, destitute, & voide of all Comfort.[176]

Margery Sagar was not in the best position to instil 'awe' in her husband, or to bring him into 'subjection'. His sixty-three-year-old father – who would have handed over 'rule' to his adult son decades ago – was now forced to resume the mantle of authority. When an adult male fell frantic, it often precipitated this sort of rapid reshuffle of the domestic hierarchy.

When no father figure was available, the situation was even worse. Akihito Suzuki's survey of English Quarter Sessions papers suggests that 'lunatic' husbands brought to court outnumbered wives by nine to five.[177] Those wives whose cases *did* reach court had been abandoned or no longer lived under the same roof as their spouses, while eight of the nine 'lunatic' husbands still lived with their wives. Suzuki concludes that the patriarchal ideology which structured English households also 'seems to have imposed different roles on the husbands and wives whose spouses became insane: powerful husbands had to be able to maintain and govern their lunatic wives, but feeble and dependent wives were put into a difficult situation because of their raging husbands'.[178] In practice, families' attempts to manage an adult male sufferer usually boiled down to his symbolic subjugation to a brother, father, or master. This was why many more wives than husbands ended up at their nearest Quarter Sessions, pleading for assistance.

The problem was worsened by the financial double bind in which many families found themselves: not only had the household lost the sufferer's income, but also the income of whoever was tasked with 'keeping' and 'watching' them. As such, the justices of the peace usually responded by arranging to pay for the hiring of extra attendants. But bringing more hands on deck was not necessarily enough to restabilize the domestic hierarchy. In early modern England, the vast majority of those who were willing to 'keep' and 'watch' the sick in return for a fee were women, many of them maidservants, spinsters, or widows. And they were no better placed to keep a frantic man 'in some awe, & subjection' than was Margery Sagar. In fact, as hired hands and outsiders to the family, they were in an even weaker position to check his behaviour. In 1676, for

176 Preston, Lancashire Archives, QSB/1/245/55.

177 Akihito Suzuki, 'Lunacy in Seventeenth- and Eighteenth-Century England: Analysis of Quarter Sessions Records Part I', *History of Psychiatry* 2(8) (1991), 437–456.

178 Ibid., p. 444.

example, a glover named John Griffes wrote to the king complaining that his neighbours had decided he was 'a frantick man', after which

> I was watched for divers nights with divers of my own neyghbours namly Elizabeth Fox daughter of John Fox mary Sagar alis Kenderik: a servant mayd of gregor waymans baker a servant maid of moses hartleys blacksmith and forbiden medling with my wife in bed after the maner of a husband ... but in no name I obeyed not: But being thus Charged a servant in his magiestyes behalfe before these above named witnesses I do make it my buisness but the virtue of the same Charge to demand all Kings Rights whatsoever.[179]

It is hard to disentangle fact from fiction in Griffes's account, but what is clear is that he would not obey his watchers because he believed he outranked them. The best that a woman in this position could do was to invoke a higher authority. The Suffolk yeoman John Piers, who was in the habit of leaving his maidservant to watch his frantic brother Arthur while he was out at work, reported that, on the day of Arthur's death, she 'did ... intreate him (because he had eate no meate [food] in divers daies before) to eate somethinge & she telling him that this defendant [John Piers] would have him eate something'.[180]

At best, these frantic charges' resistance to rule must have been wearying for their keepers; at worst, it could be downright dangerous. Occasionally, it led to the sort of situation described by the London draper Sir William Capell, who had been sued for reneging on his contract with an apprentice named Thomas Green. Capell claimed that, while under his roof, Green had fallen into 'a fransy and was clerely from his minde'. Out of tenderness towards 'his seid apprentice and to his father', Capell claimed, he had prepared for Green 'a close chamber and therin keped him and hired a woman to wait uppon him both night and day, and the seid apprentice in his seid frandesy had all most strangled her and she durst no longer kepe him without more helpe'.[181] Capell responded by hiring a male attendant to help the woman. The draper was evidently a man of means, and could afford to pay the second keeper's wage.[182] But many could not. In 1657, the widow Ellen Faulkner told the Manchester Quarter Sessions that her 'frantike' son Thomas was so unruly that she had 'been enforced to keep a

179 Kew, TNA, SP 29/382, f. 159r. 180 Kew, TNA, STAC 8/1/6, m. 1r.

181 Kew, TNA, C 1/94, m. 23.

182 This male keeper would have been paid a higher wage than his female counterpart. See Jane Humphries and Jacob Weisdorf, 'The Wages of Women in England, 1260–1850', *Journal of Economic History* 75(2) (2015), 405–447.

maidservant continually and now likewise a man servant'. She had been paying these keepers' wages on credit which she could now no longer repay. Faulkner begged the justices 'to grant an order that your petitioners son may be provided for in some way (or otherwise that your petitioner may receiue something weekly for the providing of Sustanance for herself and [her] Sonn)'.[183] To judge by the wording, Faulkner's preference was to have her son's keeping taken out of her hands altogether.

This option was probably never on the table. For crown officials outside of Middlesex, committal to Bethlem (then the only dedicated hospital for the mad) or even to a local bridewell was considerably more expensive than keeping them at home. They generally reserved it only for lunatics who had harmed their neighbours or committed arson (or had threatened to do the same).[184] When such a committal order *was* made, the intention was clear; as Jonathan Andrews puts it, the house's 'regime would supplant and reinstil an alternative (and, often, harsher) internal regime to that adjudged to have failed within the individual's original household'.[185] Sadly, there is evidence that other householders and neighbours often positively longed for this to happen. But their petitions speak not of callousness but of exhaustion: Faulkner reported that her son had 'puld to peeces all his backe and bed clothes and euerie thinge else he can come neare'.[186] This was not enough to merit his committal to gaol, but nor can it have been easy to live with.

The gender hierarchy of the early modern household no doubt made it uniquely difficult for women to govern male charges. Yet, given that frenzy could give sufferers (of either gender) uncharacteristic strength, maintaining rule was also a numbers game.[187] Napier's comment of his frantic patient Mercy Fish, that she 'doth so strugle that 3 or 4 can scarce rule her', was typical. Of another similarly afflicted patient, he marvelled, '7 not able to kepe her downe'.[188] Few English households had either the social or

183 Preston, Lancashire Archives, QSP 144/19.

184 Akihito Suzuki, 'Lunacy in Seventeenth- and Eighteenth-Century England: Analysis of Quarter Sessions records Part II', *History of Psychiatry* 3 (1992), 29–44.

185 Jonathan Andrews, 'The Politics of Committal to Early Modern Bedlam', in Andrews et al. (eds.), *The History of Bethlem*, p. 23. I have not been able to discuss institutional confinement in the full depth that it deserves. Fortunately there are many classic works on the subject. See, in the bibliography, works by Bynum et al. (*Anatomy of Madness*, vols. 1 and 2), Andrews ('Bedlam Revisited'), Suzuki ('Lunacy' I and II), Porter ('Madness and Its Institutions'), and Neely (*Distracted Subjects*).

186 QSP 144/19.

187 For unusual strength, see e.g., Timonthy Bright, *A treatise of melancholie* (London, 1586), p. 53; Willis, *Two discourses*, pp. 182, 205; Royal Society, Boyle Papers, RB/1/8/30.

188 Kassell et al., *Casebooks*, cases 66415, 53258.

financial credit to retain that many people on hand long-term. And those who could afford to hire a team were not necessarily keen to do so. Many poor and middling householders would have taken the same conservative approach as Capell and Faulkner: hiring a single female keeper, and taking on more only when it became evident that she could not cope alone.

Taken together, these sources suggest that the glorious restoration of rule envisioned by moralists, philosophers, and physicians was rarely realized. Frantic men had been socialized as rulers, and – no matter how unfit for duty – they were not about to submit to their womenfolk. Women who did try to 'wear the breeches' were ignored, rebuffed, or physically hurt by their charges. Aged fathers were obliged to treat their adult sons as disobedient children. Husbands and masters were happy to outsource the job of ruling to single women and widows. In short, these domestic arrangements often bore a closer resemblance to a 'world turned upside downward' than a 'great chain of being'. On the ground, the friends, kin, and keepers of frantic persons were often too exhausted to keep issuing the reminders of rule – whether verbal or physical – which were supposed to restore them to their wits. And those who did earnestly try to keep their frantic relatives 'in awe & subjection' were rarely rewarded with any such Nebuchadnezzar-style transformation. Nor could 'threatenings and blows' be counted on to restore rule. If Napier did not condemn Elizabeth Piddington's husband for beating his unruly wife, his offhand comment 'the more they strive with her the worse she is' was hardly a ringing endorsement of the method.[189] Even Bartholin had to admit that while 'some are returned to their senses by blows . . . others are made even more brutelike'.[190] And both the treatment and the rationale *were* 'brutalizing', stemming as they did from the notion that sufferers – having lost the use of their rational faculties – had slipped down a rung on the ladder of nature. No wonder that the therapy designed to hoist them back up could just as easily push them further down.

Cooling Agents

If neither blows nor threats nor blandishments served to return frantic persons to themselves, this left only the hope of an inward transformation, a metamorphosis of 'nature' or 'disposition'. This was why hopes had run so high in the winter of 1667/68; physicians had long aimed to artificially cool and compose the blood of their frantic patients, and transfusion

[189] Ibid., case 41459. [190] Bartholin, *De usu flagrorum*, p. 9.

promised to take this kind of therapy to a new level. And yet, in the end, it did not deliver. The virtuosos immediately blamed Coga: he 'consulted his instinct rather than the interests of his health, and completely eluded our expectations', huffed Lower in 1670.[191] Coga might justly have replied that – if they wanted a 'rational', level-headed subject – they should not have chosen him.

In truth, it was not the test subject but the procedure itself which had eluded the virtuosos' expectations. In February 1668, Lower's Parisian rival Denis had re-entered the race with a claim to have cured 'an Inveterate Phrensy by the Transfusion of Bloud'.[192] But the affair had ended in ignominy; the patient had later 'expired under his hands, while he was Tranfusing Blood into him'.[193] Denis had ended up on trial for murder, and although his name was cleared – the court found that the test subject's wife had been poisoning her husband with arsenic – it was hardly good press. The Paris *parlement* banned the procedure in 1670, and – although there was no equivalent ban in England – the Royal Society dropped the research programme for good.[194] But hopes died hard. In 1707, Salmon finished the *Praxis Medica*'s chapter on frenzy on an optimistic note:

> some Authors of considerable reputation advise to Venesection ... Tis admirable to think how calm and quiet the enraged animal spirits do become thereby, and how they are reduced to their Pristine state. And to this Authors have added other Chirurgick Operations, as ... transfusion of Mans, Calfs, Lambs, or Sheeps-blood into the Veins of the Diseased Person, &c.[195]

Nobody had performed this procedure (on record) for forty years, but the dream of restoration lived on.

Meanwhile, medical practitioners were obliged to fall back on the same old roster of cooling, moistening drugs which had been prescribed to frantic patients for centuries. And this brings us to another juncture at which principle and practice seem to have parted ways. As we saw earlier, a similar rule of thumb obtained for the prescription of both bloodletting

[191] Lower, *Tractatus de corde*, p. 200.

[192] Jean-Baptiste Denis, 'An Extract, of a Letter, written by J. Denis, ... touching a late Cure of an Inveterate Phrensy by the Transfusion of Bloud', *Philosophical Transactions* 2(32) (1668), 617–624.

[193] [Anon.], 'A Letter Written by an Intelligent and Worthy English Man from Paris, ... concerning some Transactions there, relating to the Experiment of the Transfusion of Blood', *Philosophical Transactions* 4(54) (1669), 1076.

[194] Peter Sahlins, *1668: The Year of the Animal in France* (New York: Zone Books, 2017), pp. 244–246.

[195] Salmon, *Praxis medica*, p. 177.

and opiates. Both therapies had their place, but they were to be adjusted carefully so as not to outstrip the strength of the patient. In particular, practitioners were supposed to think twice before prescribing narcotics to 'weaker' patients – women, children, and the elderly. The dangers of overdosing were all too well-known.

Although Napier's casebooks are the only sample I have found which is large enough to sustain a quantitative analysis (and a sample of sixty-six patients is too small to draw definite conclusions), the pattern of his prescriptions does provide a revealing data point. As I mentioned earlier, thirty-nine (59 per cent) of those he diagnosed with frenzy were male, and twenty-seven were female. And yet Napier prescribed opiates to six male patients (15 per cent of the male total) and to ten female patients (37 per cent of the female total). The same skewed gender ratio is visible in the number of repeat prescriptions: five women later received a second dose, as opposed to only two men. The people who were seen as most at risk of the cooling, moistening, stupefying effects of opiates were also the ones who were prescribed them most frequently.

The rector was not so meticulous about detailing his phlebotomy instructions, and as such, it is hard to make an equivalent cross-comparison. Overall, he does seem to have taken a more conservative approach to bloodletting; he tended to follow the medical authors' advice about letting women's blood only from the ankle vein.[196] But they did not always get off so lightly. One of his most physically and verbally unruly patients, Mercy Fish, was given the sort of regime usually reserved for men: 'Was let blood on her forehed in her temples [four ounces] 2 in her armes [twelve ounces] her blood was very bad', he wrote on 2 June 1628, before proceeding to prescribe further bloodletting from her ankle and under her tongue. Four days later, he updated his notes: the patient had now 'beene let blood arm boath her browes. boathe her armes & under the tongue & hed', and 'had also a blystering playster yet talketh much'.[197] All the blood removed from Mercy's body had failed to tame her tongue.

Conclusion

What are we to make of one seventeenth-century medical practitioner's apparent overprescription of narcotics to women? Although I cannot claim to know the answer, I hope that this book has offered at least two possible lines of interpretation. The first, which has been explored in this chapter,

[196] Kassell et al., *Casebooks*, cases 23753, 66415, 75687. [197] Ibid., cases 66253, 66283.

runs as follows. The inhabitants of early modern England lived in a world in which an individual's place in the 'natural', domestic, and political order was (in theory) set by the degree of reason they possessed. And that degree of reason found expression not only in the individual's soul, but also in his or her body–both in its anatomical structure, and its temperament.

This qualitative framework could be made to account for every known variegation of human and non-human 'nature', including sex difference. Whether this was explained in terms of the quantity of choler in the gall bladder or the quantity of 'fermentative particles' in the blood, the result was the same. Moral philosophers, divines, and physicians (all of them male) returned the same report: women were (on average) colder, wetter, weaker, less spirited, less aggressive, and less rational than men. This was what made them (in the eyes of these men) unfit for rule, but it also offered some natural protection against diseases like frenzy. It was also a positive help to men who fell frantic: a woman's milk could temper the patient's choler and quench his heat, bringing his temperament back towards the golden mean.

But if women were less likely to succumb to frenzy, those who *did* succumb seem to have unsettled onlookers more deeply than their male counterparts. A man who raged, shouted, brawled, bragged, soliloquized, or tried to seduce strangers was taking the available models of 'manhood' too far. In a woman, the same sort of behaviours amounted to what Forman had called a 'Reuoltion of Nature'. Forman himself seems to have been most troubled by the 'over lecherous' demeanour of these female patients (proving a solid commitment to the double standard).[198] But even the staid academic physician Oxenbridge found such behaviour alarming: he remarked of one mad patient that she 'ran up and down the Streets, bare-footed, Cloaths torn, hair loose, was ready to pull up her Cloaths to everyone'.[199]

If Napier was ever subjected to such a display, he passed over it in silence. But his descriptions of his seriously ill female patients suggest many moments of unease. Anne Syred, he wrote, was 'a strange mad filthy creature'; she would 'runne a dosen myles', 'teare rent burne any thinge', go 'into the rivers & wash her [self]', 'defile her self', and byte & scratch'.[200] Frideswide Pain was 'wilfully mad & froward' and 'very strong'.[201] Elizabeth Conyers had 'growen yet more furious cursing

198 MS Ashmole 355, pp. 133–134.

199 Oxenbridge, *General Observations*, p. 9.

200 Kassell et al., *Casebooks*, case 44800.

201 Ibid., cases 73340, 74199.

swearing fighting & talking more then before'.[202] Despite the bleeding and blistering, Mercy Fish continued to rage 'longe' and 'sorely'. After another consultation with her, he wrote simply: 'her diab*olic* frensy continued long'.[203] To be clear, Napier did not reserve this sort of remark for his female patients. But it is possible that he felt the need to get them to *stop* – to stop whatever it was they were doing – more urgently than he did with their male counterparts. Women were already seen as liable to let their passions and appetites get the better of their reason. This (in the minds of early modern patriarchs) was why they needed ruling. The sight of a woman who had lost all capacity for self-rule was bad enough, but one mounting a campaign of sustained resistance to the rule of others was hard to bear.

This is one possible explanation for Napier's greater readiness to prescribe opiates to women, and it certainly squares with this chapter's argument. But I would like to finish by suggesting another line of interpretation, one which draws on Chapter 1's discussion of causes. Looking at the ten frantic women in this sample who were prescribed opiates, some commonalities emerge. Mercy Fish's frenzy began just under a month after she had given birth; at his first consultation Napier had described her as hot, sweating, 'very aguish', and 'Sick as life will hold'. The same was true of Anne Syred; her troubles had started about six months after giving birth. 'Ever uppon childbearing [she] falleth into her mad fit', Napier wrote three years later. Elizabeth Conyers, too, was 'Worse in her childbed'. In total, four of these ten women were suffering from postpartum illness or injury, and three from the 'new ague' (one of whom died within the week). Another 'had taken grefe touching a badd husband that had a bastard & was put out of his living by his landlord & hath spent all & beateth her'. Although Napier diagnosed frenzy most often in men, his female patients were probably likelier to be suffering in body as well as in mind. Some of them were at death's door. His sedation of these patients could be read as an act of silencing; it could also be read as an act of compassion.

202 Ibid., case 58025. 203 Ibid., cases 66223, 66253, 66415.

CHAPTER 6

Pathologizing Politics

Introduction

'O intollerable mischiefe! and neuer heard of frency to runne away with such madnes against God and his truth!' exclaimed the anonymous author of *A gagge for the Pope, and the Iesuits* in 1624.[1] This English pamphleteer was only the latest in a long line of religious polemicists to use frenzy to defame his enemies. And the title of his pamphlet was no coincidence: a diagnosis of the disease was remarkably effective as a 'gagge'. As the last chapter suggested, it merited the use of 'bit' and 'bridle', whether in the form of whipping, restraint, confinement, or sedation. But it also served to gag those who received the diagnosis in a subtler but more irreversible way: once an individual had been labelled 'frantic', nothing he or she said needed to be taken seriously. This chapter explores how the disease was mobilized politically – both as a literal diagnosis and as a figure of speech – to silence, undermine, and confine its recipients.

There are four sections to this chapter, and they unfold in chronological order. The first three sections explore how frenzy was deployed in the first century after the Henrician Reformation (c. 1540–1640); the fourth turns to consider its use during the religious and political upheavals of the mid-seventeenth century (1640–1660). The first section asks why frenzy found such widespread favour among sixteenth- and early seventeenth-century religious polemicists. Focusing on skirmishes between English Catholics and Protestants – and between Protestants of different persuasions – it explores how and why the diagnosis was repurposed as a piece of religio-political polemic. The following section looks at how frenzy was deployed in the very different stories which the standard-bearers of both confessions told about their country's recent religio-political past. We then explore how the conferral or refusal of a frenzy diagnosis was weaponized by

[1] [Anon.], *A gagge for the Pope, and the Iesuits* (London, 1624), p. 12.

England's crown officials, and why – over time – they became increasingly hesitant to use it. Finally the chapter turns to consider the new 'frenzy' epidemic which broke out during the civil wars and Interregnum. By the late 1640s–a time of bitter conflict over the question of where sovereignty lay–the time-honoured tactic of allowing figurative and literal 'frenzy' to collapse into one another became political dynamite. It could be used to justify the deposition and incarceration of a king; it could be used to justify a military coup. Yet the same drawback which had led previous regimes to abandon the diagnosis remained: taken too literally, it would turn its recipients into innocents. In the 1650s, I argue, this led some Anglican polemicists – still fighting a rearguard action against religious non-conformity – to develop a new and improved diagnosis: 'melancholy enthusiasm'.

Metaphor

Heat

If an early modern English physician had been asked to name a quintessentially hot, dry disease, frenzy might easily have been the first to spring to mind. As we saw in Chapter 1, it was defined as a hot, burning abscess in the brain or meninges, caused by the hot, dry humour choler. Unlike the other forms of madness, it was always accompanied by an acute fever. The naturally choleric person was irascible, 'hot-blooded', or 'hot-tempered'. Frenzy caricatured the same picture: its sufferers fell into hot fits, senseless paroxysms of 'raging', 'raving', and 'railing'. Choler's elemental counterpart was fire, and the morbific bodily processes of burning and inflammation made this link explicit.

This brought frenzy into alignment with another inflammatory condition: religious zeal. While the burning heat of frenzy was desired by nobody, however, many English Protestants positively yearned to 'burne in the spirit'.[2] They knew from scripture that when the Spirit of the Lord made himself manifest, it was usually in the form of fire. In Matthew 3:11, John the Baptist explained that while he baptized with water, his successor would baptize 'with the holy Ghost, and with fire'.[3] In *A coal from the altar, to kindle the holy fire of zeale* (1615), Samuel Ward explained that 'Baptisme of water, is but a cold proofe of a mans Christendome . . . but if

[2] Samuel Ward, *A coal from the altar, to kindle the holy fire of zeale* (London, 1615), p. 5.
[3] KJV, Matthew 3:11.

any be baptised with fire, the same is sealed vp to the day of Redemption'.[4] For Ward, the lukewarm water of nominal Christianity stood in stark contrast to the 'heauenly fire' which burned in the hearts of all those touched by the Holy Spirit.[5] This condition, Ward explained, was 'zeal', a word which in 'plaine English' meant 'nothing but heate'.[6] It was not a single passion, or a mixture of passions, but rather a 'hot temper, higher degree or intension [intensity] of them all'. By the same logic, 'the opposites of zeale, keye-coldnes and luke-warmenesse . . . are no affections, but seuerall tempers of them all'.[7] As Alec Ryrie's work has shown, this thermogenic language became central to the affective lives of English Protestants.[8] Typical in this vein was Thomas Sorocold's prayer that God would 'Kindle, o kindle my desires . . . with the fire of zealous loue to burne alwayes, and flame vpon the Alter of my hart'.[9] Concomitant to this longing, of course, was a perpetual dread of 'keye-coldnes'.[10] The godly were renowned for taking their own spiritual temperature daily, if not hourly. Comforting those who despaired at low readings, the minister Daniel Dyke counselled: 'if thou feele at any time, that thy heart is warmed with good motions . . . doest thou feele any sparkled of the heauenly fire; take thou the bellowes presently, blowe till they flame'.[11]

As Ward noted indignantly, however, not everybody viewed zeal in such glowing terms.[12] The word still retained its association with the militant Jewish sect of the 'zealots', and thus with religious radicalism, sectarianism, violence, and revolt against 'the lawfull magistrate'.[13] The figure of heat was easily turned against those whose were judged *too* fervent in matters of religion. Those, like Ward, who saw themselves as the 'small remnaunt of the godlye' were especially vulnerable to this line of attack.[14] In 1580, the

[4] Ward, *A coal from the altar*, p. 29.

[5] Another touchstone for English Puritans was Revelation 3:16, in which God tells the Laodiceans that 'because thou art lukewarme, and neither cold nor hot, I wil spew thee out of my mouth'. In the Puritans' estimation, England easily matched Laodicea in spiritual tepidity. Ward warned his audience that 'if wee take not warning, or warming, we may I feare in time come to be spued out of Gods mouth'. Ibid., sig. A3v.

[6] Ibid., pp. 1, 5. [7] Ibid., pp. 4–5.

[8] Alec Ryrie, *Being Protestant in Reformation Britain* (Oxford: Oxford University Press, 2013), pp. 65–70.

[9] Thomas Sorocold, *Supplications of saints* (London, 1612), p. 121.

[10] Ryrie, *Being Protestant*, p. 69.

[11] Daniel Dyke, *The mystery of selfe-deceiuing. Or A discourse and discouery of the deceitfullnesse of mans heart* (London, 1614), p. 352.

[12] Ward, *A coal from the altar*, p. 2.

[13] Henry Hammond, *Of resisting the lawfull magistrate under colour of religion* (Oxford, 1644), p. 1.

[14] George Gifford, *A godlie, zealous, and profitable sermon vpon the second chapter of Saint Iames* (London, 1582), sig. B6v.

Jesuit Robert Persons snidely referred to them as 'the hotter sorte of Protestantes, called the Puritayns'.[15] One of their number, the divinity lecturer Percival Wiburn, fired back. In his writings, Persons had displayed a 'hot & too immoderate a zeale', typical of 'the hot sect of your puritane Jesuits'.[16] There was a 'hotter sort' of Catholic, too, he insisted, and Persons was among their number.[17] Heat came to stand for persecutory precisionism and fanaticism.

Seeking to rescue zeal from this negative cast, Protestant divines set about distinguishing between its 'true' and 'false' presentations. It was in depicting the latter that frenzy came into its own. In a sermon preached at Paul's Cross on 5 February 1616, the minister of St Southwark's, Thomas Sutton, expressed his fervent wish that his hearers would 'adde burning zeale to Christian profession'.[18] Yet 'because there is no point wherein a man may sooner ouer-shoote himselfe then in this', he cautioned, it was vital to check for the hallmarks of 'true zeale'.[19] First, the matter had to be 'good',

> or else it is not zeale but deuillish and fleshly heate, a frenzie, and madnesse, counterfeiting the name of zeale, like the zeale of those Idolaters that mangled and cut them selues, 1 Kings 18. Like the zeal of the Scribes and Pharise who compasse Sea and Land to make Proselites: Like the zeale of Paul before his conuersion: Like the zeale of ignorant Papists and Brownists at this day ... They are like bittes of lime neuer so hot and smoaking as in cold water, neuer earnest but in euill causes.[20]

If true zeal was a spiritual heat, the inward breath of the Spirit, counterfeit zeal was an inflammation of the 'flesh' by the devil. Sutton's differentiation between truth and falsity rested on a series of symbolic oppositions: sanity and madness, health and disease, fire and quicklime. The sickly, preternatural heat of frenzy provided the symbolic antithesis of the salvific, supernatural heat of the Holy Spirit. In turn, the outward signs of holy zeal – 'the glowing of the eares ... the wringing of the hands ... the beating of the breasts ... the sparkling of the eyes' – stood in stark contrast to the frothing tirades and self-mutilations of the frantic.[21] As the tone of his *Second Summons* may suggest, Sutton was himself unquestionably a Protestant of the 'hotter sort'. Tellingly, in his account, the Protestant

[15] Robert Persons, *A brief discours contayning certayne reasons why Catholiques refuse to goe to church* (East Ham, 1580), f. 39v.
[16] Percival Wiburn, *A checke or reproofe of M. Howlets vntimely shreeching in her Maiesties eares* (London, 1581), ff. 8r–v.
[17] Ibid., f. 9r. [18] Thomas Sutton, *Englands first and second summons* (London, 1616), p. 194.
[19] Ibid., p. 196. [20] Ibid., pp. 196–197. [21] Ibid., pp. 194–195.

'lunatic fringe' is populated not by 'Puritans', but by the radical dissenters known as the 'Brownists'.[22] It was the 'Brownists', in their 'hot frenzies', who were 'the imposthumes that disease the wombe of our mother'.[23] A caricature of radical separatism served to offset Sutton's flattering portrait of godliness. The former's 'hot frenzies' made the latter's 'zeal' look like a well-tempered warmth.

Two decades later, in a sermon preached before the royal justices of the assizes, the Church of England divine Thomas Drant returned to the same theme. It was March 1637, and William Laud's programme of ecclesiastical reform had dangerously repolarized English Protestantism. Confessional polemic was reaching a new fever pitch. Like many divines before him, Drant described the 'flashes of holinesse' experienced by sinners as sparks 'enkindled' by the 'Spirit of grace'. Yet there was also

> a *Spirit* of *giddinesse,* it rules much in some brainesick *hot-spurs,* whom it doth possesse at once with a zealous phrensie, and cast them, as that *dumbe* One did the childe in the *Gospell,* now into the *water*, sullen and rheumatick *drivelings*, spitting against the Church, vvhose Hierarchy they beate downe, that their owne braines may sway; anon into the *fire*, so hot a contention about Ceremonies, though enjoyn'd vvith equall modestie and right, as if Heaven and Earth vvere to little to bee mingled in the quarrell.[24]

Thirteen years earlier, the Laudian cleric Richard Montagu had written scathingly of 'the frantick fitts and froth of every Puritan paroxym'.[25] Now, following official guidance, Drant was systematically tarring all objectors to Laud's reforms with the same brush.[26] Whether 'in a Church-parlour at *Amsterdam*, abroad there, or an uncharitable conventicle of our Zelots, at home here', what these people had in common was that they had mistaken the heat of their own sick brains for the fire of the Holy Spirit.[27]

[22] 'Brownism', like 'Puritanism', was a name coined by enemies of the movement. Its founder, Robert Browne, had been much influenced by the Puritan Thomas Cartwright. 'Brownists' sought the right to separate from the Church of England and to form self-governing congregations. Browne had returned to the fold in 1585, much to the dismay of his fellow separatists, but the name stuck. See Gordon Campbell, *The Oxford Dictionary of the Renaissance* (Oxford: Oxford University Press, 2005), s.v. 'Brownists'.

[23] Sutton, *Englands first and second summons*, p. 233.

[24] Thomas Drant, *The royall guest* (London, 1637), p. 30.

[25] Richard Montagu to John Cosin, in George Ornsby (ed.), *The Correspondence of John Cosin, D.D., Lord Bishop of Durham*, 2 vols. (Durham: Andrews & Co., 1869), vol. 1, p. 32.

[26] The same motif recurs in other sermons printed in these years. See, for example, Humphrey Sydenham, *Sermons vpon solemne occasions* (London, 1637), pp. 124, 258–267.

[27] Drant, *The royall guest*, p. 31.

Violence

Of all of frenzy's signs, physical violence was perhaps the easiest to turn to polemical ends. We have already seen self-injury used in this way, in Sutton's reference to the worshippers of Baal 'that mangled and cut them selues', and in Drant's adaptation of Matthew 17:15. Railing against papists in 1630, the Church of England minister John Squire preached that '[m]ad men will wound themselves, and feele not: and the franticke will run into the fire, and feare not. So, those men . . . ranne out of their wits, when they ran out of the Church: and this makes them like Bedlems, to be so couragious, indeed so outragious in their heresies'.[28] The self-injury of the frantic provided a visceral metaphor for the state of the unredeemed, too 'senseless' to feel the mortal wounds they inflicted upon their own souls. If papists seemed courageous, Squire argued, this was not the result of divine fortification, but of a deadly loss of inhibition. Similarly, when Persons asked why English recusants were willing to give up so many worldly advantages for their faith, Andrew Willet shot back that 'some are possessed with a spirit of phrenzie . . . The *Donatists* did throw themselues headlong into the fire and water, and from the tops of hils'.[29] Willet was not about to let the Catholics package their pointless self-destruction as godly self-sacrifice.

Even more common than the theme of self-harm was that of violence against others. Sufferers of frenzy had a reputation for attacking their caregivers, and this common knowledge had long been put to polemical ends. Augustine of Hippo made ample use of it in his writings. If the Jews of Christ's day 'had been sick in a milder way, they would not have killed their doctor like phrenetics', he wrote.[30] On the cross, Christ had seen them 'roaring around him', 'and since he knew of their diseases, like a doctor who recognised the *phrenesis* in which their minds had become lost, directly addressed the father: "father, forgive them, because they don't know what they are doing"'.[31] Augustine's physician-slaying phrenetic was the natural polemical counterpart to his figure of *Christus medicus*, Christ

[28] John Squire, *A plaine exposition vpon the first part of the second chapter of Saint Paul his second epistle to the Thessalonians* (London, 1630), p. 25.

[29] Andrew Willet, *An antilogie or counterplea to An apologicall (he should haue said) apologeticall epistle published by a fauorite of the Romane separation* (London, 1603), p. 134. This was the same Andrew Willet who, at the age of twenty-two, had written a refutation of Galen's *Quod animi mores*. I am grateful to Reader C for drawing my attention to this earlier treatise.

[30] Augustine of Hippo, 'Enarrationes in Psalmos', *PL*, vol. 36, col. 0789.

[31] Augustine of Hippo, 'Sermo LXXX', *PL*, vol. 38, col. 0496.

the physician. This extended allegory was alive and well in early modern England. Thomas Adams lamented of 'the Church of *Israel*' that 'When her disease grew too frenzy, and her *sicknesse* so excluding from it selfe all recouerable hope, that shee had slaine her Physitian, and killed him that should haue carried her'.[32]

Predictably enough, in the hands of Protestant divines, the role which Augustine had given to the first-century Jews was soon reassigned to the papists. In the published proceedings of his 1581 'conference' with the recusant John Hart, John Rainolds described how 'the Church of Rome being taken with contagious diseases & a frensy, did put her counsellers to the fyer, frends to the sword, [and] brethren to cruell death'.[33] The 'Church of Rome', like the 'Church of *Israel*' before it, had caught the disease of idolatry, fallen into a frenzy, and slain its caregivers. This trope was grist to the mill of post-Reformation polemicists, for by the end of the century each confession could point to the other's mounting body count. Those who were executed for their faith were crowned as martyrs by their co-religionists; those ordering the executions were cast as 'frantic' killers.

Unreason

In his pamphlet *The execution of iustice in England*, the Lord Treasurer William Cecil defended the harsh measures which the Elizabethan state had taken against certain Catholics who had heeded the Pope's call to remove their 'heretic' queen from the throne. The Jesuits who had crept into England and Ireland were 'sedicious seedemen and sowers of rebellion', Cecil wrote, and the Northern and Irish rebellions of the preceding decades were the fruits of their labour.[34] The leading architect of the Jesuits' mission, William Allen, soon published a refutation of Cecil's tract, one which turned the spotlight back on the radical Protestants. Catholics, Allen admitted, 'agree with thother in the point of deposing and resisting kinges for Religion; but yet doe differ in the maner, as far as reason and conscience differ from furie and phrensie'.[35] The disease served to distance the cool-headed 'reason' of the Catholics from the febrile passions of the Protestants.

[32] Thomas Adams, *Englands sicknes, comparatively conferred with Israel* (London, 1615), p. 54.
[33] John Rainolds, *The summe of the conference betwene Iohn Rainoldes and Iohn Hart* (London, 1584), p. 179.
[34] William Cecil, *The execution of iustice in England* (London, 1583), sig. A4r.
[35] William Allen, *A true, sincere and modest defence, of English Catholiques* (Rouen, 1584), p. 85.

The fault was not in the doctrine, Allen insisted, but the interpreters' soundness of mind. Catholics were duty-bound to recognize the supreme pontiff's prerogative in spiritual matters, and this did include his right to excommunicate a heretic prince. Yet they were also capable of interpreting his bulls in the light of their own reason, common sense, and good conscience. For radical Protestants, it was the other way round: they deferred to no authority except their own will, and they obeyed its orders with an unthinking, unfeeling bloody-mindedness. The true phrenetics amongst the queen's subjects, Allen insisted, were the Protestant advocates of popular sovereignty. Of course, for Protestants, the Catholics' blind adherence to the pope's decrees was just as clear a sign that 'an holy phrensie hath distracted [their] minds'.[36]

The role of the phrenetic in Augustine's exemplum was thus open to endless recasting. 'Papists' diagnosed the disease in 'Puritans', 'Puritans' diagnosed it in 'Papists', and moderate Protestants saw it in both of them. This invertible allegory summed up the state of England's fractured confessional landscape. Each side maintained that it had access to the truth; the opposition was necessarily deluded. Yet the stubbornness with which the latter clung to its collective delusion – despite all proofs and persuasions to the contrary – still needed explaining. As we saw in the first three chapters, delusion was a sign that some war waged within the human individual was being lost. The mind had been overwhelmed by the inflamed brain; the intellective powers by the sensitive; the sensitive powers, perhaps, by the Devil. The reason had yielded to the corruptible organ-dependent powers: the imagination, the fantasy, and the passions. Catholics were not immune to this disease, Allen insisted. And yet, 'here is the difference betwene Catholique Christians, and rebellious Heretiques; that thes good-fellowes, folowing their owne deceiptful wils, and vncertaine opinions, without rule or reason, doe adiudge by their priuate follie and phantasie, that thing to be errour or idolatrie, which indeed is true Religion'.[37]

The Protestants' problem was twofold: they had abandoned both 'reason' and 'rule'.[38] The frailty of fallen Adam guaranteed occasional lapses in reason, and Catholics knew to expect them. This was why, distrusting 'their owne particuler imaginations or partial affections', they committed 'the direction of matters so important to the Church and to the

[36] Leonel Sharpe, *A looking-glasse for the Pope* (London, 1616), p. 175.
[37] Allen, *A true, sincere and modest defence*, p. 84.
[38] See Shagan, *Rule of Moderation*, pp. 111–184.

cheefe gouernours of their soules'.[39] Rejecting the latter's authority, the radical Protestants had thrown away the one compass which had stood the test of time. Now, when the sensitive powers began to steer them off course, they had no infallible rule to alert them to the fact. This was a theme to which, fifty years later, Laudian polemicists warmed. The Puritans' convictions were 'grounded upon a disturbed passion', John Featley preached in 1635. It was no surprise, then, if they mistook a will-o'-the-wisp – 'the *Ignis fatuus* of an unhallowed zeale' – for holy fire.[40]

The metaphor of spiritual frenzy was an apt analogy for several sins, but it was tailormade for heresy. The essence of heresy was not error, but the dogged embracing of error. This could only be explained by an impaired reason, for it was the nature of this God-given faculty to recognize and love the truth. As John Squire put it, 'to be *in an errour*, is to be *out of our wits* . . . We must not forget it: *Such as are out of the truth, are out of their wits*'.[41] The second-century church father Irenaeus, as we saw, had coined the *phrenesis* inversion in his treatise *Against Heresies.* In his attack on the Gnostics, he assured his readers that,

> in proportion as they vehemently maintain and rejoice in their fictitious doctrines, so much the more should we be convinced that they are under the influence of wicked spirits . . . just as those persons who fall into a fit of frenzy, the more they laugh, and imagine themselves to be well, and do all things as if they were in good health [both of body and mind], yea, some things better than those who really are so, are only thus shown to be the more seriously diseased.[42]

When a whole community fell en masse into this vicious circle, heresy was the inevitable result. Incited by Satan to spiritual pride, and rejecting the authority of the church, apostates trusted in their own powers of reason. When the reason was taken captive by its inferiors – the passions, the imagination, and the fantasy – they grew delusional. The further they drifted from reality, the likelier they became to believe the lies fed to them by Satan. The reason grew ever more attenuated, and the diseased imagination stronger. Eventually, they were totally incapable of recognizing the truth, no matter how clear the proofs laid before them. In Andrew Willet's words, those who were 'deluded of Sathan' were ultimately 'giuen ouer of God to be deceiued by him to beleeue lies, because they receiued not the

[39] Allen, *A true, sincere and modest defence*, pp. 84–85.
[40] John Featley, *Obedience and submission* (London, 1636), p. 11.
[41] Squire, *A plaine exposition*, p. 28.
[42] Irenaeus, 'Contra haereses', cap. 16, in *PG*, vol. 7, part 1, col. 635.

loue of the truth'.[43] If spiritual frenzy was endemic to the heretic community, it explained why they remained so unresponsive to the medicine of true church and the ministrations of its doctors. They were too far gone in their own fantasies. In Latin and the vernacular, the phonetic resonances between 'fanatic', 'phantastic', 'phrenetic', and 'heretic' encouraged this semiotic elision. These labels were typically applied in combination, each intensifying the other. The next section explores how they were used to narrate the lives and deaths of key figures in England's religious reformations.

Narrative

Cautionary Tales

The godly Protestants of early modern England were keenly alive to the workings of providence.[44] They expected see God's writing on the wall even in the most apparently banal events of their everyday lives, and they considered it their duty to decode his meaning. At its crudest, this strain of providentialist thinking tended to equate health and prosperity with divine blessing and misfortune with punishment.[45] It found expression in the new print anthologies of God's judgements upon sinners, a genre which found a voracious readership in early modern England. And frenzy – a natural disease with devastating effects on the soul – made for an especially good tale of divine judgement. It was naturalistic enough for the sceptics, shocking enough for the thrill-seekers, and symbolically rich enough for the connoisseurs of the wrathful deity's ingenuity.

The greatest English craftsman of these tales was the Protestant martyrologist John Foxe, whose magnum opus, the *Actes and Monuments of these latter and perillous dayes, touching matters of the Church*, was first published in 1563. Recounting the 1555 martyrdom of the former bishop John Hooper, Foxe recorded that the judge presiding at the trial, Sir Richard Morgan, had begun 'to rayle at M. Hooper a long time, with many opprobrious & fowle words'. Foxe noted in the margin that 'This Morgan shortly after fel into a phrensy, and madnes and dyed of the same'.[46] Later in the *Actes*, Foxe restaged Morgan's fall into frenzy, this

[43] Willet, *An antilogie or counterplea*, p. 134.

[44] Alexandra Walsham, *Providence in Early Modern England* (Oxford: Oxford University Press, 1999), pp. 1–64.

[45] Ibid., p. 95.

[46] John Foxe, *The first volume of the ecclesiasticall history* (London, 1576), p. 1432.

time placing it immediately after the trial of Lady Jane Grey: 'the Iudge Morgan who gaue the sentence of condemnation against her, shortly after hee had condemned her, fell mad, and in hys rauing cryed out continually to haue the Lady Iane taken away from him, and so ended hys lyfe'.[47] Foxe revelled in the poetic justice of God punishing a judge by removing his judgement. Like an unredeemed Nebuchadnezzar, Morgan had been stripped of 'reason' and 'understanding'. These were the God-given gifts which had set him on high as a magistrate, and which he had abused in condemning Hooper and Grey to death.

This narrative template was too good to resist, and it soon circulated beyond the pages of the judgement books. In December 1574, it was used by one of the crown's foreign correspondents to narrate the death of Charles de Lorraine, the Catholic cardinal and uncle of Mary Queen of Scots. The newly anointed king of France, Henri III, had insisted on joining 'the *batues* at Avignon ... men who whip themselves as they go for a manner of penance' on a nocturnal procession. The cardinal had gone with the king 'in this solemn procession welnigh all the night and the next daie he said Masse for a solmnitie wherewith he took a great cold and vppon this a contynual feuer which in contynuance brought him into a frenesie ... and so died the xviij daie after he first fell sick'.[48] There was a perfect poetic justice to the cardinal's fate: he had been a fierce enemy of Protestantism, and both he and Henri III were suspected to have had a hand in the political assassination which had led to the 1572 St Bartholomew's Day Massacre (in which thousands of Huguenots had lost their lives).[49] Although no mention of the massacre was made in this report, it was easy to read between the lines: both the king and the cardinal had Protestant blood on their hands, and their pantomimic performance of penance had done nothing to wash them clean. Self-flagellation was in itself a sign of spiritual frenzy: it showed, as Sutton would put it, a 'counterfeiting ... zeale, like the zeale of those Idolaters that mangled and cut them selues'.[50] And it did nothing to appease God's wrath; in fact, He had chosen the very moment of the cardinal's canting mass to strike him down.

As Alexandra Walsham has noted, these cautionary tales show 'a growing tendency for providence to work internally through the malefactor's

[47] Ibid., p. 1352. [48] TNA, Kew, SP 70/132, f. 165r.

[49] Mark Greengrass, *Christendom Destroyed: Europe 1518–1648* (London: Penguin, 2012), pp. 201–202.

[50] Sutton, *Englands first and second summons*, pp. 196–197.

own conscience and for divine retribution to take the more intangible form of mental torment'.[51] Madness was the logical endpoint of this character arc. The story of a born 'papist' dying in a state of frenzy was deeply satisfying to Protestant readers, but it was an even better fit for an apostate. Apostates had knowingly abandoned the true religion for the false, and the burden of guilt was – Protestants imagined – enough to drive anyone mad. The favourite template in Protestant England was the story of the Italian lawyer Francisco Spira (1502–1548). Having publicly recanted his Protestantism in May 1548, Spira had heard a voice sentencing him to eternal damnation. He descended into wild despair, attempted suicide, and ultimately died from self-starvation. The story was told time and time again, circulating throughout Europe in plays, broadsheets, ballads, and sermons. It was told afresh in times of Protestant persecution, serving as a touchstone for those who faced the temptation to apostatize.[52] Throughout the sixteenth and seventeenth centuries, Protestants continued to identify those who abjured the faith and returned to Catholicism as 'Second Spiras'.[53] In January 1587, for example, the English soldier Sir William Stanley, previously knighted by Elizabeth I for his service in Ireland, unexpectedly defected to the side of the King of Spain, Philip II.[54] In one fell swoop, the war hero had turned apostate and traitor. Six weeks later, one of Francis Walsingham's spies in the Netherlands reported that 'by letters from Deventer the wryt that the Traytor Standley groweth franticque; a Just punishment of god'.[55] 'If this be true (as yt is so reported)', wrote another, 'as he was known for a Traitor, so he may be noted for a foole'.[56]

Sometimes, it was the self-identified apostate who shaped his or her story to fit this mould. This was evidently the case for the sailor Francis Collingwood, who was arrested in December 1606 after declaring that the newly crowned king was a 'Traytor, a Cuckold, and some saye, a Bastard'. Collingwood and his hearers were immediately sent for examination by the bishop of Winchester. In a covering letter to the Lord Chancellor Robert Cecil, the bishop explained that Collingwood had

51 Walsham, *Providence*, p. 89.
52 Michael MacDonald, '*The Fearefull Estate of Francis Spira*: Narrative, Identity, and Emotion in Early Modern England', *Journal of British Studies* 31(1) (1992), 32–61; M. Anne Overell, 'The Exploitation of Francesco Spiera', *Sixteenth Century Journal* 26(3) (1995), 619–637.
53 MacDonald, '*The Fearefull Estate of Francis Spira*', p. 38.
54 Rory Rapple, 'Stanley, Sir William (1548–1630), Soldier', *ODNB*, 4 October 2008, https://doi.org/10.1093/ref:odnb/26283.
55 Kew, TNA, SP 84/13, f. 80v.
56 SP 84/18, f. 304r.

> seemed to the standers by, to have spoken in a frensie . . . but vpon his appearance before mee, he spake so soberly and advisedly in his owne defence, pretending only that he was then possessed with a spirite, that I thought my dewtie to enter into the examination of the whole course & cariage thereof, as far as I could comme by any light.[57]

Collingwood's story was consistent, and it was corroborated by six eyewitnesses. Three days earlier, on 20 December, he had been

> strangely possessed in the sight of the beholders, with a sudden passion of furie, seeking by all means to destroye himself, as stabbing, hanging and drowning, with other violences against himself; and lastly sayed, if nothing els will prevayle to take away my life; then he would speak woords which should doe it: And those were: That the king (meaning the king of England our soveraigne) is a Traytor and a Cuckold.[58]

In speaking these words in a busy taproom, in front of both the local sheriff and the town constable, Collingwood had been trying to commit the early modern equivalent of 'suicide by cop'. On examination, he insisted that he had uttered these speeches while 'invaded and corporally possessed with a divell'. But the suicidal despair which had made him vulnerable to diabolic attack had begun much earlier. The hostess of the tavern at which he was lodging deposed that, on first announcing his possession 'with a spirit', he had declared that 'vnles he might presently haue a Jesuite to resolue him, he was but a damned man: for that he was somme yeeres since confessed and absolued by a Priest in the low Countries and receaued the sacrament therevpon, and sithence [since] hath fallen from it'.[59] Collingwood had come to see himself as a Catholic Spira, and was determined either to rejoin 'the true Churche', or to die trying.[60]

Pseudo-martyrs

Thus far, we have seen several instances of Catholics and Protestants battling to monopolize the meanings of their opponents' lives – and sometimes their *own* lives – through storytelling. The fiercest struggle of all, however, was over the lives of the martyrs. Often, the battle was waged over one and the same life: one side's holy martyr became the other's 'pseudo-martyr'. Foxe's Protestant martyrology was vulnerable to just such a rewriting, and, at the turn of the seventeenth century, the Jesuit master

[57] SP 14/26, f. 36r. [58] Ibid., f. 38r. [59] Ibid., f. 41r. [60] Ibid., f. 38r.

polemicist Robert Persons rose to the challenge. His *Treatise of three conuersions of England from paganisme to Christian religion* (1603–1604) offered a blow-by-blow refutation of Foxe's *Actes*. The 'braines of Iohn Foxe', Persons wrote, 'were knowne to be out of tune for many years, before he died', and this much he had in common with his so-called martyrs.[61] Unashamedly elitist, Persons made much of their humble rank and lack of learning. Typical was Rawlins White, a 'simple vnlearned ould fisherman' from Cardiff. Illiteracy was no barrier to White's becoming a theologian, Persons sniped, for what other qualification was needed than 'the gyft he had receyued of interpretation'?[62] Won over by peddlers of false doctrine, rustics of this sort fell all too easily into false zeal. Their 'visions' were delusions; the so-called 'feruour of each ones spiritt . . . the different fancy of each ones brayne'.[63] In the end, Rawlins White had become so fixed in his 'phantasticall opinions' that he ended his days 'more than half franticke with heresy'.[64] These examples showed all too clearly 'the spiritt of heresy, how dangerous and desperate a phrensy yt is, when yt taketh deep roote. Especially in ignorant people, who commonly are more incureable, then others'.[65] Once heresy had infected this sort, he lamented, 'nothing can cure or moderate the same'.[66]

In Persons's hands, the metaphor soon took an unsettling turn. Among the Protestants executed under Mary was the ironmaker Richard Woodman, to whom Foxe had referred as 'this blessed Woodman, or rather goodman'. Woodman's reasonableness under examination was contrasted with 'the grosse ignorance and barbarous cruelty of his aduersaryes, especially of D. White B. of Winchester'.[67] Responding to the passage, Persons marvelled

> And yet is yt notoriously knowen how learned and myld man this Doctor White was . . . And he that shall read the examinations and conferences wrytten by Woodman himself, will easily see, that the Ironmaker bare himself like a true woode or maddman indeede, and the other like patient and pittifull pastors ouer a sheepe put out of his true sense & witts by the phrenesy of heresy.[68]

[61] Robert Persons, *A treatise of three conversions of England from paganism to Christian religion* (Saint-Omer, 1603), vol. 1, p. 294.
[62] Robert Persons, *The third part of a treatise, intituled: of three conuersions of England* (Saint-Omer, 1604), vol. 2, p. 390.
[63] Ibid., p. 214. [64] Ibid., p. 391. [65] Ibid., p. 505. [66] Ibid., vol. 3, p. 200.
[67] Foxe, *Actes and monuments* (1570), Book 12, p. 2194.
[68] Persons, *The third part of a treatise*, vol. 2, p. 514.

Once again, the persecutor and the persecuted change places. Here, Persons's insistence that the 'phrenesy' of heresy was 'incureable' began to lose its comfortably figurative padding. His 'patient and pittifull' pastor was a variation on Augustine's loving physician, but with an important difference. If a phrenetic sheep was incurable, the good shepherd had little choice but to put it out of its misery. Persons elaborated on the same theme in his defence of the burning at Rome in 1581 of an English nailsmith named Richard Atkins. On a visit to St Peter's, Atkins had fallen into a paroxysm of anti-papal rage, seizing the priest's chalice from his hands and hurling it into the crowd. Attacked by a sheep with a such a patently terminal case of the 'phrenesie of heresie', Persons argued, the Roman church had had no other choice.[69]

Foxe had played into Persons's hands with his inclusion in his 1563 saints' calendar of some questionable candidates for martyrdom. These included a law student named Collins, who, falling mad after discovering his wife's infidelity, and 'beynge beside his wyttes seynge the priest hold vp the host ouer his head, and shew it to the people, he in like manner counterfaytinge the priest, taking vp a litle dogge by the legges, holdinge him ouer his heade, shewed him vnto the people'.[70] This was not the kind of behaviour expected of a holy martyr, and Foxe clearly had second thoughts about the placement of Collins among their ranks. The same was true for another new addition to the calendar, William Cowbridge, who had put forth 'opinions and Articles' which were undeniably 'erroneous'.[71] Foxe inserted into all later editions an embarrassed defence of his inclusion of Collins and Cowbridge. The latter was 'a man mad, and destitute of sense and reason'.[72] He did not count either of them 'in the number of Gods professed martyrs', he insisted.[73] Rather, 'these two miserable examples' served to reveal the true colours of the church of Rome, for they

> rather should haue bene pitied, and all wayes conuenient sought, hoe to reduce the seely wretches into their right myndes agayne, according as the true Pastours of Israell be commaunded by the spirite of God, to seeke agayne the thynges that be lost, to bynd vp the thynges that be broken &c. and not so extremely to brust the thyngs that be bruised before.[74]

[69] Robert Persons, *The copie of a double letter sent by an English gentilman from beyond the seas* (Rheims, 1581), p. 10.

[70] Foxe, *Actes and monuments* (1563), Book 3, p. 570.

[71] Foxe, *Actes and monuments* (1570), Book 8, p. 1331. [72] Ibid., p. 1331. [73] Ibid., p. 1330.

[74] Ibid., p. 1331.

The deaths of these unfortunates exposed the 'crueltie and madnesse' of these false 'Pastours'.[75] Foxe was uncomfortable with the mad martyrs he had made, but he couldn't let go of the chance to cast the Catholics as frantic tyrants. It was a clumsy save, and Persons pounced on it:

> John Foxe, blushing thereat, hath somewhat (as the saying is) pulled in his horns, and albeit out of willfull obstinacy he would not put them out quite of his calendar of martyrs yet is forced to abate them so much in this his last narration as with farre less shame might he have left them out wholly.[76]

Collins and Cowbridge were not mad, Persons argued, or at least, no madder than the rest of Foxe's motley crew.[77] All without exception were delusional; it was simply that the behaviour of Collins and Cowbridge was so egregious that even Foxe was forced to admit the fact. The same was true of Richard Atkins. Observers had first 'thought best he should be put into the Hospital of the *patzí* which is for the cure and keeping of mad men and fooles', but 'after the rulers of that howse . . . had by good triall discerned him not to be distracted, they refused plainly to take charge of him'.[78] Persons alternately collapsed and reinstated the distinction between corporeal and spiritual frenzy to suit his purposes. Heretics were spiritually frantic, but not literally brainsick – after all, they had been well enough to give Satan their full and informed consent. Some heretics were so desperately deranged that killing them was an act of mercy; but the Protestants were not to be allowed to use that fact to distance themselves from their own zealots.

Protestant polemicists were, of course, capable of playing the same game. The Catholic cause had plenty of its own diplomatic embarrassments, especially after the papal bull of 1570, when scores of loyal vigilantes took it upon themselves to depose Elizabeth I. Among their number was the Warwickshire recusant John Somerville, who had been sentenced to death in December 1583 after publicly announcing his intention to assassinate the queen.[79] In *The execution of iustice*, published that year, Cecil suggested to the Catholics that, if they wanted 'to increase their Kalender of the popes martyrs', they could 'adde a furious yong man of Warwickeshire, by name Someruile who of late was discouered and

75 Foxe, *Actes and monuments* (1576), Book 8, p. 1128.
76 Persons, *The third part of a treatise*, vol. 3, p. 196.
77 Persons, *A treatise of three conversions*, vol. 1, p. 521.
78 Persons, *The copie of a double letter*, p. 10.
79 See William Wizeman, 'Somerville, John (1560–1583), Convicted Conspirator', *ODNB*, 3 January 2008, https://doi.org/10.1093/ref:odnb/26022.

taken in his way, comming with a ful intent to haue killed her Maiestie'.[80] William Allen fired back:

> he is malitious in bidding vs enroule Somerfild in the number of our Martirs; as perhaps before God he is, if he were distract of his wittes, or furious (as al men say, and the Libeller confesseth) to whom can not be imputed what so euer he did in alienation of mind; and to his enimies shalbe imputed murther what so euer was done against him in that his state.[81]

Allen's move echoed the one made by Foxe fourteen years earlier regarding Collins and Cowbridge. It was the Elizabethan regime, the Jesuit insisted, which had innocent blood on its hands. As we saw in Chapter 4, English law held that the 'furious' were not to be held accountable for their crimes. It is unlikely that Cecil had intended the word to be taken in its full medico-legal sense. Nevertheless, by invoking it, he had invited the accusation that Somerville's death was not lawful execution, but murder.

Strategic Diagnosis

This brings us to the English crown's use of the frenzy diagnosis as a strategic political measure. The heads of church and state knew from experience that there was no better lightning rod for popular unrest than a self-styled martyr, displaced heir, or messiah. Over the course of the sixteenth and seventeenth centuries, they had become increasingly skilled at diagnosing frenzy in religious and political dissidents. This section looks at how it was used to silence, discredit, and deter potential agitators.

Labelling

The crown's most effective strategy was also its quietest. No evidence of it remains today except a single volume of petitions. First sent to Cecil between the 1570s and 1590s, around the turn of the eighteenth century they were discovered by the historian John Strype, who dubbed them 'Letters of Several Madmen to Lord Burghley'. Strype, however, was only the last in a line of amateur diagnosticians to examine these letters; in fact, he was often echoing the assessments of an earlier team. These two or three Elizabethan readers, who referred to Cecil as 'my L.', were probably administrative clerks tasked with wading through the drifts of petitions

[80] Cecil, *The execution of iustice*, sig. D3v. [81] Allen, *A true, sincere and modest defence*, p. 49.

which amassed daily on the Lord Treasurer's desk. Most of these letters bear a summary in one of their tidy hands. On the back of a letter which opened 'My lord I am sent an embassador from god the father vnto the quenes highnes to declare unto her that I am the sonne of them both', for example, was written 'Emanuel Plantagenet alias John Frye, who semes to be distempred in his wytts . . . Giving out himself to bee þe Son of God & Q Eliz. taken fro her by the Ang. Gabriel & carried to Mrs Fry'.[82] The effect was to pour cold water on the petitioner's painstakingly crafted opening address. An introit 'To Her Most gracious and excellent highnes', for example, bore in one corner the remark 'One Johnson a franticque person to þe Qs. Maty'.[83]

The contents of these letters vary greatly, and who chose to group them together – and why – remains unclear. They do share features in common: there is a general tendency to florid prose, grandiose self-presentation, and high-pitched religious feeling. Some – like John Frye's claim to be Elizabeth's lost heir – clearly beggared belief. But the insinuation that the virgin queen had given birth was probably a surer sign of Frye's folly than the appearance of the Angel Gabriel. In early modern England, an encounter with an angel did not automatically signal madness; many contemporaries who were perfectly well in their wits had had one. Richard Napier, for example, sometimes asked one of the archangels for a second opinion on difficult cases, and he usually received a reply.[84] As present-day readers, we are not best-placed to judge why some early modern letter writers were labelled 'frantic', and others were not.

Reports of encounters with invisible spirits were not necessarily implausible, and vice versa, reports that today sound basically plausible were summarily dismissed as the products of fevered brains. In a letter listing '30 treasons against her majesty', for example, the Huguenot Jean Gerare warned that he had heard reports that the Pope had sent men to infiltrate the English army. They had been instructed to poison the country's supplies of meat, flour, and beer, to kill the queen and her officials, and to do everything within their power 'to make easy the Pope's victory over this kingdom'.[85] Gerare was clearly a conspiracy theorist, but these were decades in which conspiracies to overthrow the English crown sometimes turned out to be real. Indeed, a vast intelligence

82 Lansdowne MS 99/6, f. 13v. 83 Lansdowne MS 99/13, f. 31v.

84 See Peter Marshall and Alexandra Walsham (eds.), *Angels in the Early Modern World* (Cambridge: Cambridge University Press, 2006); Ofer Hadass, *Medicine, Religion and Magic in Early Stuart England* (Philadelphia: Penn State University Press, 2018), pp. 96–104.

85 Lansdowne MS 99/21, ff. 54r–59v, quotation at f. 55v.

service was dedicated to the task of their discovery and eradication. For whatever reason, however, Gerare was sent to the same pile as Emmanuel Plantagenet. He was, according to the recipient, merely 'A frantik French man'.[86]

To judge by the laconic comments of Cecil's clerks, they had grown accustomed to such tales. Typical was the response to the letter of John Richardson, who had 'a message or errand from God Almighty, sent by revelation of the Holy Ghost, to none but the Queen. He would persuade her Majesty, for the "rareness and strangeness of it", not to refuse the same'.[87] The dorse read simply '7 June, 1601. A frantic man'. If the clerk responsible for the endorsement had been intrigued by the letter's 'rareness and strangeness', he showed no sign of it. Richardson was not to be brought in on suspicion of heresy, but he most emphatically was not to be allowed anywhere near the queen.

Despite the many-hued variegation of their letters, these authors did share a common aim: they wanted their voices to reach the monarch's ear. As far as we know, none of the authors whose petitions ended up in Strype's collection of 'Letters of Several Madmen' ever achieved this goal. Flooded by correspondence of every conceivable kind, the crown had evidently developed a highly efficient vetting system. The clerks reading these letters were not – in the first instance – looking to identify deserving petitioners, nor even to gather useful intelligence; their first task was to decide which petitions needed to be taken seriously and which could be summarily dismissed. They knew how to sieve the wheat from the chaff: the vital intelligence from the visions of imminent apocalypse, personal messages from God, conspiracy theories, and claims to long-lost titles. And the default course of action – in case of letters whose authors sounded 'frantic' – was inaction. There is no suggestion that any one of these petitioners to Elizabeth I ever gained the audience they craved. Their letters were met with stony silence, and this, in turn, silenced them. Some wrote again, but their subsequent letters were trapped and absorbed by the same bureaucratic filter.

Few comparable petitions survive from the interregnum period (for obvious reasons), but the restoration of Charles II saw a new influx of post. This trend was no doubt encouraged by the new king's careful self-

86 Ibid., f. 59v.

87 John Richardson, 'John Richardson to the Queen', in Richard Arthur Roberts (ed.), *Calendar of the Manuscripts of the Most Honourable Marquis of Salisbury preserved at Hatfield House* (Dublin: HMSO, 1906), vol. 11, p. 219.

fashioning as a charismatic, personally available monarch, acted out in rituals like the 'royal touch'.[88] The extent to which Charles II had succeeded in encouraging his subjects to develop intimate (if one-sided) attachments to him is evident in a 1676 letter sent to Whitehall by the Birmingham glover John Griffes, addressed 'to his magiest King Charles . . . or in his absence to his speiciall trust to be deliuered to his Right honoured queen Katherine'.[89] Griffes explained that, having been appointed 'a servant in his magiestyes behalfe', 'I do make it my buisness by the virtue of the same Charge to demand all Kings Rights whatsoever with all Chargg lands and ogmentations also scool lands in birmingham gon from the Right poors land Builded upon by the Rich and \So/ inhabited Contrary to the Right'.[90] Despite his efforts to restore justice, the glover complained, 'I am looked upon as a frantick man and as a Rebell . . . and that of [by] my own townsmen and townswomen'. What Griffes wanted was for the king to summon these townspeople before him, 'to make apear in what i Rebel'. If innocent, he demanded 'to be freed acordind [sic] to his magiesties lawes and if a Rebell . . . to Sufer therby'. The prospect of even one 'Rebel' sharing controversial opinions with his neighbours would ordinarily have been enough to make crown officials sit up and take notice. And yet no recorded response to Griffes's letter survives.

Silencing

Many would-be Robin Hoods and John the Baptists were successfully ignored, but not all did the crown the courtesy of advertising their activities. Some simply went out and shared the word they had been given, whether in pulpits, marketplaces, homes, or in print. And early modern prophets, like their Old Testament forebears, had a bad habit of criticizing their betters. One such thorn in Elizabeth I's side was David Black, a Scottish schoolmaster who had settled in Cornwall in the 1580s. Black was first summoned before the English high commission in 1584, charged with preaching without a licence, inveighing against 'the state ecclesiasticall of this realme', denying the queen's ecclesiastical supremacy, and refusing to pray for her.[91] Around 1590, Black fled to Scotland, where he was

[88] Schaffer, 'Regeneration', pp. 85–88; Andrews, 'Politics of Committal', in Andrews et al. (eds.), *The History of Bethlem*, pp. 20–21.

[89] TNA, SP 29/382, f. 159v. [90] Ibid., f. 159r.

[91] London, Lambeth Palace Library, CM XII/16.

appointed the minister of St Andrews. English agents were keeping close watch on the contents of Black's sermons, however, and in October 1596 they reported that he had 'said that her Maiestie was an Atheist'.[92]

The fact that these words had been broadcast from a Scottish pulpit was deeply embarrassing for James VI. He was anxious to prove to Elizabeth that he had tamed the Presbyterian kirk; now one of its leading ministers was slandering her name. Black was immediately arrested on the charge of treason. The following March, Elizabeth wrote to James in conciliatory tones. She was pleased with how he had handled the recent disorders in his realm, she assured him. And '[a]s for that franticke man that shewed in Pulpytt the hedlenes off his Hedd, I owe you most thankfullnes, for taking it so evyll, but of him I disdayned my selfe to make mention of, but did referre both his punishment and all els to your best disposing'.[93] Labelling Black as frantic was a delicate diplomatic manoeuvre on Elizabeth's part, intended to de-escalate the situation and to put James's mind at rest. Black was not a typical representative of James's ecclesiastical polity, she implied, but a half-crazed lone crusader. A sane monarchomach nestling in the kirk's bosom would have been a major security threat, one which would have cast serious doubt on James's competence as king. A 'franticke man', on the other hand, was scarcely worth mentioning. He merited pity, 'disdayn', or perhaps punishment, but not alarm. In addition, if treason transcended borders, madness was a strictly *local* matter: arrangements were typically made by county justices, town mayors, or aldermen. This was James's business; Elizabeth trusted him to choose the best course of treatment.

Diagnosing, discrediting, and ignoring dissidents was the safest course of action, but sometimes it was not enough. This was ground, however, on which monarchs knew they had to tread with extreme caution. To shut the mouth of a self-proclaimed visionary by force was to risk playing into the hands of polemicists, for it was easily construed as religious repression. The last thing monarchs and their councillors wanted was the creation of a new 'martyr'. Worse, if the individual in question did turn out to be genuinely brainsick, cruelty towards pitiable innocents could be added to the charge of religious persecution. It was on these grounds that Allen had castigated the Elizabethan regime for the execution of Somerville, just as Foxe had done for the Marian executions of Cowbridge and Collins.[94]

[92] TNA, SP 52/59, f. 71r. [93] TNA, SP 52/52, pp. 159–160.

[94] Monarchs were supposed to care for their frantic subjects, not murder them. See William Staunford, *An exposicion of the kinges prerogative* (London, 1567), f. 36v; McGlynn, 'Idiots, Lunatics', p. 2; Richard Neugebauer, 'The Treatment of the Mentally Ill in Medieval and Early

Putting a frantic person to death was very bad for a monarch's public image.[95]

The question of what to do with a self-publicizing prophet caused headaches for lesser crown officials, too. Among them was the Essex justice of the peace Arthur Herrys, who on 22 October 1586 wrote to the Lord Chancellor Thomas Bromley to ask for his advice. The previous day, his constables had brought before him a shoemaker named John White, alias Snellyng, whom they had arrested making speeches at a local shoemaker's shop.[96] According to the apprentice George Young, White had come to his master's shop the preceding Friday, announcing himself with the words 'I come to do you goode'. In what followed, White managed to hit on almost every conceivable raw nerve in the Elizabethan body politic, endorsing antinomianism, epicurism, polygamy, and sexual license. Accused by Young of being an Anabaptist, he responded 'if ye had sayd, A John of Baptiste, ye had said right, for there was but one before Christ, and another after'.[97] Even more damning than this grandiose claim was the content of his prophecies. Two witnesses deposed that they had heard him declare that 'our quene shall lyue but a lytle whyle, she wil be gone ere somer come'.[98] Herrys professed himself uncertain what to make of White, but he was inclined to think him 'a man overstudyed with Annabaptystycall Conceyptes, & therwith all partlye entered into Lunacye or Frensye'. He asked the Lord Chancellor to direct him as to 'what shalbe done with hym, for he resteth as yet in the warde of the Constables'.[99] It would usually have been the local justice's task to make arrangements for a frantic man. Herrys might have made new parish-level care arrangements, or sent the man to a local spital, poorhouse, or bridewell. If the sufferer was not from the locality – and White was not – he might have had him sent to his birthplace. But if White was faking madness, as Herrys feared, then he was convictable on charges of blasphemy and *lèse-majesté*. Bromley's reply does not survive, but it is

Modern England: A Reappraisal', *Journal of the History of the Behavioural Sciences* 14 (1978), 158–169, p. 159.

95 This is evident in the fact that Henry VIII had to update the Treason Act in 1541 in order to legitimate his execution of Jane Boleyn, Lady Rochford. She had fallen 'mad' during her trial for high treason, but Henry suspected this was a ploy to escape the scaffold. The new statute made it legal to execute 'mad' traitors, as long as they had been sane 'at the tyme of doinge their treason'. As Owen Williams notes, 'The fact that Henry covered himself with the sanction of law indicates that he or his advisors considered it a politically unpopular action'. Owen Williams, 'Exorcising Madness in Late Elizabethan England: The *Seduction of Arthington* and the Criminal Culpability of Demoniacs', *Journal of British Studies* 47 (2008), 36.

96 Kew, TNA, SP 12/194, f. 87r. 97 Ibid., f. 88r. 98 Ibid., f. 88v. 99 Ibid., f. 87r.

likely that he would have approved of Herrys's decision to 'keep' White in the interim. The first priority was to take such a person off the streets. A prophet holding forth at a shoemaker's stall was infinitely more dangerous than a prophet who rambled quietly in Lord Burghley's ear.

For the louder sort, the obvious choice of detention centre was Bethlem. The optics of committal were much better; it was after all the monarch's prerogative to provide care for all persons non compos mentis. And the hospital's walls trapped and contained such persons' 'lewd words' just as effectively as any prison. This aim was sometimes made explicit; in 1551, the London Court of Aldermen ordered that a merchant named Richard Brady 'beyng frantyk . . . for his raylyng & other condyggne causes shalbe commyted to Bedlem there to be closely kept & cheyned that no man speke with hym'.[100] Five years earlier, a Surrey man named Richard Cheeseman had been 'committed to bedlem for certayne Lewde wordes in tyme of his frenesy spoken against the kings Majestie'.[101] Frenzy was not always the diagnosis of choice, but these warrants belong to a larger series of politically motivated state committals.[102]

Bethlem made political quarantine possible; although solitary confinement was very hard to achieve anywhere in early modern England, committal to the hospital went some way in halting the spread of the individual's 'Lewde words'.[103] This was another reason why this option was preferable to arraignment – the former required only a discreet letter to the hospital's governors; the latter required a public recitation of the charges levelled against the accused. Regarding Francis Collingwood, the bishop of Winchester asked Cecil 'What is fitt to be done with him, and whether it be meete that soe haynous slaunders against his Majestie should be repeated openly in the peoples eares at his arraignment here in the Countrie'.[104] Whether or not such an individual were 'frantic' mattered little; there was no sense in letting his or her words spread further among the common sort.

This tactic was even more noticeable in the years of Charles I's personal rule. In April 1636, two weavers named John Bull and Richard Farnham were arrested in London after staging a re-enactment of Christ's entry to Jerusalem. Farnham was reported to have claimed that he 'hath the very spirit of God, which revealeth unto him all secrets whatsoever: and that he

[100] Cambridge, Cambridge University Library, Repertories of the Court of Aldermen (microfilm), 12/2, f. 323r.
[101] London, BL, Add MS 5476, ff. 181r, 252v.
[102] Andrews, 'Politics of Committal', pp. 12–18.
[103] Ibid., p. 15.
[104] SP 14/26, f. 36r.

is moreover Anointed, and can predict and foretell whatsoever is to come'.[105] He was sent to Bethlem. Although the staff observed that the 'new prisoner did not appeare either by words or gesture to be made [sic] or Lunatique', he remained at the hospital until August 1638.[106] The preceding year, the Privy Council had issued a warrant 'to the Master, Governors and keeper of Bethelem to receive into their charge the person of William Ellis, an Anabaptist, [who] beinge distract and madd hath expressed much ill affection by lewde and scandalous wordes against his Majestie's sacred person, and to keepe him safe their [sic] in chaynes vntill further order'.[107] The prophetess Eleanor Davies also spent these years in Bethlem. She had first been arrested in 1633, after presenting Laud a handwritten paper 'to give him a taste or warning of his judgment at hand'.[108] The heads of church and state had learned that there was no more reliable way to silence a politically inconvenient prophet than to literally shut them up.

The point should not be overstressed. Bethlem was far too small to contain all of England's political dissidents, and its fees were high. An ordinary gaol was much the cheaper option. On 29 August 1638, Farnham was deemed 'not soe distracted but that he is well able to worke and get his living', and was sent to Bridewell 'to be safely kept at hard Labour and not live idly uppon that which may serve for the necessary releife of distracted impotent persons'.[109] Many, like the 'fanatique franticke' James Hunt, who 'tooke it upon him to preach & expound the Scriptures', were sent straight to Bridewell.[110] As Jonathan Andrews has shown, although crown officials did on the whole try to respect Bethlem's status as a hospital for the genuinely mad, there were plenty of borderline subjects who ended up being transferred from Bridewell to Bethlem, or vice versa.[111]

Confinement in either of these institutions cannot have been a pleasant experience, but 'hard rule' and 'correction' was a deliberate policy in gaols. In the minds of those issuing the warrants, this wasn't necessarily a bad thing; it might weed out a dissembler, or even restore a genuinely frantic

[105] Thomas Heywood, *True discourse of the two infamous upstart prophets, Richard Farnham weaver of White-Chappell, and John Bull weaver of Saint Butolphs Algate, now prisoners, the one in Newgate, and the other in Bridewell* (London, 1636), p. 9.

[106] Kew, TNA, SP 16/379/96, f. 176r. [107] Kew, TNA, PC 2/29, p. 213.

[108] Esther S. Cope, *Handmaid of the Holy Spirit: Dame Eleanor Davies, Never Soe Mad a Ladie* (Ann Arbor: University of Michigan Press, 1992), p. 65; Diane Watt, 'Davies [née Touchet; other married name Douglas], Lady Eleanor (1590–1652), Prophetess', *ODNB*, 3 January 2008, https://doi.org/10.1093/ref:odnb/7233.

[109] SP 16/397/86, f. 151r. [110] SP 16/434A, f. 31v.

[111] Andrews, 'Politics of Committal', p. 18.

person back to their senses. When, on 28 August 1545, a man named Thomas Yemans was apprehended wandering around Oxfordshire 'seming to be in a frensie, and declaring that he was sent from God with a message to the Kinges Majeste', his case was sent straight to the Privy Council. Yemans was detained in gaol while the Council commissioned reports 'of his father . . . [those] with whom he had only dwelte, his conversacion, and with whom he had used to conferre'.[112] The flurry of intelligence gathering proved unnecessary; on 14 September, it was reported that, after a fortnight in 'the Colehouse here at Windesour, [he is] nowe come to himself and repenting his foly, declaring to have been seduced for the love of a woman'. Yemans received some form of corporal 'correction' before his release; he 'was with a good Lesson put to libertie', the clerk noted with relish.[113] As we saw in the last chapter, hard usage was widely understood to have therapeutic as well as punitive uses, and frantic persons – especially those whose behaviour threatened to cause civil unrest – were not always spared.

Gaols were a viable alternative to Bethlem, but even these buildings could only hold so many. The cheapest and most effective way to pathologize nonconformists, statesmen knew, was the richly descriptive polemic we explored in the first section. Only the loudest and most stubborn merited confinement. It is worth leavening our suspicion a little, however, if not towards men like Cecil or Laud, then towards the thousands of local administrators of the justice system. Faced with bizarre self-sabotaging displays of civil disobedience, some may have had no agenda other than determining the appropriate course of action. Herrys's exhaustive investigation of White's case, and his observation that White seemed 'of Imperfect sence, but whether so indede, or but feyned, I knowe not certaynly', suggests an honest effort on his part to ascertain whether the shoemaker was a criminal or genuinely ill.[114] He ultimately leaned towards the latter view; if Bromley listened, his diagnosis might have saved White from gaol or from the gallows.

Nor was Herrys the only crown official who sought to spare frantic persons from undeserved punishment. When one William Williams, who had been sent to the 'common gaole of Glocester' in 1580 'for certain unduetifull speaches uttered againste her majesty', was found to have been 'at the time of the speaches uttered, and yet is, franticke', the Privy Council ordered for him to be released into the custody of his former guardian, and for the gelding and other property which had been confiscated at his arrest

[112] London, BL, Add MS 5476, f. 64r. [113] Ibid., f. 73r. [114] SP 12/194, f. 87r.

to be restored to him.[115] Even the bishop of Winchester, on hearing report of the 'vild, infamous and trayterous speeches' which Collingwood had made, was willing to agree with the witnesses that if the man really had been 'distracted of his witts . . . therevpon [he] was like to haue been freely dismissed, as rather worthie of pittie then punishment'.[116]

Punishment

If frenzy had immense political utility, it had one major risk. If the level of threat which an individual posed to the state was gauged wrongly, there was no going back to correct the mistake. Labelling a self-proclaimed visionary as a 'frantic' man stripped him of credibility, but also of responsibility for his actions. If it later transpired that he was modelling himself not just on the Old Testament prophets, but also on its divinely appointed assassins, the label became a sticking point. In the eyes of Elizabeth's councillors, a would-be regicide was simply too dangerous to be allowed to live. But a 'frantic' one could not be executed, for he or she could not be convicted. By the 1580s, Elizabeth's secretaries of state knew better than to back themselves into this corner. If a detainee was considered a real threat to national security, they studiously overlooked the possibility of frenzy. Burghley had made a mistake in 1583 when he had publicly referred to the Warwickshire recusant John Somerville as 'furious', but he did not repeat it. Allen's assertion that 'al men' said of the young man that he was 'distract of his wittes' contrasts with the state papers' silence on the matter.

John Somerville had first attracted notice on 25 October 1583, while lodging overnight at an Oxfordshire inn. Several witnesses present at the inn reported having heard him say that 'his purpose was to goe to London wher he was in hope to se the Quenes Majestie and he ment to shoute [stab] her thoroe with his dagg[er] and hopt to se her head to be set uppon a pole for that she was a serpent and a viper'.[117] Somerville was apprehended and brought before the local justice, Sir John D'Oyley, and sent to London three days later. In his first examination in London, he was asked 'whan were you fyrst moved to attempt the most wycked and desperate act by you intended'.[118] The question was framed in terms of cold-blooded

[115] Kew, TNA, PC 2/13, f. 306v. Custody of persons non compos mentis technically fell to the monarch; it formed part of the package of legal rights and duties known as the 'royal prerogative'. In practice, few if any monarchs elected to become the personal guardians of their frantic subjects. Instead, the crown treated them much as it treated underage heirs: it transferred the guardianship of their bodies and estates to a private individual. See McGlynn, 'Idiots, Lunatics'.

[116] SP 14/26, f. 36r. [117] Kew, TNA, SP 12/163, f. 57r. [118] Ibid., f. 54r.

premeditation, and was evidently designed to elicit an admission of the same. Yet Somerville did not, at first, comply. He claimed that he had 'never had any motion before that nyght he was commyted by mr doylye to the cvstody of an constable at what tyme thorrowghe the mysvsage of thos to whos cvstodye he was commytted he was put besydes him self'.[119] This version of events was instantly let drop by the examiners, and never allowed to resurface. On 31 October, the question was put to him again, possibly after torture.[120] This time, he replied that he had given 'assent to that motion the tewsday before his departure'.[121] All the further papers kept on his case stressed Somerville's capacity for calculation, resolve, and consent: the plot was a 'wicked enterprice', a 'traiterouse resolution'.[122] He was convicted of high treason on 16 December 1583, and found strangled in his cell three days later.

The approach taken by Cecil and Walsingham in Somerville's case had been worked out at least a decade earlier. In October 1573, a student of the Middle Temple named Peter Birchet had stabbed the naval commander John Hawkins on the Strand. Birchet had mistaken Hawkins for his target Sir Christopher Hatton, a favourite of the queen and a bitter enemy of the Puritans. After Birchet's arrest, two of his fellow legal students, Edward Aylworth and John Spenser, provided the inquiry with a lengthy account of the weeks they had spent in his company before the attack. The three young men had travelled to Dorsetshire to stay at the house of a mutual acquaintance named James Dackombe, 'for pleasures sake'. At the start of their trip, they recalled, Birchet had been 'in very good case greatlye delightyng hym self in the plesantnes of the countrye'.[123] After a few days, Aylworth and Spenser continued their circuit of the countryside, leaving their friend at Dackombe's for some days. When they returned, they were met with relief by Dackombe's wife. Birchet, she told them,

> had fallen sodenly distract, duryng which tyme as they sayd he could not sleepe nor would not come downe to dynner or supper but oftentymes being in his chaumber alone, he would walk up and downe strikyng hym self vppon the brest, throwing his handes abroad, philliping with his fyngers, and speaking to hym self soe softlye as they could not well heare what he sayd.[124]

The list of 'frantick gestures' which the household had witnessed went on and on. Aylworth and Spenser had laughed when first told of 'berchetes

[119] Ibid., f. 56r. [120] Wizeman, 'Somerville, John'. [121] SP 12/163, f. 67r.
[122] Ibid., ff. 67r, 138r. [123] London, British Library, Lansdowne 16/84, f. 191r.
[124] Ibid., f. 193v.

sodayne frensey', but when he came down from his chamber, they recalled, 'euen at our first seing of Berchet we demed that all thing was not well with hym, and partlye beleued all that before the gentlewomen had towld vs'.[125] Something in Birchet's changed demeanour rang alarm bells. In the days that followed, his behaviour confirmed the truth of the gentlewomen's account. Dackombe was desperate to be rid of his troubled lodger, and Birchet's peers eventually persuaded him to return to London with them. On the morning of their departure, they reported, a local preacher who had come for breakfast 'perceyung his madd behauyour, thought hym to be cleane owt of his wittes, as Mr Dackombe, and the rest of his house did'.[126] The three law students arrived back in London on Thursday 8 October; Birchet stabbed Hawkins six days later.

According to Aylworth's and Spenser's testimony, at least six people had judged Birchet to be mentally unsound in the week leading up to the attack. As in Somerville's case, however, this was not a line of inquiry which the examiners had any interest in pursuing. On 27 October, they asked Birchet

> Whether a pryvate man beinge perswaded in his owne conseyte that one is a willfull papist and hindereth the glory of god so moche as in him lyeth, may of his owne authoryty in the fervency of his zeale, kyll the same persone, And whether the same Acte is to be warraunted by the worde of god or no.[127]

He had not acted 'of his owne authority', Birchet insisted, but upon God's 'assured perswasions'. Like the Old Testament killers Joab, Ehud, or Phineas, he was an assassin by divine appointment. If 'I had killed him', the answer went on, the 'Acte had bene lawfull by gods lawe yf not by mans lawe. And I wold not haue repented me of the same ded'.[128] This answer alarmed Elizabeth so much that she ordered his execution by martial law. Cecil managed to dissuade her; the last such executions had been of the Wyatt rebels under Mary Tudor. Circumventing due process in this way did not look good. Birchet was sent to the Tower instead, awaiting trial on charges of heresy. Days later, he made the Privy Council's work a good deal easier by killing one of his keepers with a firebrand; a verdict of homicide was swiftly procured.[129] A serious assessment of

[125] Ibid., f. 195r. [126] Ibid., f. 195v. [127] Lansdowne 17/88, f. 192r. [128] Ibid., f. 192r.
[129] William Camden, *Annales rerum Anglicarum*, et Hibernicarum, regnante Elizabetha, ad annum salutis M.D. LXXXIX (London, 1615), pp. 242–243.

Birchet's mental health was not – and had never been – on the table. A second Elias could be laughed off; a second Ehud had to hang.

When, in July 1591, the Puritans Edmund Coppinger and Henry Arthington mounted an upturned cart in Cheapside to announce the Second Coming – this time, in the person of the Northamptonshire maltmaker William Hacket – the Privy Council was well prepared. All three men were arrested the same day and sent to Bridewell. By this point, many observers had already reached the conclusion that Hacket and his prophets were mad. Hacket had had several previous run-ins with the Northamptonshire magistrates, and they had reportedly attributed his 'outrages' to 'some spice of phrenesie' rather than to 'any setled and aduised malice'.[130] On his arraignment, Walsingham's spy Thomas Phelippes came to a similar conclusion, referring to the maltmaker as a 'madde foole'.[131] There were some at court, he wrote on 28 July, who 'pittyed theyr follye, which is like to cost them theyr lives; though they be but in the ranke of madde men, it is thought the state must be satisfied [touching] the proffett of vengeance at least, for that he hath deprived the Quene, & sayth she is not to raigne any longer'.[132] Phelippes's judgement was astute. Convicted of high treason, Hacket was hanged, drawn and quartered within a fortnight of his arrest. At the trial, the question of Hacket's mental soundness was raised by someone in the jury. The Attorney General's response was firm: 'howsoeuer these men vz. Hackett & the reste fained them selues as thoughe they were franticke yet this matter was determined Amongeste them by ther common consente att what tyme ther was no suspicion of frencye in him, or any of them'.[133] The culprits were not to be allowed to slip the noose with their 'franticke humoures of late contriued', for they had 'with greate consultacion resolved upon this course'.[134] This was the same language applied to Somerville and Birchet: their actions were the result of 'resolution', 'consultacion', and 'consent'. Stressing the suspects' capacity for reasoning, willing, and remembering, this language blocked the exculpatory verdict of non compos mentis.[135] In the official account, published that September, the civil lawyer Richard Cosin explained the reasoning for his lay readers. 'In wants of understanding and reason', he declared, 'there are noted divers degrees'; if Hacket *had* been disturbed, this was at most 'a kind of

130 Richard Cosin, *Conspiracie, for pretended reformation* (London, 1592), p. 8.
131 Kew, TNA, SP 12/239, f. 123v. 132 Ibid., f. 124r.
133 Preston, Lancashire Archives, DDKE/Box 122/1, f. 159v. 134 Ibid., f. 159v.
135 Cosin, *Conspiracie*, pp. 73–74.

Inconstancy voide in deede of perfite soundness of mind, yet such, as that he which hath it can observe and doe the common offices of this life among men, in some reasonable and tolerable sort'.[136]

The coming of the Puritan pseudo-messiah had been a special gift to Cosin and his ally, the bishop of London Richard Bancroft. Hacket's actions and words, Bancroft insisted, were not illogical: on the contrary, they were the logical consequences of Presbyterianism.[137] The argument made by Persons – that a 'frantic' Protestant was not sick at all, but only an extreme representative of his heretical brood – was easily adapted to the anti-Puritan cause. As Bancroft's colleague Matthew Sutcliffe put it, 'if all that have talked of the overthrow of Bishops and the Ecclesiasticall government, were to bee reputed as madde men, Bedlem if it were thrise so great would not holde them'.[138] Either all Puritans were frantic, or none of them were.

The various uses of frenzy which this chapter has explored converged – and clashed – in the case of William Hacket. As Walsham has shown, each faction with a stake in the episode struggled to wrest control of its interpretation. If the civil and ecclesiastical authorities differed somewhat in their objectives, their methods dovetailed. Burghley's first priority was to secure the safety of the queen; Bancroft's was to harness the full anti-Puritan potential of the affair. Both, however, were united in their efforts to deny the conspirators a diagnosis of frenzy. The Presbyterians, meanwhile, continued to insist upon that diagnosis. It was grossly unfair that the case of 'FranticK Hacket' had been 'thrust into the ballance of their false accusation against us', Josias Nicholls complained.[139] In its broad outlines, this pamphlet war bears traces of previous campaigns waged over 'martyrs' like Collins, Cowbridge, Atkins, and Somerville. Polemicists seized upon the other confession's most embarrassing members and packaged them up as figureheads; the other side did its best to have the package returned to sender. A frenzy diagnosis was singularly effective here. It was not the professors of the invalid's faith who were put to shame by his behaviour, it implied, but the 'physicians' who had killed him.

Over the course of the long Reformation, monarchs, bishops, and their counsellors became increasingly aware that the disease's power to exonerate its sufferers could work against them. Diagnosis – or its refusal – was a

[136] Ibid., p. 74. [137] Walsham, '"Frantick Hacket"', p. 58.
[138] Matthew Sutcliffe, *An ansvvere vnto a certaine calumnious letter published by M. Iob Throkmorton* (London, 1595), f. 8r.
[139] Josias Nichols, *The plea of the innocent* (London, 1602), p. 112.

calculated risk. By the turn of the seventeenth century, they had become well-practised in the art of producing sanity. In the case of the mariner Francis Collingwood, for example, who had declared the king 'a Traytor, a Cuckold, and . . . a Bastard' in 1607, the bishop of Winchester had already made up his mind when he wrote to Cecil. At the time, the bystanders had asserted that Collingwood had spoken these words 'in a frensie', and had even been

> forward enoughe to haue cleered him from advised purpose to reproche his Majesty . . . but I finding that formerly he was not towched with any suche infirmitie of his braines, and that in his greatest pretended furie, he had the witt to save himself from all harme, and within an hower [hour] or somewhat more fell to his meate, speaking verie soberly and remembering most things past in his counterfeit madnes, and laughing at them that bound him, for that he could haue hurt himself, as he sayed, for all their binding, if he had beene soe disposed; I tooke him for a dangerous & trayterous counterfeit.[140]

Every scrap of evidence served to prove that Collingwood had been faking madness at the time of making these speeches.[141] He had beaten his head against a cupboard, but 'so advisedly, that he drew no bloud from himself'; he had tried to strangle himself with 'the string of the door latche, but tyed no knott, nor was the string long enough to be tyed'.[142] He had threatened to kill his hostess, but had not, 'though he had a knife abowt him'.[143] Even the gaoler into whose keeping he had been committed deposed that

> Euer since his commitment he hath behaued himself soe civilly and advisedly, as the Examinate since he came to keepe the gaile, neuer saw any prisoner behaue himself so well . . . [as] for any shewe of madnes, he hath been so farre from it; That this Examinate taking special notice & observation of his cariage could neuer perceave any spark or inclination that way: And that for proof of his patience, this Examinate hath putt score of Irons on him & given him hard lodging yet could neuer finde any suche thing by him.[144]

Not only was Collingwood not mad, he was a good deal saner than the average prisoner. No amount of goading could produce signs of his former 'furie', and this was proof that the original bout was counterfeit. The sheer

[140] SP 14/26, f. 36r.
[141] The question of how to detect and deal with feigned insanity had long been discussed by legal theorists, especially within the civil law tradition. For civil lawyers, the starting point was Justinian's *Digest*. See *Digest* 1.18.13–14, 27.10.6; Richard Zouch, *Cases and questions resolved in the civil-lavv* (London, 1652), p. 254.
[142] SP 14/26, ff. 39r–v. [143] Ibid., f. 41r. [144] Ibid., f. 40r.

self-sabotaging illogicality of his conduct was ignored; Bilson even briefed Cecil that 'From himself I could haue heard muche in his excuse which I beleeved not, . . . [and was] not mentioned in his examination because it was tedious, partial, and impertinent'. Nothing the suspect could have said – no matter how deranged – would have exculpated him; Bilson had already decided that he had 'witt enough to cozen & dissemble', and that was that.[145]

New Polemics

Frantic Spirits

The strategy of conferring (or refusing) a diagnosis of frenzy did not die out entirely in the later seventeenth century, but it was resorted to less frequently and with more care.[146] And yet, in the 1640s, its decline coincided with a new efflorescence of frenzy as a polemical weapon. This was not a coincidence: the machinery of royal government which had produced the diagnosis was crumbling, and its loss of control over the press unleashed a tide of religio-political polemic. In the decades of the civil wars and the Interregnum, nobody lacked enemies, and words did to enemies what swords could not: they questioned their sanity.

The metaphor of 'spiritual frenzy' – developed in the 1580s by the English Jesuits and their opponents, and later perfected by Puritan and Laudian preachers – was an especially apt barb for the new sects of radical Protestantism that were emerging in these decades. It seemed that every night saw the birth of some new and more dangerous strain: first 'Ranters, Seekers, Shakers, Quakers, and now *Creepers*', fulminated one Presbyterian minister in 1651.[147] The publication of several new histories of the sixteenth-century Anabaptists – one provocatively titled *A warning for England especially for London in the famous history of the frantick Anabaptists their wild preachings and practises in Germany* (1642) – only added fuel to the fire.[148] It was 'these frantick and seditious men', English readers were reminded, who had betrayed the Protestant cause, by exalting

[145] Ibid., f. 36r. [146] See, for one example, Kew, TNA, ADM 77/2, no. 144 (1685).

[147] Thomas Hall, *The pulpit guarded with XVII arguments proving the unlawfulness, sinfulness and danger of suffering private persons to take upon them publike preaching, and expounding the Scriptures without a call* (London, 1651), p. 15.

[148] [Anon.], *A warning for England especially for London in the famous history of the frantick Anabaptists their wild preachings & practises in Germany* (London, 1642).

their 'wicked and franticke opinions, above Gods holy Word'.[149] Attacks on the 'frantick' Quakers, 'frenzy-conceited men of the Fifth Monarchy', and all 'home-spun Dissenters of frantick and fanatick brain' soon proliferated.[150] The trope found new purchase when applied to these nonconformist sects, not just because they placed the revelations of the spirit of God above all other sources of authority, but because their members had a reputation for manifesting the inward workings of that spirit in signs easily interpretable as symptoms of brain disease: trembling, swooning, seeing visions, and entering trance states.[151]

But no one was safe from attack. In 1654, a mouthpiece for the newly established Protectorate, identified only as 'E. M.', published a pamphlet 'proving' three propositions – that Oliver Cromwell was 'the aptest, ablest and most worthy person for place of Lord PROTECTOR', that 'the people, by the laws of God and man are obliged to loyalty and obedience to his Highness [Cromwell]', and that 'all Opposers are Enemies to the publick Peace and Safety, and deserve exemplary punishment'.[152] In an uncanny echo of Laud's polemicists, the pamphleteer advised those who considered themselves 'Gods Ministers' to take care, 'lest the pulpit which should be the chair of sound verity, seem to be the chair of insane vanity to vent the *frenzied* folly of phantastick Brains'.[153] This was not a condemnation; it was a warning. Any minister who raised objections to the new regime could expect – at best – to have his words written off as brainsick raving. If unqualified acceptance of the established religious and political order had not been a precondition of sanity in the 1640s, it was now.

Overruling the Ruler

Among the many qualities which – in the eyes of this author – made Cromwell worthy of the title Lord Protector, not least was 'his humility of Spirit, meekness and mildnes, in patient and Gentle passing by the Ignomy of some ignorant wretches . . . rather pittying their weakness than

149 Friedrich Spanheim, *Englands vvarning by Germanies vvoe* (London, 1646), pp. 8, 21.

150 Christopher Wade, *Quakery slain irrecoverably by the principal Quakers themselves* (London, 1657), pp. 8, 14, 23, 43; [Anon.], *The downfall of the Fifth Monarchy* (London, 1657), title page; Kew, TNA, SP 29/435, ff. 166–169.

151 See Kate Peters, 'Ranter and Quaker Stereotyping in the English Revolution', in Koji Yamamoto (ed.), *Stereotypes and Stereotyping in Early Modern England* (Manchester: Manchester University Press, 2022), pp. 150–183.

152 E. M., *Protection perswading subjection: or A word of peace to the well-affected* (London, 1654), frontispiece, sig. B1.

153 Ibid., p. 28.

punishing their frenzied folly and wickedness'.[154] Like many a polemicist before him, E. M. was returning to one of Augustine's time-honoured allegories: that of the frantic patient attacking the loving physician. It was Cromwell, this time, who was assigned the latter role, standing in for *Christus medicus*. The Lord Protector would have been well within his right to take his opponents' 'wickedness' at face value, E. M. implied; it was lucky for them that his 'patient' and 'pittying' nature had won out.

As we have seen, polemicists had long reworked Augustine's trope to fit their purposes. But there was one version which was too subversive to ever have become a commonplace. In 1561, the Scottish reformer John Knox had been bold enough to put it to Mary Stuart, Scotland's newly arrived queen. If a 'Father may be stricken with a Phrenzie, in the which he would slay his owne Children', he hypothesized,

> if the children arise, joyn themselves together, apprehend the Father, take the Sword or other Weapon from him, and finally, binde his hands, and keepe him in Prison till that his Phrensie be over-past, Thinke ye (Madame) that the children do any wrong? . . . It is even so (said he) Madame, with Princes that would murther the children of God, that are subject unto them. Their blinde zeale is nothing but a very mad phrenzie; and therefore to take the sword from them, to binde their hands, and to cast them into prison, till that they be brought to a more sober minde, is no disobedience against Princes, but just obedience, because that it agreeth with the Word of God.[155]

Knox had developed this analogy as a Marian exile, and he had had a quite specific scenario in mind: a Catholic queen (illegitimate in the first place on account of her sex) persecuting her Reformed subjects.[156] Yet events like the 1572 St Bartholomew's Day Massacre would push others to develop their own more systematic versions of resistance theory.[157] One of the most radical was advanced by the humanist scholar George Buchanan, tutor to the young prince James VI, in his *De jure Regni apud Scotos* (1579).[158] A tyrant was so far from being a true king, Buchanan declared, that his or her reign was to be brought to an end by any means

[154] Ibid., p. 15.

[155] John Knox, *The history of the reformation of religioun within the realme of Scotland* (London, 1587), unnumbered page. Quotation from Knox, *The historie of the reformation of the Church of Scotland* (London, 1644), p. 313.

[156] Robert M. Kingdon, 'Calvinism and Resistance Theory, 1550–1580', in J. H. Burns (ed.), *The Cambridge History of Political Thought, 1450–1700* (Cambridge: Cambridge University Press, 1991), pp. 194–200.

[157] Ibid., pp. 207–214. [158] Ibid., pp. 216–218.

necessary, even – if it came to it – assassination.[159] *De jure* was written as an explicit justification of the Scottish peers' 1567 overthrow of Mary Stuart, but there was nothing to stop readers applying its conclusions to other circumstances.[160] On assuming personal rule in 1584, James VI moved swiftly to have the book banned.[161]

In the reigns of Elizabeth I and her Stuart successors, any English subject espousing these views in public would have been sent to the gallows (or, if they were lucky, to Bethlem). But that world had been turned 'upside down' in 1642, and Knox's inversion of the old Augustinian trope had become not only thinkable, but sayable.[162] It was voiced anew by the Puritan lawyer William Prynne (1600–1669), in *The soveraigne povver of parliaments and kingdomes* (1643):

> If then a King in an angry franticke passion (for Ir. brevius furor est;) shall take up Armes against his loyall Subjects, and assault their persons to murther them and spoyle their goods; if they (by common consent in Parliament especially) shall forcibly resist, disarme or restraine his person, till his fury be appeased, and his judgement rectified by better councells; shall this be Treason, Rebellion, or Disloyaltie? God forbid: I thinke none but mad men can or will averte it.[163]

On the face of it, this picture looks very similar to the one painted by Knox. But there is one important difference: where Knox was happy to leave open the question of which of the frantic father's 'children' had the right to restrain him, Prynne was at pains to stress that, whoever it was, they were to proceed only after having sought and received Parliament's 'common consent'. In fact, this had always been the majority view among the sixteenth-century resistance theorists; most had been willing to entrust the task only to the 'inferior magistrate' – or failing that, an assembly of godly men, acting on behalf of 'the people'.[164]

The irony was that even this qualified version of resistance theory did not sit right with Prynne.[165] He had always been a committed religious

[159] George Buchanan, *Rervm Scoticarvm historia … Accessit De iure regni apud Scotus Dialogus* (Edinburgh, 1583), sig. C2v.

[160] Ibid., sigs. a2r–v.

[161] Jenny Wormald, 'James VI and I, *Basilikon Doron* and *The Trew Law of Free Monarchies*: The Scottish Context and the English Translation', in Linda Levy Peck (ed.), *The Mental World of the Jacobean Court* (Cambridge: Cambridge University Press, 1991), p. 44.

[162] [Anon.], *The world is turned upside down* (London, 1646).

[163] William Prynne, *The third part of The soveraigne povver of parliaments and kingdomes* (London, 1643), p. 15.

[164] Kingdon, 'Calvinism and Resistance Theory', pp. 200–206, 209–214.

[165] William Lamont, 'Prynne, William (1600–1669), Pamphleteer and Lawyer', *ODNB*, 19 May 2011, https://doi.org/10.1093/ref:odnb/22854.

reformer (before the war he had been imprisoned, mutilated, and branded for portraying the Caroline court as a den of iniquity), but even afterwards he had remained a royalist.[166] Plus, he was a lawyer, and – unlike Knox – he needed a resistance theory which accorded with the law and not just the 'Word of God'. He found it in the pages of the Dutch lawyer Hugo Grotius's *De jure belli ac pacis* (1625). 'The first cause of a justifiable war' Grotius had written, 'is an injury not yet inflicted, which menaces either person or property'.[167] A monarch like Charles, who had shown himself ready to 'deliver up possession of all or any part of his Realm to another forraign power' could 'lawfully be resisted with force by his subjects'.[168] With this Grotian principle of self-preservation as his template, characterizing the king as 'franticke' was technically superfluous to Prynne's needs: Parliament's actions were defensible because they were acts of self-defence. Perhaps his invocation of frenzy served another purpose; perhaps it was to help him (and other former royalists) to swallow what was – despite everything – still a bitter pill.

Prynne's *The soveraigne povver of parliaments* has been justly (if unflatteringly) described as 'a series of *post hoc* justifications of actions taken by the parliamentary army during the campaign itself'.[169] As far as we know, the generals who commissioned the treatise had no complaints about the results. If any of the Presbyterians among them – the natural heirs to Knox – felt that Prynne's argument was not quite as expected, they said nothing. But the gulf between them and Prynne soon became impossible to ignore. For Prynne, Charles was guilty of many wrongs – mostly, of listening to papists – but the fact that he had stained the mantle of his absolute sovereignty did not mean that it could be thrown into the fire.[170] By 1645, the Scottish Presbyterian Robert Baillie was comparing Prynne to the *remora*: the little fish whose suction was fabled to bring even the greatest ship to a halt.[171]

In 1648, still desperately trying to negotiate a settlement with the king, Prynne returned to the familiar legal definition of non

166 'Prima igitur causa justi belli est injuria nondum facta, quae petit aut corpus, aut rem.' Hugo Grotius, *De jure belli ac pacis* (Amsterdam, 1632), pp. 91–92. Quotation from Stephen C. Neffe (trans.), *Hugo Grotius on the Law of War and Peace* (Cambridge: Cambridge University Press, 2013), p. 82.

167 Quotation from Neffe (trans.), *Hugo Grotius*, p. 73.

168 Quotation from William Prynne, *The soveraigne povver of parliaments and kingdomes* (London, 1643), p. 103; Grotius, *De jure*, p. 83. 'Si tamen rex reipsa etiam tradere regnum aut subjicere moliatur . . . ei resisti in hoc possit.'

169 Lamont, 'Prynne'.

170 Ibid.; William Lamont, *Marginal Prynne, 1600–1669* (London: Routledge & Kegan Paul, 1963), pp. 108–109, 116–117.

171 Lamont, 'Prynne'.

compos mentis. There were several historical precedents, he pointed out, in which

> the Parliaments of England and Scotland (as well as of most other Kingdomes) have during the Minority, absence, sickness, frenzie, dotage, or other naturall, accidentall, or criminall disabilities of their Kings to discharge their Royall Office, and Dutie usually constituted a Viceroy, Regent, Protector, or Custos Regni ... to guard both their Persons and Realms, and execute all Regal Acts belonging to the King himself.[172]

Again, Prynne's offhand equation of 'natural, accidentall, or criminal disabilities' was perhaps more soothing than necessary: rhetoric aside, none of the conditions on this list applied to Charles. It was a way of holding out an olive branch to the imprisoned king: 'frenzie, [or] dotage' preserved the possibility of innocence, and with it the hope of restoration. A king rendered temporarily non compos mentis by sickness might recover; even Nebuchadnezzar had regained his reason in the end. But Charles I never did – or not, at least, to the satisfaction of the radicals in Cromwell's New Model Army. For many, the news that he had invited a Scottish army to invade England was all the proof they needed that his 'disabilities' were beyond cure.[173] But not for Prynne. He would never forgive those responsible for bringing about the king's execution; in fact, by 1647, he had come to see them as crypto-papists, conspiring with the Jesuits to sever the head from England's body politic.[174]

Unfortunately, like many an anti-Catholic polemicist before him, Prynne was soon to find that he had no monopoly on the figure of the frantic tyrant. In 1648, it was picked up and repurposed by one of his bitterest enemies: the Independent minister John Goodwin (c. 1594–1665). In his pamphlet *Right and Might Well Met* (1648), Goodwin asked his readers to imagine a 'Pilot, or Master of a Ship at Sea', unexpectedly 'disabled, as through a phreneticall passion, or sicknesse in any kinde, so that he is uncapable of acting the exigencies of his place'. In this situation, Goodwin continued, was it not permissible for 'anyone, or more of the inferiour Mariners, having skill ... [to] very lawfully assume and act according to the interest of a Pilot, or Master, and give orders and directions to those with them in the Ship accordingly'? This was not just a

[172] William Prynne, *A plain, short, and probable expedient, to settle the present distractions of both kingdomes* (London, 1647).
[173] Mark Kishlansky, *A Monarchy Transformed: Britain, 1603–1714* (London: Penguin, 1996), pp. 181–185.
[174] Lamont, *Marginal Prynne*, pp. 124–134.

right but a duty, both 'for the preservation of the Ship, being now in present danger, either of running upon a quick sand, or splitting against a rock', and the saving 'of the lives of all that are in it'.[175] Goodwin backed the point up with a verbatim quotation from the relevant 'passage in Master Prynne':

> Seeing then (as Plato saith) TYRANNY IS A CERTAIN *PHRENSIE* ... [if] there is one of the Nobles, which considers the incroaching tyranny, and detests it from his soule: what think'st thou is now to bee done against him by this man? ... [he] shal preserve the Kingdome even against the Kings wil and resistance, by WHICH HE HIMSELF BECOMES A KING and shall cure the King himselfe as a frantique man, by BINDING HIS HANDS AND FEET, if he may not otherwise doe it.[176]

The two pamphleteers had been at each other's throats since at least 1644, and it is hard not to detect a note of waspish triumph in this passage.[177] Goodwin had hoisted Prynne with his own petard.

Adding insult to injury was the fact that the 'frantique man' whom Goodwin had in mind was not the king. He had written *Right and Might Well Met* to defend what would become known as 'Pride's Purge': the expulsion of a full third of the Long Parliament's eligible members from the House by a regiment of the New Model Army, led by the colonel Thomas Pride.[178] Most of the targets had recently voted to continue the negotiations which – if successful – would lead to Charles's restoration; for the Army, this was no longer an acceptable outcome.[179] Goodwin was writing to win over those who accepted the reasons for Pride's Purge, but balked at the methods. The words of 'Mr. Prynne', Goodwin claimed, were 'full far enough to justifie whatsoever is said in these papers for the justification of the Army in their binding the hands and feet of some frantique Parliament men (as [Prynne] himself ... phraseth those, who either thorough malice, or slothfulnesse, shall betray those, whom they have undertaken to protect)'.[180] Prynne had argued that Parliament had a duty to prevent a 'frantic' tyrant from harming his subjects. What he had *not* said was that, if some 'Parliament men' succumbed to same

175 John Goodwin, *Right and Might Well Met* (London, 1648), p. 9. 176 Ibid., p. 10.

177 See John Goodwin, *Innocencies triumph* (London, 1644); John Goodwin, *Calumny arraign'd* (London, 1645); William Prynne, *Truth triumphing over falshood, antiquity over novelty* (London, 1645).

178 Tai Liu, 'Goodwin, John (c. 1594–1665), Independent Minister', *ODNB*, 3 January 2008, https://doi.org/10.1093/ref:odnb/10994.

179 Kishlansky, *A Monarchy Transformed*, pp. 180–186.

180 Goodwin, *Right and Might Well Met*, pp. 10–11.

disease – then the same responsibility defaulted to 'the Army'. Goodwin's extension of the metaphor had disturbing implications, and they did not go unnoticed. Another London minister shot back: 'An easie, and readie way to de-throne all Authoritie, if saying they be mad will serve the turne, when they are neither in drinke, passion, nor under any other symptome of such unnaturall distemper'.[181] Goodwin was not only willing to conflate figurative and literal frenzy; he was content to leave it to the military to track the spread of the disease, and to restrain its victims. There was no telling where this cycle of ruling and overruling – of binding and being bound – would end.

The Flaws in the Figure

As a polemical device, frenzy was hard to resist. Yet ultimately the parliamentarian pamphleteers fell foul of its one major flaw – the same flaw which had caused problems for its sixteenth-century users. It worked well as a pretext for many coercive measures: restraint, imprisonment, silencing, even corporal 'correction'. But, in the end, none of these measures was enough for the king's captors. Cromwell and his generals had become convinced that their captive was a criminal, guilty of 'a more prodigious treason than any that had been perfected before'.[182] And the punishment for treason was death. The army's spin doctors now found themselves in a similar situation to their crown predecessors, tasked with stage-managing the trials of Somerville, Birchet, and Hacket. Labelling an individual as 'frantic' had its purposes, but – if a death sentence later became necessary – it had to be made clear that it had never been meant literally. Putting a man to death for deeds done while non compos mentis was not lawful execution; it was murder of a pitiable innocent. It was, in other words, the act of a tyrant. Collapsing the divide between literal and figurative frenzy – as Goodwin had done – risked accidentally exculpating the target of the polemic. Any hint that the king had ever suffered from lapses of reason was now a positive liability. The moment he had signed the treaty with the Scots in December 1647, Charles had become perfectly, terribly sane.

[181] John Geree, *Katadynastēs: might overcoming right. Or a cleer answer to M. John Goodwin's Might and right well met* (London, 1649), p. 18.

[182] Oliver Cromwell to Robert Jenner and John Ashe, 20 November 1648. 'Letter LXXXII', in Thomas Carlyle (ed.), *The letters and speeches of Oliver Cromwell* (London: Methuen, 1904), p. 387.

The risk of unintended exculpation may be one reason why, in the 1650s, frenzy began to lose ground to another polemical diagnosis. In his 1621 *Anatomy of melancholy*, Robert Burton had written of the 'peculiar sects' that 'their religion takes away not spirits only, but wit and iudgement, and depriues them of all vnderstanding: for some of them are so farre gone with their priuate Enthusiasmes, and reuelations, that they are quite madde, out of their wits'.[183] 'Enthusiasm' was not and had never been a disease category; the word still retained its ancient Greek meaning of possession or inspiration by a deity. By the seventeenth century, however, it had acquired an incredulous cast; 'enthusiasts' merely *believed* that they were vessels of God.[184] The term had occasionally been applied to religious radicals in the sixteenth century, but, as Michael Heyd has shown, it was in mid-seventeenth-century England that it came into its own. Heyd charts a progressive 'medicalization of enthusiasm' in this period, beginning with Burton's *Anatomy* and culminating with Meric Causabon's *A treatise concerning enthusiasme* (1654) and Henry More's *Enthusiasmus Triumphatus* (1655).[185] Both Causabon and More were avid readers of Burton, and they followed him in identifying black bile as the cause of all such spurious raptures, visions, and prophecies. By the 1660s, melancholy enthusiasm was steadily becoming the favoured diagnosis for those seeking to discredit religious nonconformity.[186]

Offering a literalistic, naturalistic medical explanation for religious nonconformity was still controversial at the time, not least because it seemed to let sufferers off the hook. In an addendum to the second edition of *Enthusiasmus Triumphatus*, More defended himself from this charge. If he had not dealt directly with 'the wilfull wickedness of the Mind of man' and had instead 'resolved all into Complexion, or present temper, or rather distemper, of the body arising from natural causes', readers were not to judge his 'Discourse as well an excuse for, as a Discovery of, this Disease of Enthusiasm'.[187] On the contrary, he insisted that 'the Enthusiast, though he be necessarily assaulted by his own Complexion, yet not irresistibly; and that therefore the guilt of his extravagancies lies at his own door'.[188] More thus mobilized the longstanding legal distinction

[183] Burton, *The anatomy*, p. 757.
[184] Michael Heyd, *Be Sober and Reasonable: The Critique of Enthusiasm in the Seventeenth and Early Eighteenth Centuries* (Leiden: Brill, 1995), pp. 11–23.
[185] Ibid., esp. ch. 3. [186] MacDonald, 'Insanity and the Realities of History', 11–25.
[187] Henry More, 'Enthusiasmus Triumphatus', in *A collection of several philosophical writings of Dr Henry More* (London, 1662), p. 47.
[188] Ibid.

between partial and total madness (*furor*): it was total madness, not 'every melancholy or hypochondriacal distemper', which exonerated sufferers from wrongdoing.[189] Melancholy enthusiasm *could* be resisted, and thus its onset signalled a failure of self-government. It was the enthusiast's 'own fault' that he was 'not *temperate*, *humble*, and *attentive to Reason*'.[190] The natural distemper wrought by melancholy was not so severe as to incapacitate the soul's rational faculties: the reason, the understanding, and the will. Frenzy – known to deprive the sufferer of the use of all of these faculties – had never been a perfect fit. Once a favourite shorthand for 'false zeal', by the Restoration, it was steadily losing ground to melancholy enthusiasm. Perhaps the risk of giving the target the accidental gift of legal immunity had become too well known. Or perhaps England's polemical writers and their readers were simply growing tired of frenzy; perhaps it had been weaponized so often that it was starting to lose its edge. It must have lost it eventually; today, the words 'frenzy' and 'frantic' have retained their hyperbolic quality, but nothing of their former power.

Conclusion

The strategic diagnosis of frenzy was a delicate balancing act for the ruling elites of early modern England. Done right, it stopped up the mouths of self-proclaimed visionaries with the lightest of touches. It consigned their letters to the oblivion of the archive; failing that, it persuaded the recipients not to listen. It legitimated the use of physical force, coercion, and confinement without trial. Yet one substantial risk had to be weighed against these benefits. The frantic could not be held responsible for their own actions; heretics, traitors, tyrants, and would-be assassins had to be shown to have acted 'wilfully' and 'advisedly'. Any previous allusion to frenzy threatened to jeopardize a conviction. And even if a death sentence *was* successfully procured, it left the prosecutors open to future accusations of shedding innocent blood. For William Allen, it was the presence of 'corporal frenzy' which had made John Somerville's execution an unlawful murder. An insistence on its absence was ultimately what had sent Birchet and Hacket to their deaths.

Polemicists were often a good deal less careful than crown officials in their invocations of frenzy, and it continued to be recycled as a figure of speech long after it had been abandoned as a strategic diagnosis. Not that

189 Hale, *Historia placitorum coronae*, vol. 1, p. 412.
190 More, 'Enthusiasmus Triumphatus', p. 48.

the polemicists liked to be too exact about their meaning; neglecting to signal the register in which they wrote encouraged an associative slippage between literal and figurative frenzy. This made the latter sort of diagnosis just as dangerous as the former (and, to life and limb, probably more). In Persons's account, it was the incurability of some cases of 'spiritual frenzy' which justified the killing of sick 'sheepe' by the 'pittiful pastors' of Rome. A diagnosis of the '*PHRENSIE*' of tyranny was enough to justify a civil war, a king's incarceration, and a military coup. The less the reader remembered the fact that there were a few obvious differences between literal and figurative frenzy, the more powerful the effects became. But the flaw in the figure remained: if the conflation was allowed to continue for too long, or was pressed too hard, it threatened to turn the guilty party into a pitiable innocent. 'Melancholy enthusiasm' – preserving as it did a remnant of the sufferer's 'reason' and 'will' – circumvented this problem. Whether brought about by humoral distemper, poor self-governance, spiritual pride, or diabolic manipulation (and More and Causabon usually detected a combination of all four), the enthusiast could and should have done a better job of guarding the citadel of the rational soul.

Conclusion

A Disease of the Person

On 31 October 1698, the non-conformist minister Oliver Heywood performed the last rites for a neighbour named Mercy Stocks, who had fallen into a frenzy some months before. It was seventeen years since he had first been summoned to the sickbed of the frantic young man Joshua Bates. Just as Bates had been 'a godly young man' before the onset of his illness, Stocks had been 'a gracious woman that had sate down with us at the Lords supper'.[1] Yet in her frenzy she had grown

> very unruly [so] that they were forced to bind her, she rambled about and talked very idly and extravagantly, so that the neighbours were greatly disturbed with her both day and night, often naming the dead, and expressed such shameful words, that many wondred at her, where she should learn them, thus she continued night and day a great affliction to her husband and family ... many means were used, blooding severall times, physick, all did no good, at last we resolved to keep a solemn fast with her.[2]

Stocks was beyond the help of medicine, Heywood guessed, but she was not beyond God's mercy. And 'god graciously heard prayer', for at the end of the day-long fast, she

> had more exercise of her reason, talkt sensibly, I prayd with her, thankt god for her, Oct 27, blessed be god, tho her body is weaker, declining ... [she] desired me to pray with her which I did, put her into the hands of god, she thankt me was sensible, on Tuesday night Nov 1 she departed about 12 a clock in the night.[3]

God's answer to prayer was not to cure the disease, or to spare the sufferer's life, but to restore to her the 'exercise of her reason'.

[1] Heywood, 'Objects and Observations', pp. 31, 161. [2] Ibid., p. 161. [3] Ibid., p. 161.

That Stocks had died a good death was some comfort to Heywood. Yet her behaviour during the last months of her life must have resurrected the questions which he had asked back in 1681: 'Doth our Lord give them grace and then deprive them of the use of Reason?'[4] Reflecting on Bates's death, he had concluded:

> god giues and takes away the order and regular use of the soules most noble facultys, to teach us rightly to improue that talent to gods glory, the good of others, and if the Lord see good to restore them ... when these black clouds are blown over and their understanding returnes – we praise and honour him that liveth for ever – the inhabitants of the earth are reputed as nothing – none can stay his hand or say unto him what doest though [thou]?[5]

There was no jubilation in this Job-like submission to divine authority; this was a hard lesson, learned by 'sad spectators'.[6] In his habit of seeking to discern God's providential purposes in the events of his own life, Heywood had more in common with his sixteenth- and seventeenth-century predecessors than his more urbane, 'Enlightened' peers. His reactions to frenzy touch on the key themes which lie at the heart of this book: the status of the rational soul, its fraught relationship with the body, the nature of its faculties, and the meaning of their loss. In what follows, I review each of these themes in turn, before offering a short summary of the book's larger argument.

Ensouled Brains

In *Being Brains*, Vidal and Ortega argue that the identification of the self with the brain 'predated reliable neuroscientific discoveries and has all the appearance of having been a motivating factor of brain research'.[7] This book's findings offer full support to this claim: it was the belief that the brain was somehow integral to the self which prompted the study of the organ's structures and functions, and not vice versa. If I have queried Vidal and Ortega's account of the rise of the 'cerebral subject', it is only on account of its chronology. The acquisition of 'knowledge about the brain' – they imply – began in earnest only in the late seventeenth century, when the decline of humoral psychophysiology marked a 'turn to "solidism"'.[8] This narrative relies on an overemphasis on the total explanatory power of fluids (including spirits) in pre-1660s medical theory. As Jennifer Wright

[4] Ibid., p. 33. [5] Ibid. [6] Ibid. [7] Vidal and Ortega, *Being Brains*, p. 31.
[8] Ibid., p. 31.

has elegantly shown, it does not do justice to pre-Enlightenment understandings of the brain.[9] Wright's argument relates to late antiquity, but it can easily be extended to early modernity. Like late antique *phrenitis*, early modern frenzy was a disease which arose in the decidedly solid parts of the brain or meninges, and which announced itself through alarming changes in the sufferer's speech, demeanour, and behaviour. Long before 1660, it had prompted observers to connect the presence (or absence) of personhood to the health (or sickness) of the brain.

Nor were learned anatomists the only ones to make this connection. Whatever Napier knew about the contents of the skull, he had gleaned it from the vernacular *practica*; if he had any working model of brain–mind relations, it was the old ventricular one. And yet in his casebooks he used 'brain' as a synecdoche for the whole: Anne Syred was 'soarli distracted in her brayne', John Quarrell 'frentick & distemperd . . . in his brayne'.[10] And Napier was not the only one to use the word in this way. The witnesses to Collingwood's 1607 outburst had chalked up his outrageous speeches to the 'infirmitie of his braines'.[11] The 'braines of Iohn Foxe', Persons wrote in 1603, 'were knowne to be out of tune for many years, before he died'.[12] These non-specialists may have had a less thoroughly worked-out model of the brain and its diseases than their medical peers (and this is still true of non-specialists today), but this does not mean that nobody living before 1660 saw the organ as integral to personal identity. If this were the case, insults like 'frantic' and 'brainsick' would surely not have hit as hard as they did.

Up until the close of the seventeenth century (and beyond), this was principally a conversation about an ensouled brain: the rational soul was the musician, and the whole mass inside the skull (in all of its solid, liquid, and spiritous parts) was its instrument. Substance dualism, mechanism, and atomism made it easier to imagine prising the two apart, but – for the vast majority of late seventeenth-century Europeans – doing away with the musician was a prospect too horrible to bear thinking about. I have argued that what made brain disease so unsettling was its capacity to disable all this soul's 'noblest' operations in one fell swoop. I have also argued that frenzy spurred those who had witnessed its effects to map out those operations on the internal structures of the brain. Many of these early brain cartographers had never witnessed a dissection, and those who had (Thomas Willis

[9] Wright, 'Ventricular Localization in Late Antiquity', esp. pp. 3–11.
[10] Kassell et al., *Casebooks*, cases 23753, 70899. [11] SP 14/26, f. 36r.
[12] Persons, *A treatise of three conversions*, vol. 1, p. 294.

included) were often obliged to fall back on speculation. Although it is impossible to deny that Willis's anatomical findings were more accurate (by present-day standards) than those of his predecessors, the impetus behind his research project was anything but 'empirical'. Willis's fascination with cerebral anatomy stemmed from his fascination with diseases of the mind, and this in turn was driven by pressing metaphysical concerns. Frenzy bothered Willis because it threatened to erode the certainties of Christian doctrine: the immortality of the rational soul, the inalienability of its faculties, and the integrity of the divide which separated it from the souls of 'brutes'.

Willis's solution was twofold. First, he reintroduced the ontological divide between the rational and sensitive souls, and quarantined diseases 'of the Brain and nervous stock' to the latter. Second, he moved the seat of the disease from the meninges to the animal spirits, redefining it as a 'burning or inflammation of the whole sensitive soul'.[13] Iatrochemistry, mechanism, and atomism equipped him with the conceptual tools to tailor the disease mechanism to size. Willis claimed that this redefinition of frenzy was prompted by his post-mortem findings, and we have no reason to disbelieve him. Yet it also helped to explain how it was that – if human souls could never lose their God-given rational faculties – frantic souls made it look so much like they had. In life, the rational soul relied on accurate input from its sensitive counterpart to exercise its faculties; no wonder it was unable to do so when its closest collaborator was on fire.

As a medical diagnosis, frenzy emerged from the profound social, cultural, and religio-political upheavals of the early modern period remarkably intact. In his 1746 *Treatise on phrensy*, the German physician Peter Frings announced that he had 'exploded' the Galenic account of the disease.[14] Yet his version bore a more than passing resemblance to the one he claimed to have just blown to bits. Frenzy was caused by the spread of a noxious, inflammatory substance (not burnt choler but 'nitro-sulphureous . . . Particles') from the vital spirits in the blood to the animal spirits in the brain.[15] Following in Willis's footsteps, Frings was translating an old humoral story into a new chemical language. *Mutatis mutandis*, the organic pathways of the disease looked much like they always had. It was precisely this adaptability to new medical philosophies which helped the disease category to endure for as long as it did.

It was only at the turn of the nineteenth century that medical theorists began to abandon frenzy. In *A treatise on mortal diseases*, published in

[13] Willis, *Two discourses*, p. 183. [14] Frings, *A treatise on phrensy*, title page.
[15] Ibid., pp. 22, 25.

1798, the Dutch physician Conrad George Ontijd announced that 'I have changed the indeterminate and vague appellations of phrenitis and paraphrenitis for those of encephalitis and diaphragmatitis'.[16] In 1817, the English nosologist John Mason Good followed suit, writing of '*Emprésma Cephalitis*' (encephalitis) that 'this word is preferred to phrenitis, as more descriptive of the organ affected'.[17] Good was of the opinion that there was no point in creating two distinct disease categories – one for the inflammation of the meninges and one for the substance of the brain – for in practice the symptoms were indistinguishable.[18] Early modern physicians would have agreed: their *phrenitis* had covered exactly the same ground as Good's *cephalitis*. But not all of Good's contemporaries were of the same mind: by the 1820s, the term meningitis had been coined to describe the inflammation of the *arachnoid* and the *pia mater*.[19]

The timing of *phrenitis*'s disaggregation into diaphragmatitis, encephalitis, meningitis, and delirium is revealing. In 1985, Theodore M. Brown argued that it was only in the nineteenth century that 'neoclassical conceptions' began to be

> abandoned and broadly replaced by views based instead on anatomical localism, cellular pathology, and microbiological etiology – each fragmenting the notion of organismic totality implicit in humoral and post-humoral physiology. Specialization further fragmented the object of medicine into separate and compartmentalized organs and systems.[20]

In Brown's view, it was modern biomedicine which had produced modern mind–body dualism, a crime which its twentieth-century critics would later pin on René Descartes.[21] Brown's account does risk replacing one 'before and after' story with another; as Thumiger has shown, 'anatomical localism' had shaped the definition of *phrenitis* since classical antiquity.[22] Yet there is no doubt that the nineteenth century wrought some decisive

[16] Ontijd, *A treatise on mortal diseases*, p. 223.
[17] John Mason Good, *A Physiological System of Nosology, With a Corrected and Simplified Nomenclature* (London, 1817), p. 167, n. 1.
[18] Ibid. Good cited the Scottish physician William Cullen as the author of this opinion. Cullen had chosen 'phrenitis' as the umbrella category which Good would replace with 'cephalitis'. See William Cullen, *Synopsis nosologiae methodicae* (Ticino, 1787), p. 48.
[19] Abercrombie, *Pathological and Practical Researches*, p. 51.
[20] Theodore M. Brown, 'Descartes, Dualism, and Psychosomatic Medicine', in Bynum et al. (eds.), *The Anatomy of Madness: Essays in the History of Psychiatry*, vol. 1, p. 52.
[21] Ibid., pp. 52–57.
[22] See Thumiger, *Phrenitis*, esp. chs. 2, 5. Thumiger also argues for coeval ebbs and flows of delocalization. Her book gives a much fuller account of the lives and afterlives of ancient *phrenitis* than I have been able to offer here.

changes: the refinement and 'rationalization' of nosology, the development of histology and cellular pathology, and an increasing move towards professional specialization. Brown's argument offers a persuasive rationale for the fractionation and ultimate expiry of *phrenitis*. In an era of tissue samples and literal-minded labelling, it was no longer acceptable for an inflammation of the brain to be named after its effects on the soul. Thus when, in 2013, the medievalist Luke Demaitre wrote of frenzy 'the label is now obsolete and replaced by two distinct ones, namely, "encephalitis" and "delirium"', technically speaking he was not wrong.[23] Nor was the classicist Peter Pormann exactly wrong when, in 2017, he glossed ancient *phrenitis* as meningitis.[24] Yet, as this book has shown, these nineteenth-century diagnoses are fragments of an inherited nosology. Each offers only a distant likeness of the early modern disease.

Embodied Souls

Fernando Vidal has described early modern Europe not only as the cradle of 'brainhood' but also of the discipline of 'psychology'.[25] The shift from an Aristotelian 'soul-form' to a post-Aristotelian 'soul-mind', which he traces over the course of the late seventeenth century, also finds ample corroboration in this book.[26] Willis's solution to the problem posed by Galen's *Quod animi mores* looked radically different to that of Willet, written eighty years earlier. And yet, although tensions between different visions of the human soul–body composite may have ratcheted up in the sixteenth and seventeenth centuries – most of them had ancient roots.[27] Some (like Augustine's dualism) had inherited the Platonists' tendency to polarize soul and body. Some (like Aquinas's dualism and Ockham's pluralism) had been engineered to make Aristotle's soul-form compatible

[23] Luke Demaitre, *Medieval Medicine: The Art of Healing from Head to Toe* (Santa Barbara, CA: Praeger, 2013), p. 134.

[24] Peter Pormann, 'Medicine on the Different Shores of the Mediterranean: Scientific Discourse Beyond Country and Creed'. Lecture given at the Alwaleed Centre, University of Edinburgh, 6 December 2017.

[25] Fernando Vidal, *Les sciences de l'âme: XVIe–XVIIIe siècle* (Paris: Honoré Champion Editeur, 2006). Published in English as *The Sciences of the Soul: The Early Modern Origins of Psychology*, trans. Saskia Brown (Chicago: Chicago University Press, 2011). See also Mengal, *La naissance de la psychologie*.

[26] Vidal, *Les sciences de l'âme*, p. 78.

[27] Ibid., pp. 23–25, 339–342; Serjeantson, 'The Soul' pp. 119–141; Porter, *Flesh in the Age of Reason*, ch. 2; Michael, 'Renaissance Theorics', pp. 147–172; Angus Gowland, 'Melancholy, Passions, and Identity in the Renaissance', in Brian Cummings and Freya Sierhuis (eds.), *Passions and Subjectivity in Early Modern Culture* (Farnham: Ashgate, 2013), pp. 75–95.

with Latin Christian doctrine. These two conflicting views of the soul's relation to the 'flesh' – on the one hand, a marriage made in heaven, and on the other, a high-risk and hopefully temporary hostage situation – had always co-existed within Christianity.[28]

Reinstating a distinctively Augustinian soul/body dualism, England's post-Reformation divines had reopened the delicate 'seam between soul and body' which previous generations of Christian metaphysicians had taken pains to close.[29] Frenzy drew unwelcome attention to this seam, for whatever was susceptible to organic corruption was necessarily mortal. The traditional scholastic solution to this problem was to argue that what had been damaged by the disease was not the rational soul, but only its 'next instruments': the brain, nerves, and animal spirits. But it was also the rational soul's demonstrable independence from these instruments – in at least *one* of its operations – which was supposed to furnish proof of its immortality. To admit that a brain disease could put a stop to *all* of these operations – even the reason – was to scupper this proof.

The only alternative was to accept plural souls, and for most early modern Christians this was not a palatable idea. An orthodox Anglican, Willis chose it only for want of a better option. His anxiety about this uncharacteristic departure from the fold is evident in his dedication of *De anima brutorum* to Gilbert Sheldon, Archbishop of Canterbury: in claiming 'a Man (as the Mad-man in the Gospel possess't with a Legion) to be indued [endowed] with many distinct Souls' – he admitted – he had cause to 'fear the Censures of the Church'.[30] 'Altho I have a place of Safety, in that the Arguments and Reasons fight on my Side, and that I have got the Suffrages of the ancient Philosophers, and the holy Fathers', he wrote plaintively, 'yet suffer your Grace for my greater Safety, to extend your help to me'.[31] Willis need not have worried; he was never subjected to open censure by the Anglican establishment, although few readers openly endorsed his reinvention of pluralism.[32] Those who *did* subscribe to it found themselves obliged to continually redraw the boundary between the

[28] Caroline Walker Bynum, *The Resurrection of the Body in Western Christianity, 200–1336 CE* (New York: Columbia University Press, 1995); Caroline Walker Bynum, 'Why All the Fuss about the Body? A Medievalist's Perspective', *Critical Inquiry* 22(1) (1995), 1–33.

[29] Michel de Montaigne, 'De la force de l'imagination', in Pierre Villey and Verdun L. Saulnier (eds.), *Les Essais* (Paris: Presses Universitaires de France, 1992), 1.21, p. 104.

[30] Willis, *Two discourses*, sig. A2v. [31] Ibid.

[32] It did win a few converts; see, e.g., M. S., *A Philosophical Discourse of the Nature of Rational and Irrational Souls* (London, 1695); John Turner, *A phisico-theological discourse upon the Divine Being* (London, 1698), p. 53.

two souls of 'Man'.[33] In 1746, for example, Frings interrupted his *Treatise on phrensy* to remind his readers that he was discussing only 'the Sensitive Soul, not the Human Soul, which is not subject to Diseases'.[34] The possibility that the rational soul *was* harmed by frenzy was still unsettling enough to prompt fresh refutation. At the turn of the eighteenth century, the battle to save the immortal soul from the encroach of brain disease was very far from over.[35]

The Will

It was the debilitating effect of frenzy on the rational faculty known as the will which placed the disease at the centre of early modern assessments of moral and legal accountability. Medieval legal theorists had recognized that the degree to which these faculties were alienated could differ, and they had come up with a list of codified 'madness words' which could be used to locate sufferers on a gradated scale of culpability. Only those who were utterly bereaved of their mental faculties were to be counted innocent. Frenzy *could* confer this status, and it was used in several contexts to make a bid for absolution. The 'partially' mad, by contrast – those who suffered only from a 'distemper' or 'inconstancy' of mind – were denied a non compos mentis verdict. Whatever the nature of their illness, they were judged to have reason and will enough to be capable of crime. Those of them who killed themselves 'by the instigation of the devil' were guilty, for they had been able to understand his words, and had chosen to obey them.

What was true of Satanic temptation was not true of possession; a diabolic siege of the body (and by extension the sensitive soul) was understood to disable the will just as completely as a bout of frenzy.[36] In fact, these varying degrees of diabolic interference meshed perfectly with the degrees of madness set out by the common lawyers. The tempted were to blame for their actions; the possessed were not (not while the invading spirit remained in them). The witnesses to Collingwood's outburst had tried to save him by invoking 'frensie', but Collingwood himself had begged his innocence on account of his possession: the 'iniurious slaunderous & impious woords' which he had spoken 'he most seriously detesteth

[33] Willis, *Two discourses*, sig. A3v. [34] Frings, *A treatise on phrensy*, p. 50.
[35] For the continuation of these debates in the eighteenth century, see Thomson, *Bodies of Thought*.
[36] See David Harley, 'Explaining Salem: Calvinist Psychology and the Diagnosis of Possession', *American Historical Review* 101(2) (1996), 310–311.

and abhorreth from his hart: and thinketh he could never haue vttered them or the like, but being invaded & corporally possessed with a divell'.[37]

The same bid for innocence was made in 1592, by William Hacket's former 'prophet of judgment' Henry Arthington. As we saw in Chapter 6, the magistrate (and Cosin) had worked hard to establish the sanity of Hacket, Arthington, and their accomplices. Arthington, however, had friends in high places, and he was ultimately pardoned and released. His public apology, published as *The seduction of Arthington by Hacket* (1592), was carefully stage-managed by the Privy Council.[38] If Arthington was to be pardoned for treason, he needed to show that he had been non compos mentis at the time. But a plea of brainsickness was off the table; to allow it would have been to lend credence to the rumours of Hacket's frenzy.[39] Possession offered the only viable way out. Satan, working through Hacket, 'dyd my scenses for the tyme controll', Arthington claimed. He had 'had no power nor grace to resist, being sore bewitched and possest with his diuelish spirit, to be led like a drunkard which way he would'.[40] The message was clear: diabolic possession had immobilized Arthington's will as completely as any bout of natural frenzy would have done. Neither diagnosis was without stigma, but this was the price to be paid for innocence.

The Reason

Throughout this book, we have seen early modern writers visualize several different conceptual domains in the same way, as a top-down, hierarchical 'chain of being'. Both the human body and the soul were arranged in this order; Willis even saw its outlines in the anatomy of the brain. God had allotted each living being its rung on the 'ladder of nature', the noblest at the top and the humblest at the bottom. And he had intended human beings to govern themselves in the same way. These blueprints had been layered one on top of the other so often that – for early modern readers – the equivalences were intuitive. God, the head, the 'soul-in-chief', the human being, the husband, the father, and the prince all shared the same attributes: a superior reason, and the right to rule its inferiors which that faculty bestowed. The problem was that frenzy was just as capable of disabling this faculty in husbands, fathers, and princes as it was in anyone

[37] SP 14/26, f. 38r. [38] Walsham, '"Frantick Hacket"', p. 29.
[39] Williams, 'Exorcising Madness', pp. 30–52.
[40] Henry Arthington, *The seduction of Arthington by Hacket especiallie with some tokens of his vnfained repentance and submission* (London, 1592), sigs. E2r, K2r.

else. It could leave a household or a nation functionally 'headless', and this – for many – was a terrifying prospect. At the level of the household, it left its functioning members short on income, labour, time, and legal and social capital. And yet, as we saw in Chapter 5, it was the frenzy of subjects – and especially of women – which seems to have disturbed observers the most. A frantic husband left his family without a ruler, but a frantic wife showed the world that her husband had failed to maintain 'rule'.

At the level of the nation, a mad prince could be counted on to cause political instability (England was spared from this fate until the reign of George III, but other European monarchies were not).[41] Yet it was precisely the hypothetical scenario of the frantic father (or captain) which, in the sixteenth century, allowed Protestant resistance theorists to develop a justification for what was otherwise unthinkable: the overthrow of an anointed monarch. For Knox, a queen who had become deaf to the voice of God had also become deaf to the voice of reason, and could not therefore be trusted to act in the best interests of her subjects. In 1643, William Prynne resurrected the same allegory to justify the parliamentarians' revolt against Charles I. Unfortunately, as Prynne would soon learn, it was easier to tell the story than to contain its meanings. What for him had served as a limited justification of 'self-defence' was soon repurposed to justify something else entirely. For Goodwin, it was the leaders of the New Model Army whose rational faculties remained intact (and who had thereby acquired the right to rule). If they also happened to possess the strength to overpower a few 'frantique Parliament-men', this was simply a coincidence (or rather, a provision of Providence). But not everyone was convinced by this happy convergence of sanity and firepower. What Goodwin called 'Might and right well met', his critics called 'might overcoming right'.[42]

To be classed as irrational was to be transformed from a ruler – of oneself, of one's property, of one's inferiors – into a subject in need of rule. For a monarch, the fall was especially precipitous, but the effects were devastating no matter how humble the sufferer's status. Given no solid

[41] In 1562, for example, Elizabeth I's ambassador to Spain received the news that Philip II's eldest son and heir apparent, Don Carlos, was showing signs of taking after his 'phreneticall' great-grandmother. Thomas Challoner to Elizabeth I, 11 May 1562, draft copy. SP 70/37 f.75v. For German examples, H. C. Erik Midelfort, *Mad Princes of Renaissance Germany* (Charlottesville: University of Virginia Press, 1994).

[42] Goodwin, *Right and Might Well Met*; Geree, *Katadynastēs: might overcoming right.*

food for days on end, James Carkesse felt 'reduce[d] . . . again to a *Child*'.[43] The relatives of Thomas Sagar – once a dutiful husband, father, son-in-law, and schoolmaster – had resorted to chaining him up in an outhouse. Arthur Coga was recruited as an experimental subject, not just because it was hoped that blood transfusion would cure his frenzy, but because the death of 'a frantic man' seemed like less of a tragedy than the alternative.[44] This was a period in which the faculty of reason was widely seen as humanity's finest possession. For a human being, created only a little lower than the angels, to live without it was to be truly pitiable.[45]

Sometimes, of course, humiliation was exactly what the Almighty had in mind. If 'god calls out to be his souldiers in some personal conflicts of a strange nature', Heywood ventured, 'not only to fight against principalitys and powers but . . . with beastly passions, imaginations, astonishing phrenzys . . . [it is] to teach them humility, self-denyall and with restored Nebuchadnezzar an holy awe and reverence of the great god'.[46] Heywood had watched frenzy claim the lives of Joshua Bates, Mercy Stocks, and others in his community, but he had also seen some survive the disease.[47] He seems to have found God's purposes easier to discern in the recoveries than in the deaths. Like Nebuchadnezzar, these individuals were being subjected to the 'correction' of a loving father. He had taken away their reason in order to demonstrate their utter helplessness and wretchedness without it. Leaving them at the mercy of their own 'beastly passions' and 'imaginations' gave them a taste of what it was like to live as a beast. The humiliating nature of the experience was a check to vainglory, and a lesson in how to 'improue that talent [the gift of reason] to gods glory'. This was the rationale given for all such 'corrective' measures: hard rule was supposed to remind sufferers of their lost rationality.

Heywood was not the only divine who seems to have prized the return of a sufferer's reason more highly than her bodily recovery. When the 'phrentick daughter' of one of Napier's clients died a week after jumping 'out of a window to breake her necke', he still found cause to thank God:

43 Carkesse, *Lucida intervalla*, p. 14.

44 Anthropologists use the term 'social death' to describe this diminishment of value. See Dana Walrath, *Aliceheimer's: Alzheimer's Through the Looking Glass* (University Park: Penn State University Press, 2016), pp. 4–5; Jana Králová and Tony Walter (eds.), *Social Death: Questioning the Life–Death Boundary* (London: Routledge, 2017).

45 The definition of 'man' as a 'rational animal' was a scholastic commonplace, based on Aristotle's writings but not coined by him. See Christian Kietzmann, 'Aristotle on the Definition of What It Is to Be Human', in Geert Keil and Nora Kreft (eds.), *Aristotle's Anthropology* (Cambridge: Cambridge University Press, 2019), pp. 25–43.

46 Heywood, 'Objects and Observations', p. 33.

47 Ibid., pp. 31–32.

she 'dyed coming to her wits by gods grace', he wrote, 'and well in memory, the lords name be blessed for it'.[48] The return of the young woman's wits was a gift from God, one perhaps more precious than her bodily survival. Neither Napier nor Heywood said as much, but others did. In 1682, Richard Baxter's anonymous correspondent declared that a truly rational soul would prefer to 'desert its being' than 'degrade its self by . . . bruitish acts'. Although 'death (before due time)' was a terrible prospect, the physician John Archer reflected in 1673, 'Distraction or Madness' was 'worse then death while they live'.[49] If these comments sound callous, it is worth remembering that their authors expected a full restoration of all such persons to their right wits after death. Frenzy was a horrible prospect because – for as long as it lasted – it shrouded the 'image of God' in darkness. But 'when these black clouds are blown over . . . their understanding returnes', Heywood reassured his readers. If the clouds did not blow over in this life, they would in the next.

Whether or not Heywood and Archer meant well, their comments remind us that 'personhood' was never fashioned, found, lost, or regained by the individual sufferer alone. Sometimes frantic people *did* intuit that something had changed in them, and not for the better. Of his 'frentick' patient Ferdinando Burgess, Napier wrote, '[he] sayeth I hope I shal doe well & is there noe good man that can helpe me'. Yet, in practice, it was rarely individual sufferers who decided when the essential attributes of human personhood – reason, understanding, and will – had left them. Nor was it the sufferers who decided when the associated prerogatives of personhood – the right to self-rule, to manage one's affairs, to make a will – needed to be taken away. As the anthropologists Sharon Kaufman and Lynn Morgan have put it, 'producing persons is an inherently social project'.[50] Nowhere was this more evident in early modern England than in the conferral of a frenzy diagnosis.

Personhood

How far frenzy altered the subjective experience of 'being an *I* or having a self' must ultimately remain guesswork; I have yet to find a single first-person account written by a self-diagnosed sufferer.[51] What *is* clear is that

48 Kassell et al., *Casebooks*, cases 37423, 37424, 37425.

49 John Archer, *Every Man his Own Doctor, Compleated with an Herbal* (London, 1673), p. 120.

50 Sharon R. Kaufman and Lynn M. Morgan, 'The Anthropology of the Beginnings and Ends of Life', *Annual Review of Anthropology* 34 (2005), 320.

51 Vidal and Ortega, *Being Brains*, p. 25.

it mattered to personhood, in the sense intended by Kaufman and Morgan. This book has suggested that, despite never having had the pleasure of reading John Locke, most of the inhabitants of sixteenth- and seventeenth-century England *did* equate personhood with 'memory, consciousness, and self-awareness'.[52] Nowhere is this more apparent than in their reactions to the unexpected alteration or loss of these faculties in others. It is apparent, for example, in their reactions to the disorders of memory wrought by frenzy. The prospect of memory loss troubled philosophers and divines much less than the loss of the reason; for them, the memory was an organ-bound, sensitive faculty, and as such its impairment posed no threat to the rational soul. But this did not mean that it was not vital to personhood. Sir Thomas More reported with satisfaction that the recipient of his beating had 'gathered hys remembraunce to him, and begann to come agayne to hym selfe'.[53] Memory was important enough to common lawyers that they were content to let it stand in for all the other mental faculties; to call a person *non sanae memoriae* was to call him or her non compos mentis. The fact that, soon after his fit, Francis Collingwood was capable of 'remembering most things past' was proof that his frenzy was 'counterfeit'.[54] It mattered to Napier that Elizabeth Piddington was capable of 'remember[ing] when she has done evil'.[55] He mourned that one of his frantic patients had 'lost her remembrance', and praised God that another had been 'well in memory' before her death.[56] Continuity of memory was constitutive of legal, social, and spiritual personhood at the turn of the sixteenth century, just as it would be at the turn of the eighteenth.

Nor were the witnesses of frenzy untroubled by the changes which frenzy wrought to 'consciousness' and 'self-awareness' (they did not use the latter term, but then nor did their eighteenth-century successors). Nonetheless, the rational soul's awareness of its own existence was continually cited as a proof of its uniqueness. The same God which 'gave me eyes the world to view', Sir John Davies reflected, 'To view my selfe, enfus'd an inward light,/Whereby my Soule, as by a Mirror true,/Of her owne forme may take a perfect sight'.[57] For the unlearned, the loss of these kinds of awareness was signified more simply: frantic people were 'senseless', out of their 'wits' and 'senses'. When she first fell sick in 1632, Napier's patient Anne Bosworth 'her selfe did send & was then in

[52] Ibid. [53] More, *The apologye of syr Thomas More knyghte*, ff. 197r–198v.
[54] SP 14/26, f. 36r. [55] Kassell et al., *Casebooks*, case 41459. [56] Ibid., cases 37425, 40373.
[57] Davies, *Nosce teipsum*, p. 9.

her sences yet crazed'; three days later she was simply 'frentick. Senseless'.[58] Ferdinando Burgess was 'prating he knoweth not what'; Mercy Fish's fits made 'her to talk she knoweth not what'.[59] This refrain recurs often, and (given that Napier often consulted by letter) it is safe to conclude that sometimes it was a paraphrase of a caregiver's report. That the sufferer no longer knew what she was saying or doing *mattered* to onlookers, and not just in situations which called for an assessment of culpability.

The inhabitants of early modern England were unsettled by frenzy, above all, because of the way it changed the people whom they knew and loved. Elizabeth Allen had been 'a good woman [who] hated cursing & swearing all her life'; in her distracted state, Napier wrote, she 'rageth & curseth & sweareth. which she could neaver abyd'.[60] Heywood, too, was appalled that Joshua Bates had sworn 'many dreadful oaths, which he never did in all his life'. Hearing Mercy Stocks's 'shameful words', her neighbours 'wondred at her, where she should learn them'.[61] All the familiar signs by which individuals made themselves known – their words, looks, customs, conduct, carriage, voice – were suddenly and inexplicably altered, and not for the better. Frenzy was terrifying not just because it killed its sufferers, but because it laid bare the fragility of personhood. The decline of the immortal Christian 'soul' and the rise of the Lockean 'person' no doubt did change what it meant to be a human being (at least, among the lettered elites of 'Western modernity'). Yet there are elements of the story of early modern frenzy which, I would argue, are not best understood by setting up a gulf between then and now. This was a brain disease which made its sufferers 'enraged . . . with those whom previously [they] had most loved'.[62] It made them strangers to those who knew them best.

58 Kassell et al., *Casebooks*, cases 74761, 74801.
59 Ibid., cases 52403, 66415.
60 Ibid., case 61877.
61 Heywood, 'Objects and Observations', and 'Returns of Prayer', in Turner (ed.), *Autobiography*, vol. 4, pp. 31, 161.
62 Hall, 'Curationum', p. 142.

Select Bibliography

PRIMARY SOURCES

Manuscripts

Cambridge, King's College Library

King's MS 16 (fifteenth-century manuscript of the *Tabula medicine*, purchased by Simon Forman in 1574).

Huntingdon, Huntingdonshire Archives

HP82/9/1, f. 52v. (Great Staunton Constables' Accounts, 1690/1).

Kew, The National Archives

C 1/94/22 (Chancery proceedings, William Grene versus William Capell, c. 1486–1493).

C 1/1344/51 (Chancery proceedings, John Cowper versus Thomas Fullwood, 1553–1555).

KB 9 (Coroners' reports submitted to the Court of King's Bench).

KB 29 (Court of King's Bench controlment rolls, summarising findings of coroners' inquests).

PC 2/13, f. 306v. (Order regarding William Williams, 13 February 1580).

PC 2/29, ff. 187r, 213r. (Orders regarding William Ellis, November 1617).

REQ 2/84/12 (Court of Requests, bill of complaint of Simon Springold and Robert Lemying, 1560).

SP 12/163, f. 16r ('Examination of John Somerfeld (or Somervyle) in the Tower', 6 October 1583).

SP 12/163, ff. 54–57r (Interrogatories and depositions relating to John Somerfeld, 28 October 1583).

SP 12/163, f. 125r ('A memorial for the Queen's Majesty's learned Counsel, appointed to examine John Somerfeld's wife, sister, and servants', 5 November 1583).

SP 12/163, f. 129r ('Resolution of the Council for a commission of Oyer and Terminer for the trial of John Somerfeld and examination of the prisoners', 5 November 1583).

SP 12/163, f. 137r ('Attorney General Popham to Walsyngham', 7 November 1583).

SP 12/194, f. 87r ('Arthur Herrys to Lord Chancellor Bromley, touching certain indecent speeches uttered by John Whyte, alias Snellyng, a shoe-maker of Rayleigh, in Essex', 22 October 1587).

SP 12/239, ff. 123r–124r (Report on William Stanley, 'Thos. Phelippes to Saint Mains?', 19 July 1591).

SP 14/26, ff. 36r–42r. (Thomas Bilson, Bishop of Winchester, to Robert Cecil, Earl of Salisbury, regarding Francis Collingwood, 22 January 1606/7).

SP 16/379, f. 176r (Assessment of Richard Farnham by Bethlem physician, 'Order of Council', 26 January 1637/38).

SP 16/397, f. 151r (Order for transferral of Richard Farnham from Bethlem to Bridewell, 29 August 1638).

SP 16/434A, f. 31v (Commitment of James Hunt to Bridewell, 1639/40).

SP 29/382, f. 159r–v. (Letter from John Griffes of Birmingham to Charles II, 1676).

SP 29/435, ff. 166–169. ('Report of the speech of William Williams, Recorder of Chester, 1683).

SP 52/52, pp. 159–161 ('Queen Elizabeth to James VI', March 1596/97).

SP 52/59, f. 71r ('Mr. David Black's declaration to the King and Council of Scotland', 22 November 1596).

SP 70/37 ff. 70r–81r. (Thomas Challoner to Elizabeth I, draft copy, 11 May 1562).

SP 84/13, ff. 80r–81r ('Edward Burnham to Walsingham', 7 March 1587).

STAC 5/A24/21 (Star Chamber proceedings, Queen's Almoner versus Edmund Brice, October 1591).

STAC 8/3/14 (Star Chamber proceedings, King's Almoner versus Thomas Crompton, November 1624).

London, British Library

Add MS 5476 (Orders relating to Thomas Yemans and Richard Cheeseman, 1545–1546).

Cotton MS Caligula C/VIII, ff. 660r–v. ('The contentes of the discourse made by Mr. Walter Lindsay of Balgas', 1586).

Lansdowne MS 16/84 ('A narrative of the frantic behaviour of Peter Burchett', 16 October 1573).

Lansdowne MS 17/88 ('Peter Byrchett's case stated by himself', 27 October, 1573).

Lansdowne MS 99/3 ('Two letters of one Roger Edwardes, a religious madman, to Lord Burghley', May 1579).

Lansdowne MS 99/6 ('Miles Fry, a madman (who calls himself Emanuel Plantagenet), to Lord Burghley', 28 June 1587).
Lansdowne MS 99/9 ('Robert Dickons, a distracted Glover, requests of the Queen that he may preach repentance', 1588).
Lansdowne MS 99/13 ('One Johnson, a frantic person, tells Lord Burghley he is a nobleman born, and desires his interest with the Queen in his favour', 1591).
Lansdowne MS 99/21 ('An information of a distracted Frenchman, discovering (as he pretends) thirty treasons against the Queen', c. 1570–1597).
Sloane MS 65 (Collection of medical treatises and recipes, 1633–1651).
Sloane MS 640 (Collection of medical treatises and recipes, fourteenth–eighteenth centuries).
Sloane MS 2550 (Simon Forman, 'The groundes of physique and chirurgerie', c. 1589).

London, Lambeth Palace Library

CM XII/16 (High Commission proceedings against David Black, 9 November 1584).

London, Royal College of Physicians

MS 4143, f. 149r. (Complaint about Simon Forman, *Annals*, 25 June 1601).

London, Royal Society

CLP/12i/12 (Edmond King, 'A method of transfusing bloud into men', 1667).
RBO/3/58 (Edmond King, 'A Further Account Of some Experiments of Transfusion made by Dr King at his house', 1667).
RB/1/8/30, ff. 208–209. (Robert Boyle's list of scientific projects/desiderata, also known as his 'wish list').

Norwich, Norfolk Record Office

NCR 18d/13 (Norwich Hamper Accounts 1550–1601).

Oxford, Bodleian Library

MS Ashmole 175 (Richard Napier's casebooks, vol. 1, 26 January–6 September 1596).
MS Ashmole 182 (Richard Napier's casebooks, vol. 2, 13 February 1597–16 July 1598).
MS Ashmole 196 (Richard Napier's casebooks, vol. 24, 19 April 1615–7 August 1616).
MS Ashmole 200 (Richard Napier's casebooks, vol. 20, 12 January 1611–18 February 1612).
MS Ashmole 208 (Simon Forman, alchemical notebook XII, c. 1585–1598).

MS Ashmole 214 (Richard Napier's casebooks, vol. 52, 11 September 1632–3 April 1633).
MS Ashmole 231 (Richard Napier's casebooks, vol. 34, 1 June 1621–19 February 1622).
MS Ashmole 233 (Richard Napier's casebooks, vol. 33, 3 November 1620–31 May 1621).
MS Ashmole 240, ff. 104r–v (Letter from Simon Forman to Richard Napier, undated, 1599–1611).
MS Ashmole 355 (Simon Forman, 'Liber juditiorum morborum', 1600).
MS Ashmole 389 (Simon Forman, 'The astrologicalle judgmentes of phisick and other questions', 1606, with later additions).
MS Ashmole 404 (Richard Napier's casebooks, vol. 5, 2 January 1601–8 March 1602).
MS Ashmole 405 (Richard Napier's casebooks, vol. 44, 25 April–7 December 1628).
MS Ashmole 1429 (Medical compendium owned by Simon Forman, inscribed 'September 1611 Docter Formans booke reserved for the use of Clement his sonne').
MS Ashmole 1495 (Simon Forman, 'The grounds of arte gathered out of diverse authors', 1594–1595).

Preston, Lancashire Archives

DDKE/Box 122/1 (Memorandum book, 'Memorandum of the arraignment, at Newgate, of William Hacket, of Northamptonshire, for high treason', 1591).
QSB/1/245/55 ('The humble peticion of Margerie Sagar wiffe of Thomas Sagr [sic]', 1641).
QSP 144/19 ('The humble petition of Ellin Faukner of Manchester widdowe', 1657).

Printed Books

A., B. *The sick-mans rare jewel.* London, 1674.
Abercrombie, John. *Pathological and Practical Researches on Diseases of the Brain and Spinal Cord.* Edinburgh, 1828.
Acton, George. *Physical Reflections upon a Letter… Concerning a New way of Curing sundry Diseases by Transfusion of Blood.* London, 1668.
Adams, Thomas. *The deuills banket described in foure sermons.* London, 1614.
Englands sicknes, comparatively conferred with Israels. London, 1615.
Mystical bedlam, or the vvorld of mad-men. London, 1615.
Diseases of the sovle: a discovrse diuine, morall, and physicall. London, 1616.
A divine herball together with a forrest of thornes. In five sermons. London, 1616.
The happines of the Church. Or, a description of those spirituall prerogatiues vvherewith Christ hath endowed her. London, 1619.

Ainsworth, Henry. *The communion of saincts. A treatise of the fellowship that the faithful have with God, and his angels, and one with an other; in this present life.* Amsterdam, 1607.

Allen, Hannah. *A narrative of God's gracious dealings with that choice Christian Mrs Hannah Allen.* London, 1683.

Allen, William. *A true, sincere and modest defence, of English Catholiques that suffer for their faith both at home and abrode against a false, seditious and slanderous libel intituled; The exectuion of iustice in England.* Rouen, 1584.

Allwyn, Robert. *The oyle of gladnesse: or, Musicke at the house of mourning.* London, 1631.

Andrewes, Lancelot. *XCVI. sermons by the Right Honorable and Reverend Father in God, Lancelot Andrevves, late Lord Bishop of Winchester. Published by His Majesties speciall command.* London, 1629.

Anglicus, Bartholomaeus. *De proprietatibus rerum.* London, 1495.

Bertholomeus De proprietatibus rerum. London, 1535.

Batman vppon Bartholome, his booke De proprietatibus rerum, newly corrected, enlarged and amended, trans. Stephen Bateman. London, 1582.

Anglicus, Gilbertus. *Compendium medicinae.* Lyon, 1510.

[Anon.] *Prognosticacion, drawen out of the bookes of Ipocras, Auicen, and other notable auctours of physycke. . .* London, 1545.

[Anon.] *Certayne sermons appoynted by the Quenes Maiestie.* London, 1559.

[Anon.] *Articles to be enquired in the visitation, in the firste yere of the raigne of our moste dread soueraigne lady, Elizabeth by the grace of God, of Englande, Fraunce, and Irelande, Queene, defendour of the faith. &c. Anno. 1559.* London, 1562.

[Anon.] *A gagge for the Pope, and the Iesuits: or The arraignement, and execution of Antichrist Shevving plainely, that Antichrist shall be discouered, and punished in this vvorld: to the amasement of all obstinate papists.* London, 1624.

[Anon.] *A warning for England especially for London in the famous history of the frantick Anabaptists their wild preachings & practises in Germany.* London, 1642.

[Anon.] *The world is turned upside down.* London, 1646.

[Anon.] *The downfall of the Fifth Monarchy.* London, 1657.

[Anon.] *Metamorphosis Anglorum, or reflections historical and political, upon the late changes of government in England, from the death of Oliver Lord Protector, to the last dissolution of the Parliament.* London, 1660.

[Anon.] 'A Letter Written by an Intelligent and Worthy English Man from Paris, to a Considerable Member of the R. Society in London, concerning some Transactions there, relating to the Experiment of the Transfusion of Blood'. *Philosophical Transactions* 4(54) (13 December 1669), 1075–1076.

[Anon.] *Documents Relating to the University and Colleges of Cambridge.* 3 vols. London, 1852.

Aquinas, Thomas. *Summa theologiae: Pars prima.* Venice, 1477.

Archer, John. *Every Man his Own Doctor, Compleated with an Herbal. . .* London, 1673.

Arthington, Henry. *The seduction of Arthington by Hacket especiallie with some tokens of his vnfained repentance and submission.* London, 1592.

Asseline, Eustache [Eustachius à Sancto Paulo]. *Tertia Pars Summae Philosophicae Quae est Phsica, De rebus Naturalibus, in tres partes divisa.* Cambridge, 1648.

Avicenna [Ibn Sīnā]. *al-Qānūn fī l-ṭibb*, in Giovanni Costeo and Giovanni Paulo Mongio (eds.), *Avicennae Arabum medicorum principis...*[*Canon Medicinae*]. Venice, 1595.

al-Qānūn fī l-ṭibb, in Pierre Vattier (ed.), *Abugalii filii sinae, sive, ut vulgo dicitur, Avicennae, Philosophorum ac Medicorum Arabum Principis, De Morbis Mentis Tractatus*. Paris, 1659.

Bacon, Francis. *The tvvoo bookes of Francis Bacon. Of the proficience and aduancement of learning, diuine and humane. To the King.* London, 1605.

De dignitate et augmentis scientarium. London, 1638.

Bale, John. *The laboryouse iourney [and] serche of Iohan Leylande, for Englandes antiquitees geuen of hym as a newe yeares gyfte to Kynge Henry the viij. in the. xxxvij. yeare of his reygne, with declaracyons enlarged.* London, 1549.

Ball, Robert. *The mirror of pure devotion: or, The discovery of hypocrisie.* London, 1635.

Banister, Richard. *A treatise of one hundred and thirteene diseases of the eyes, and eye-liddes.* London, 1622.

Barrough, Philip. *The methode of phisicke, conteyning the causes, signes, and cures of invvard diseases in mans body from the head to the foote*. London, 1583.

Bartas, Guillaume du. *La sepmaine, ou creation du monde.* Antwerp, 1579.

Du Bartas his deuine weekes and workes, trans. Josuah Sylvester. London, 1611.

Bartholin, Thomas. *De morbis biblicis miscellanea medica*. Frankfurt, 1672.

Bartholin, Thomas, and Johann Heinrich Meibom. *De usu flagrorum in re medica & veneria.* Frankfurt, 1669.

A treatise of the use of flogging in venerial affairs... made English from the Latin original by a physician. London, 1801.

Bayfield, Robert. *Enchiridion Medicum*. London, 1655.

Tes iatrikes kartos, or, A treatise de morborum capitis essentiis & pronosticis adorned with above three hundred choice and rare observations... London, 1663.

Bayle, Pierre. *Dictionnaire historique et critique*. 2 vols. Rotterdam, 1697.

Baynes, Paul. *A letter written by Mr. Paul Bayne, minister of Gods word, lately deceased.* London, 1617.

A helpe to true happinesse. Or A briefe and learned exposition of the maine and fundamentall points of Christian religion. London, 1618.

Baxter, Richard. *The nature and immortality of the soul proved in answer to one who professed perplexing doubtfulness*. London, 1682.

Beard, Thomas. *The theatre of Gods iudgements: or, a collection of histories out of sacred, ecclesiasticall, and prophane authours concerning the admirable iudgements of God vpon the transgressours of his commandements.* London, 1597.

Birch, Thomas. *The History of the Royal Society of London*. 4 vols. London, 1756.

Blount, Thomas. *Glossographia: Or, A Dictionary.* London, 1659.

Boorde, Andrew. *The breuiarie of health*. London, 1587.

Boyle, Robert. *Some considerations touching the vsefulnesse of experimental naturall philosophy*. Oxford, 1663.

'Tryals proposed by Mr. Boyle to Dr. Lower, to be made by him, for the Improvement of the Experiment of Transfusing Blood out of one live Animal into another'. *Philosophical Transactions* 1(22) (11 February 1666), 385–388.

Buchanan, George. *Rervm Scoticarvm historia... Accessit De ivre regni apud Scotus Dialogus*. Edinburgh, 1583.

King, Edmund. 'King to Boyle, 25 November 1667', in Thomas Birch (ed.), *The Works of the Honourable Robert Boyle*, vol. 6. 5 vols. London, 1772.

Bright, Timothy. *A treatise of melancholie*. London, 1586.

Brown, John. *A compleat discourse of wounds*. London, 1678.

Browne, Sir Thomas. *Religio Medici*. London, 1642.

Bruele, Gualtherus. *Praxis medicinae, or, the physicians practice*. London, 1632.

Brunfels, Otto. *Iatrionices medicamentorum simplicium*. Strasbourg, 1533.

Brydall, John. *Non Compos Mentis, or the Law Relating to Natural Fooles, Mad-Folks, and Lunatic Persons*. London, 1700.

Bryskett, Lodowick. *A discourse of ciuill life containing the ethike part of morall philosophie*. London, 1606.

Burton, Robert. *The anatomy of melancholy*. Oxford, 1621.

Calvin, John. *Institutio Christianae Religionis*. Geneva, 1559.

The institution of Christian religion, vvrytten in Latine by maister Ihon Caluin, and translated into Englysh..., trans. Thomas Norton. London, 1561.

Camden, William. *Annales rerum Anglicarum, et Hibernicarum, regnante Elizabetha, ad annum salutis M.D. LXXXIX*. London, 1615.

Carkesse, James. *Lucida intervalla*. London, 1679.

Carpi, Berengario da. *Tractatus de fractura calue siue cranei*. Leiden, 1629.

Casaubon, Meric. *A treatise concerning enthusiasme, as it is an effect of nature: but is mistaken by many for either divine inspiration, or diabolical possession*. London, 1654.

Cawdrey, Robert. *A treasurie or store-house of similies both pleasaunt, delightfull, and profitable, for all estates of men in generall*. London, 1600.

Cecil, William. *The execution of iustice in England for maintenaunce of publique and Christian peace*. London, 1583.

Charleton, Walter. *Two discourses. I. Concerning the different wits of men: II. Of the mysterie of vintners*. London, 1669.

Cogan, Thomas. *The hauen of health*. London, 1636.

Coke, Edward. *The third part of the Institutes of the laws of England concerning high treason, and other pleas of the crown, and criminall causes*. London, 1644.

The first part of the Institvtes of the laws of England, or, A commentarie upon Littleton. London, 1656.

Copley, Anthony. *Another letter of Mr. A.C. to his dis-Iesuited kinseman*. London, 1602.

Cosin, Richard. *Conspiracie, for pretended reformation: viz. presbyteriall discipline*. London, 1592.

Cullen, William. *Lectures on the Materia Medica*, 2nd ed. Dublin, 1781.

Synopsis nosologiae methodicae. Ticino, 1787.
Dalton, Michael. *The countrey justice*. London, 1619.
Davies, Sir John. *Nosce teipsum*. London, 1599.
Denis, Jean-Baptiste. 'An Extract of a Letter, written by J. Denis, Doctor of Physick, and Professor of Philosophy and the Mathematicks at Paris, touching a late Cure of an Inveterate Phrensy by the Transfusion of Bloud'. *Philosophical Transactions* 2(32) (10 February 1668), 617–624.
Descartes, René. *Discours de la méthode pour bien conduire sa raison et chercher la vérité dans les sciences*. Leiden, 1637.
Meditationes de Prima Philosophia. Paris, 1641.
Principia philosophiae. Amsterdam, 1644.
Dixon, Robert. *The doctrine of faith, justification, and assurance*. London, 1668.
Downame, John. *The second part of The Christian warfare; or the contempt of the world*. London, 1611.
A guide to godlynesse or a Treatise of a Christian life. London, 1622.
Drant, Thomas. *The royall guest: or, A sermon preached at Lent Assises*. London, 1637.
Dyke, Daniel. *The mystery of selfe-deceiuing*. London, 1614.
Featley, Daniel. *Clavis mystica: a key opening divers difficult and mysterious texts of Holy Scripture*. London, 1636.
Featley, John. *Obedience and submission*. London, 1636.
Fenner, William. *A treatise of the affections, or, The souls pulse whereby a Christian may know whether he be living or dying*. London, 1642.
Ficino, Marsilio. *Marsilii Ficini... de vita libri tres*. Lyon, 1560.
Foxe, John. *Actes and monuments of these latter and perillous dayes, touching matters of the Church... by Iohn Foxe*. London, 1563.
The first volume of the ecclesiasticall history contaynyng the actes and monumentes of thynges passed in euery kynges tyme in this realme, especially in the Church of England principally to be noted. London, 1570.
The first volume of the ecclesiasticall history... London, 1576.
Actes and monuments... London, 1583.
Frings, Peter. *A treatise on phrensy: wherein the cause of that disorder, as assigned by the galenists, is refuted; And their method of curing the phrensy, with their various prescriptions at large, are exploded*. London, 1746.
Fuller, Thomas. *The holy state*. Cambridge, 1642.
The church-history of Britain from the birth of Jesus Christ until the year M.DC.XLVIII endeavoured by Thomas Fuller. London, 1655.
Gassendi, Pierre. *Opera Omnia*. Lyon, 1658.
Geminus, John. *A table instructiue whan and how a man may co[n]nyngly let bloude of all the necessary veynes of mans body very profitable for all chirurgeons and barbers*. London, 1546.
Geree, John. *Katadynastēs: might overcoming right. Or a cleer answer to M. John Goodwin's Might and right well met*. London, 1649.
Gifford, George. *A godlie, zealous, and profitable sermon vpon the second chapter of Saint Iames*. London, 1582.

Good, John Mason. *A Physiological System of Nosology, With a Corrected and Simplified Nomenclature*. London, 1817.
Goodwin, John. *Innocencies triumph*. London, 1644.
Calumny arraign'd. London, 1645.
Right and Might Well Met. London, 1648.
Gordon, Bernard de. *Opus lilium medicinae*. Lyon, 1559.
Hale, Matthew. *Historia placitorum coronae*, vol. 1. 2 vols. London, 1736.
Hall, John. *Select observations on English bodies*, trans. James Cooke. London, 1657.
Hall, Joseph. *The balm of Gilead*. London, 1646.
Hall, Thomas, *The pulpit guarded with XVII arguments proving the unlawfulness, sinfulness and danger of suffering private persons to take upon them publike preaching, and expounding the Scriptures without a call*. London, 1651.
Hammond, Henry. *Of resisting the lawfull magistrate under colour of religion*. Oxford, 1644.
Hart, James. *Klinike, or The diet of the diseased*. London, 1633.
Helmont, Franciscus Mercurius van. *The Spirit of Diseases; or, Diseases from the Spirit*. London, 1694.
Herring, Francis. *The anatomyes of the true physition and counterfeit mounte-banke*. London, 1602.
Heurne, Johan van. *De morbis humani capitis*. Leiden, 1594.
Heywood, Thomas. *True discourse of the two infamous upstart prophets, Richard Farnham weaver of White-Chappell, and John Bull weaver of Saint Butolphs Algate, now prisoners, the one in Newgate, and the other in Bridewell*. London, 1636.
Hobbes, Thomas. *Leviathan, or, The matter, forme, and power of a common wealth, ecclesiasticall and civil*. London, 1651.
Holland, Guy. *The grand prerogative of humane nature namely, the souls naturall or native immortality*. London, 1653.
Hooker, Thomas. *The immortality of mans soule, proved both by scripture and reason contrary to the fancie of R.O. in his book intituled Mans mortality*. London, 1645.
Huarte, de San Juan. *Examen de ingenios: The examination of mens vvits*. London, 1594.
Johnston, Nathaniel. *The excellency of monarchical government, especially of the English monarchy*. London, 1686.
Jonstonus, Joannes. *Idea universae medicinae practicae*. Amsterdam, 1648.
The idea of practical physick in twelve books. London, 1657.
Knox, John. *The history of the reformation of religioun within the realme of Scotland*. London, 1587.
The historie of the reformation of the Church of Scotland. London, 1644.
Langham, William. *The garden of health, conteyning the sundry rare and hidden vertues and properties of all kindes of simples and plants*. London, 1597.
Langton, Christopher. *An introduction into phisycke, wyth an vniuersal dyet, gathered by Christofer Langton*. London, 1545.

Layton, Henry. *Observations upon a sermon intituled, A confutation of atheism from the faculties of the soul, alias, Matter and motion cannot think*. London, 1692.
Observations upon a short treatise, written by Mr. Timothy Manlove: Intituled, The Immortality of the Soul Asserted. London, 1697.
Lemnius, Levinus. *The touchstone of complexions*, trans. Thomas Newton. London, 1581.
Locke, John. *An Essay Concerning Humane Understanding... In Four Books*. London, 1689.
Lowe, Peter. *The whole course of chirurgerie*. London, 1597.
[Lower, Richard]. 'The Method observed in Transfusing the Bloud out of one live Animal into Another'. *Philosophical Transactions* 1(20) (17 December 1666), 353–358.
Tractatus de corde. London, 1669.
M., E. *Protection perswading subjection: or A word of peace to the well-affected*. London, 1654.
Mackenzie, George. *The laws and customes of Scotland, in matters criminal*. Edinburgh, 1678.
Maplet, John. *A greene forest, or A naturall historie*. London, 1567.
McMath, James. *The expert mid-wife a treatise of the diseases of women with child, and in child-bed*. Edinburgh, 1694.
Melanchthon, Philip. *Commentarius de anima*. Wittenberg, 1548.
More, Thomas. *The apologye of syr Thomas More knyghte*. London, 1533.
More, Henry. *The immortality of the soul, so farre forth as it is demonstrable from the knowledge of nature and the light of reason*. London, 1659.
'Enthusiasmus Triumphatus', in *A collection of several philosophical writings of Dr Henry More*. London, 1662.
Divine dialogues containing sundry disquisitions & instructions concerning the attributes and providence of God. London, 1668.
Nichols, Josias. *The plea of the innocent: wherein is auerred; that the ministers & people falslie termed puritanes, are iniuriouslie slaundered for enemies or troublers of the state*. London, 1602.
[Oldenburg, Henry]. 'An Account of an easier and safer Way of Transfusing Blood out of one Animal into another'. *Philosophical Transactions* 2(25) (1667), 449–451.
'An Account of the Experiment of Transfusion, practised upon a Man in London'. *Philosophical Transactions* 2(30) (1667), 557–559.
'An Account of more Tryals of Transfusion'. *Philosophical Transactions* 2(28) (1667), 517–525.
Ontijd, Conrad George. *A treatise on mortal diseases*. London, 1798.
Overton, Richard. *Mans mortalitie*. London, 1643.
[Oxenbridge, Daniel]. *General Observations and prescriptions in the practice of physick on several persons of quality, &c. By an eminent London Physician, who was contemporary with Dr. Gifford, Dr. Ridgely, etc*. London, 1715.
Paré, Ambrose. *Les Oeuvres d'Ambroise Paré, conseiller et premier chirurgien du roy*. Paris, 1575.

Opera Ambrosii Parei, regis primarii et Parisiensis chirurgi..., trans. Jacques Guillemeau. Paris, 1582.

The workes of that famous chirurgion Ambrose Parey translated out of Latine and compared with the French, trans. Thomas Johnson. London, 1634.

Perkins, William. *An exposition of the Symbole or Creed of the Apostles, according to the tenour of the Scriptures, and the consent of orthodoxe Fathers of the Church.* Cambridge, 1595.

The first part of The cases of conscience. Cambridge, 1604.

The arte of prophecying. London, 1607.

A garden of spirituall flowers. London, 1610.

A salve for a sicke man. London, 1611.

Persons, Robert. *A brief discours contayning certayne reasons why Catholiques refuse to goe to church.* East Ham, 1580.

The copie of a double letter sent by an English gentilman from beyond the seas, to his frende in London, containing the true aduises of the cause, and maner of the death, of one Richard Atkins, executed by fire in Rome, the seconde of August 1581. Rheims, 1581.

A treatise of three conversions of England from paganism to Christian religion, vol. 1. Saint-Omer, 1603.

The third part of a treatise, intituled: of three conuersions of England... Wherunto in the end is annexed a defence of a certain trial... By N.D., vol. 2. Saint-Omer, 1604.

The third part of a treatise, intituled: of three conuersions of England... VVherunto is annexed in the end, another seuerall treatise, called: A re-view of ten publike disputations, or conferences... By N.D., vol. 3. Saint-Omer, 1604.

Place, Pierre de la. *A treatise of the excellencie of a christian man, and how he may be knowen.* London, 1576.

Platter, Felix. *Observationes in hominis affectibus plerisque.* Basel, 1614.

Platerus golden practice of physick, trans. Abdiah Cole and Nicholas Culpeper. London, 1664.

Pomarius, Petrus. *Enchiridion medicum containing an epitome of the whole course of physicke.* London, 1609.

Pomponazzi, Pietro. *Tractatus de immortalitate animae.* Bologna, 1516.

Priestley, Joseph. *Disquisitions Relating to Matter and Spirit.* London, 1777.

Primerose, James. *De vulgi erroribus in medicina.* Amsterdam, 1639.

Popular errours. London, 1651.

Prynne, William. *The soveraigne povver of parliaments and kingdomes divided into foure parts.* London, 1643.

The third part of The soveraigne povver of parliaments and kingdomes. London, 1643.

Truth triumphing over falshood, antiquity over novelty. London, 1645.

A plain, short, and probable expedient, to settle the present distractions of both kingdomes. London, 1647.

The Levellers levelled to the very ground. London, 1658.

Rainolds, John. *The summe of the conference betwene Iohn Rainoldes and Iohn Hart: touching the head and the faith of the Church.* London, 1584.

Ross, Alexander. *The philosophicall touch-stone.* London, 1645.

Leviathan drawn out with a hook. London, 1653.

Rivière, Lazare. *The practice of physick in seventeen several books*, trans. Nicholas Culpeper and Abdiah Cole. London, 1655.

S., M. *A Philosophical Discourse of the Nature of Rational and Irrational Souls.* London, 1695.

Sadler, John. *The sicke vvomans private looking-glasse wherein methodically are handled all uterine affects, or diseases arising from the wombe.* London, 1636.

Salmon, William. *Ars chirurgica.* London, 1698.

Salmon*Praxis medica. The practice of physick, or Dr Sydenham's Processus integri*, 3rd ed. London, 1716.

Scève, Maurice. *Microcosme.* Lyon, 1562.

Shakespeare, William. *M. William Shak-speare: his true chronicle historie of the life and death of King Lear and his three daughters.* London, 1608.

The tragedy of Hamlet Prince of Denmarke. London, 1611.

Sharpe, James. *The triall of the protestant priuate spirit.* Saint-Omer, 1630.

Sharpe, Leonel. *A looking-glasse for the Pope.* London, 1616.

Smith, Henry. *The Fall of King Nabuchadnezzar.* London, 1591.

Sorocold, Thomas. *Supplications of saints.* London, 1612.

Southwell, Robert. *An epistle of comfort, to the reuerend priestes, & to the honorable, worshipful, & other of the laye sort restrayned in durance for the Catholicke fayth.* London, 1587.

Spanheim, Friedrich. *Englands vvarning by Germanies vvoe.* London, 1646.

Squire, John. *A plaine exposition vpon the first part of the second chapter of Saint Paul his second epistle to the Thessalonians.* London, 1630.

Staunford, William. *An exposicion of the kinges prerogatiue.* London, 1567.

Steno, Nicolaus. *Discours de Monsieur Stenon, sur l'anatomie du cerveau.* Paris, 1669.

Stillingfleet, Edward. *A sermon preached before the King, March 13, 1666/7 by Edward Stillingfleet.* London, 1667.

Stubbe, Henry. *Legends no histories, or, A specimen of some animadversions upon The history of the Royal Society...* London, 1670.

The Lord Bacons relation to the sweating-sickness examined... London, 1671.

Sutton, Thomas. *Englands first and second summons.* London, 1616.

Swinburne, Henry. *A Brief Treatise of Testaments and Last Willes.* London, 1590.

Sydenham, Humphrey. *Sermons vpon solemne occasions preached in severall auditories.* London, 1637.

Topsell, Edward. *The history of four-footed beasts and serpents.* London, 1658.

Tralles, Alexander of. *Practica Alexandri yatros greci.* Lyons, 1504.

Trosse, George. *The Life of the Reverend Mr Geo. Trosse, later minister of the gospel.* Exeter, 1714.

Tuke, Thomas. *The treasure of true loue.* London, 1608.

The picture of a true protestant. London, 1609.

Nevv essayes: meditations, and vowes including in them the chiefe duties of a Christian, both for faith, and manners. London, 1614.

Turner, John. *A phisico-theological discourse upon the Divine Being*. London, 1698.

Vase, Robert. *Ionah's contestation about his gourd*. London, 1625.

Vesalius, Andreas. *De humani corporis fabrica libri septem*. Basel, 1543.

Vicary, Thomas. *A profitable treatise of the anatomie of mans body*. London, 1577.

Vigo, Giovanni da. *The most excellent workes of chirurgerye*, trans. Bartholomew Traheron. London, 1543.

Vives, Juan Luis. *De anima et vita libri tres*. Zürich, 1575.

Wade, Christopher. *Quakery slain irrecoverably, by the principal Quakers themselves, with a spiritual sword of their own forgery, whose names are here underwritten*. London, 1657.

Ward, Samuel. *A coal from the altar, to kindle the holy fire of zeale*. London, 1615.

Weemes, John. *The portraiture of the image of God in man*. London, 1636.

Whetstone, George. *The English myrror*. London, 1586.

Wiburn, Percival. *A checke or reproofe of M. Howlets vntimely shreeching in her Maiesties eares*. London, 1581.

Willet, Andrew. *De animae natura et viribus quaestiones quadam... in usum Cantabrigiensium*. Cambridge, 1585.

An antilogie or counterplea to An apologicall (he should haue said) apologeticall epistle published by a fauorite of the Romane separation. London, 1603.

Willis, Thomas. *Diatribae duae medico-philosophicae*. Amsterdam, 1663.

Cerebri anatome cui accessit nervorumque descriptio et usus. London, 1664.

De anima brutorum. London, 1672.

The remaining medical works of that famous and renowned physician Dr. Thomas Willis, trans. Samuel Pordage. London, 1681.

Two discourses concerning the soul of brutes, trans. Samuel Pordage. London, 1683.

Wingfield, Henry. *A compendious or short treatise, gathered out of the chyefe and principall authors of phisycke*. London, 1551.

Wirsung, Christopher. *Praxis medicinæ vniuersalis; or a generall practise of physicke*. London, 1598.

Wiseman, Richard. *A treatise of wounds*. London, 1672.

Severall chirurgicall treatises by Richard Wiseman. London, 1676.

Zabarella, Giacomo. *De rebus naturalibus libri XXX*. Cologne, 1597.

Zanchi, Girolamo. *De operibus Dei intra spatium sex dierum*. Neustadt an der Weinstraße, 1591.

Zouch, Richard. *Cases and questions resolved in the civil-lavv*. London, 1652.

Modern Editions

Alberigo, Giuseppe, Periclīs-Petros Ioannou, Claudio Leonardi and Paulo Prodi (eds.) et al. *Conciliorum oecumenicorum decreta*. Basel: Herder, 1962.

Aristotle. 'Nicomachean Ethics', in H. Rackham (trans.), *Nicomachean Ethics*. LCL 73. Cambridge, MA: Harvard University Press, 1934.

'On the Soul' and 'Parva Naturalia', in W. S. Hett (trans.), *On the Soul, Parva Naturalia, On Breath*. LCL 288. Cambridge, MA: Harvard University Press, 1936.

(attrib.). 'Problem XXX.1', in Robert Mayhew and David C. Mirhady (trans.), *Problems, Vol II, Books 20–38*. LCL 317. Cambridge, MA: Harvard University Press, 2011.

Augustine. 'Contra Cresconium', in Jacques-Paul Migne (ed.), *Patrologia Latina*, vol. 43. Paris: Migne, 1841–1857.

'Enarrationes in Psalmos', in Jacques-Paul Migne (ed.), *Patrologia Latina*, vol. 36. Paris: Migne, 1841–1857.

'Epistola XCIII', 'Epistola CXVIII', and 'Epistola CLXVI', in Jacques-Paul Migne (ed.), *Patrologia Latina*, vol. 33. Paris: Migne, 1841–1857.

'In Iohannis evangelium Tractatus CXXIV', in Jacques-Paul Migne (ed.), *Patrologia Latina*, vol. 35. Paris: Migne, 1841–1857.

'On the Free Choice of the Will', in Peter King (trans.), *On the Free Choice of the Will, On Grace and Free Choice, and Other Writings*. Cambridge: Cambridge University Press, 2010.

'Sermo LXXX', in Jacques-Paul Migne (ed.), *Patrologia Latina*, vol. 38. Paris: Migne, 1841–1857.

Aquinas, Thomas. *Sancti Thomae de Aquino Opera Omnia*. Rome: Commissio Leonina, 1888–1906. Published online by the Aquinas Institute, https://aquinas.cc/la/en/~ST.I

Bale, John. 'Kynge Johan', in J. Payne Collier (ed.), *Kynge Johan, A Play in Two Parts*. London: Camden Society, 1838.

Bartholin, Thomas. *On Diseases of the Bible: A Medical Miscellany*, ed. Johan Schioldann-Nielsen and Kurt Sørensen, trans. James Willis. *Acta historica scientiarum naturalium et medicinalium*, vol. 41. Copenhagen: Danish National Library of Science and Medicine, 1994.

Birch, Thomas. *The Court and Times of James the First, Illustrated by Authentic and Confidential Letters, from Various Public and Private Collections*. 2 vols. London: H. Colburn, 1848.

Blund, John, 'Tractatus de anima', in R. W. Hunt (ed.) and Michael W. Dunne (trans.), *Treatise on the Soul*. Oxford: Oxford University Press, 2013.

Celsus, Aulus Cornelius. 'On Medicine', in W. G. Spencer (trans.), *On Medicine. Volume I, Books 1–4*. LCL 292. Cambridge, MA: Harvard University Press, 1935.

Cromwell, Oliver. 'Letter LXXXII', in Thomas Carlyle (ed.), *The Letters and Speeches of Oliver Cromwell*. London: Methuen, 1904.

Descartes, René. 'Dedicatory Letter to the Sorbonne', in John Cottingham, Robert Stoothoff, and Dugald Murdoch (trans.), *The Philosophical Writings of Descartes*, vol. 2. Cambridge: Cambridge University Press, 1985.

'Discourse and Essays', in John Cottingham, Robert Stoothoff, and Dugald Murdoch (trans.), *The Philosophical Writings of René Descartes*, vol. 1. Cambridge: Cambridge University Press, 1985.

'Second Meditation' and 'Sixth Meditation', in John Cottingham (trans.), *Meditations on First Philosophy, With Selections from the Objections and Replies*, 2nd ed. Cambridge: Cambridge University Press, 2017.

Dewhurst, Kenneth (trans.), *Dr Thomas Sydenham (1624 –1689), His Life and Original Writings*. London: Wellcome Historical Medical Library, 1966.

Donne, John. 'A Sermon upon the fifth of November 1622', in George R. Potter and Evelyn M. Simpson (eds.), *The Sermons of John Donne*, vol. 4, no. 9. 10 vols. Oakland: University of California Press, 1959.

Fitzherbert, Dionys. 'Dionys Fitzherbert her Booke', in Katharine Hodgkin (ed.), *Women, Madness and Sin: The Autobiographical Writings of Dionys Fitzherbert*. Farnham: Ashgate, 2016.

Galen, Claudius. 'De humoribus', in Karl Gottlob Kühn (trans.), *Claudii Galeni Opera Omnia*, vol. 19. 19 vols. Leipzig: Cnobloch, 1821.

'De locis affectis', in Karl Gottlob Kühn (trans.), *Claudii Galeni Opera Omnia*, vol. 8. 19 vols. Leipzig: Cnobloch, 1821.

'De tumoribus praeter naturam', in Karl Gottlob Kühn (trans.), *Claudii Galeni Opera Omnia*, vol. 7. 19 vols. Leipzig: Cnobloch, 1821.

'De usu partium', in Karl Gottlob Kühn (trans.), *Claudii Galeni Opera Omnia*, vols. 3–4. 19 vols. Leipzig: Cnobloch, 1821.

'Quod animi mores', in Karl Gottlob Kühn (trans.), *Claudii Galeni Opera Omnia*, vol. 4. 19 vols. Leipzig: Cnobloch, 1821.

'Book IX: On the Brain', in M. C. Lyons and B. Towers (eds.), Wynfrid Laurence Henry Duckworth (trans.), *Galen On Anatomical Procedures: The Later Books*. Cambridge: Cambridge University Press, 1962.

'The Instruments of the Pneuma' and 'The Neck, Head, Encephalon, and Senses', in Margaret Tallmadge May (trans.), *On the Usefulness of the Parts of the Body*, vol. 1, books 6–8. 2 vols. Ithaca, NY: Cornell University Press, 1968.

'On the Differentiae of Symptoms', in Ian Johnston (trans.), *On Diseases and Symptoms*. Cambridge: Cambridge University Press, 2006.

'The Soul's Traits Depend on Bodily Temperament', in Ian Johnston (trans.), *On Temperaments. On Non-Uniform Distemperment. The Soul's Traits Depend on Bodily Temperament*. LCL 546. Cambridge, MA: Harvard University Press, 2020.

Gassendi, Pierre. 'Objectiones quintae', in Charles Adam and Paul Tannery (eds.), *Oeuvres de Descartes*, vol. 7. Paris: L. Cerf, 1904.

Hall, John. 'Curationum Historicarum et Empiricarum', in Greg Wells (trans.), *John Hall, Master of Physick: A Casebook from Shakespeare's Stratford*. Manchester: Manchester University Press, 2020.

Harvey, William. 'Prelectiones Anatomine Universalis', in C. D. O'Malley, F. N. L. Poynter, and K. F. Russell (trans.), *Lectures on the Whole of Anatomy: An Annotated Translation of Prelectiones Anatomine Universalis*. Oakland: University of California Press, 1961.

Heywood, Oliver. 'Objects and Observations' and 'Returns of Prayer', in Joseph Horsfall Turner (ed.), *The Rev. Oliver Heywood, B.A., 1630–1702: His*

Autobiography, Diaries, Anecdote and Event Books, vol. 4. Bingley: T. Harrison, 1882.

Hippocrates (attrib.). 'Airs, Waters, Places' and 'Epidemics 3', in W. H. S. Jones (trans.), *Ancient Medicine. Airs, Waters, Places. Epidemics 1 and 3. The Oath. Precepts. Nutriment*. LCL 147. Cambridge, MA: Harvard University Press, 1923.

Horace. 'Epistle 1.2', in H. Rushton Fairclough (trans.), *Satires, Epistles, Ars Poetica*. LCL 194. Cambridge, MA: Harvard University Press, 1926.

Hunnisett, Ralph (trans.). *Sussex Coroners' Inquests, 1485–1558*. Lewes: Sussex Record Society, 1985.

Sussex Coroners' Inquests 1603–1688. Kew: PRO Publications, 1998.

Irenaeus. 'Contra haereses', in Jacques-Paul Migne (trans.), *Patrologiae cursus completus: Series graeca*, vol. 7. Paris: Migne, 1857–1866.

Isḥāq, Ḥunayn ibn. 'Isagoge', in Gregor Maurach, 'Johannicius: Isagoge ad Techne Galieni'. *Sudhoffs Archiv* 62(2) (1978), 148–174.

Lucretius. 'On the Nature of Things', in W. H. D. Rouse (trans.), *On the Nature of Things*. LCL 181. Cambridge, MA: Harvard University Press, 1924.

Luders, Alexander, et al. (eds.). *The Statutes of the Realm: Printed by Command of His Majesty King George the Third*, vol. 3. 12 vols. London: Dawsons, 1817.

Melanchthon, Philip. 'Preface to the Commentary on the Soul', in Sachiko Kusukawa (ed.), Christine F. Salazar (trans.), *Melanchthon: Orations on Philosophy and Education*. Cambridge: Cambridge University Press, 1999.

Mildmay, Lady Grace. 'Extracts from Medical Papers', in Linda Pollock (ed.), *With Faith and Physic: The Life of a Tudor Gentlewoman Lady Grace Mildmay, 1552–1620*. London: Collins & Brown, 1993.

Montaigne, Michel de. 'De la force de l'imagination', in Pierre Villey and Verdun L. Saulnier (eds.), *Les Essais*. Paris: Presses Universitaires de France, 1992.

Montagu, Richard. 'XXI. – From the same to the same', in George Ornsby (ed.), *The Correspondence of John Cosin, D.D., Lord Bishop of Durham: Together with Other Papers Illustrative of His Life and Times*, vol. 1. 2 vols. Durham: Andrews & Co., 1869.

Oldenburg, Henry. 'Oldenburg to Boyle, 25 November 1667' and 'Oldenburg to Sluse, 25 November 1667', in A. Rupert Hall and Marie Boas Hall (trans.), *The Correspondence of Henry Oldenburg*, vol. 3. 13 vols. Madison: University of Wisconsin Press, 1966.

'Oldenburg to Boyle, 17 December 1667' and 'Oldenburg to Denis, 23 December 1667', in A. Rupert Hall and Marie Boas Hall (trans.), *The Correspondence of Henry Oldenburg*, vol. 4. 13 vols. Madison: University of Wisconsin Press, 1966.

Pepys, Samuel. Diary entries from 21 and 30 November 1667, in Robert Latham and William Matthews (eds.), *The Diary of Samuel Pepys*, vol. 8. 11 vols. London: Harper Collins, 1971.

Plato. 'Phaedo', in Harold North Fowler (trans.), *Euthyphro, Apology, Crito, Phaedo & Phaedrus*. LCL 36. Cambridge, MA: Harvard University Press, 1914.

'Charmides', in W. R. M. Lamb (trans.), *Charmides. Alcibiades I and II. Hipparchus. The Lovers. Theages. Minos. Epinomis*. LCL 201. Cambridge, MA: Harvard University Press, 1927.

'Phaedrus', in Christopher Emlyn-Jones and William Preddy (trans.), *Lysis. Symposium. Phaedrus*. LCL 166. Cambridge, MA: Harvard University Press, 2022.

Pliny. 'Naturalis historia', in John Bostock and H. T. Riley (trans.), *The Natural History of Pliny*. London: Bohn, 1855.

Richardson, John. 'John Richardson to the Queen', in Richard Arthur Roberts (ed.), *Calendar of the Manuscripts of the Most Honourable Marquis of Salisbury preserved at Hatfield House*, vol. 11. 18 vols. Dublin: HMSO, 1906.

Skippon, Philip. 'Sir Phil. Skippon to Mr Wray', in Edwin Lankester (ed.), *The Correspondence of John Ray*. London: The Ray Society, 1848.

Sydenham, Thomas. 'Anatomie, 1668', in Kenneth Dewhurst (trans.), *Dr Thomas Sydenham (1624 –1689), His Life and Original Writings*. London: Wellcome Historical Medical Library, 1966.

Tralles, Alexander of. 'Therapeutics', in Theodor Puschmann (trans.), *Alexander von Tralles, Original-Text und Übersetzung nebst einer einleitenden Abhandlung: ein Beitrag zur Geschichte der Medicin*. Vienna: Braumüller, 1878–1879.

Vesalius, Andreas. *De humani corporis fabrica* libri septem, in William Frank Richardson and John Burd Carman (trans.), *On the Fabric of the Human Body*. 5 vols. San Francisco, CA: Norman Publishing, 2009.

Ward, G. R. M. (trans.). *Oxford University Statutes*. 2 vols. London: W. Pickering, 1845.

Wood, Anthony. *Athenae Oxonienses: An exact history of all the writers and bishops who have had their education in the University of Oxford.* London: Rivington, 1813.

Willis, Thomas. *Willis's Oxford Lectures*, trans. Kenneth Dewhurst. Oxford: Sandford, 1980.

Willis's Oxford Casebook, trans. Kenneth Dewhurst. Oxford: Sandford, 1981.

Online Editions and Databases

Anglo-American Legal Tradition Online. http://aalt.law.uh.edu/.

British History Online. www.british-history.ac.uk/.

Early English Books Online. www.proquest.com/eebo.

Early European Books. https://search.proquest.com/eeb/.

Hopper, Andrew, David J. Appleby, Mark Stoyle, Lloyd Bowen, et al. (eds.). *Civil War Petitions*. www.civilwarpetitions.ac.uk/.

Jacques-Paul Migne (ed.), *Patrologia Graeca*. 1857–1866. https://archive.org/details/PatrologiaGraeca.

Jacques-Paul Migne (ed.), *Patrologia Latina*. 1841–1857. http://pld.chadwyck.co.uk/.

Kassell, Lauren, Michael Hawkins, Robert Ralley, John Young, Joanne Edge, Janet Yvonne Martin-Portugues, and Natalie Kaoukji (eds.). *The Casebooks of*

Simon Forman and Richard Napier, 1596–1634: A Digital Edition. https://casebooks.lib.cam.ac.uk.
Loeb Classical Library. www.loebclassics.com/.
Mark Greengrass, David Loades, Thomas S. Freeman, Joy Lloyd, John Wade, and Matt Phillpott (eds.). *The Acts and Monuments Online*. https://www.dhi.ac.uk/foxe/index.php.
Medieval and Early Modern Sources Online. sources.tannerritchie.com/.
Perseus Digital Library, Tufts University. https://www.perseus.tufts.edu/hopper/.
Ralley, Robert, Lauren Kassell, and Michael Hawkins (eds.). 'A Critical Edition of Simon Forman's "The Astrologicalle Judgmentes of phisick and other Questions"', in *The Casebooks of Simon Forman and Richard Napier, 1596–1634: A Digital Edition*. https://casebooks.lib.cam.ac.uk./transcriptions/TEXT5.
Sancti Thomae de Aquino Opera Omnia. Aquinas Institute. https://aquinas.cc/.
State Papers Online, 1509–1714. Gale Primary Sources. www.gale.com/intl/primary-sources/state-papers-online.
Wellcome Collection Online. https://wellcomecollection.org/works/.

SECONDARY SOURCES

Adamson, Peter (ed.). *Interpreting Avicenna: Critical Essays*. Cambridge: Cambridge University Press, 2013.
Alexander, Sally, and Barbara Taylor (eds.). *History and Psyche: Culture, Psychoanalysis and the Past*. New York: Palgrave Macmillan, 2012.
Allan, David. 'Ross, Alexander (1591–1654), Church of England Clergyman and Writer on Philosophy'. *ODNB*, 4 October 2007, https://doi.org/10.1093/ref:odnb/24110.
Allen, Phyllis. 'Medical Education in Seventeenth Century England'. *Journal of the History of Medicine and Allied Sciences* 1(1) (1946), 115–143.
'Scientific Studies in the English Universities of the Seventeenth Century'. *Journal of the History of Ideas* 10(2) (1949), 219–253.
American Psychiatric Association (ed.). *Diagnostic and Statistical Manual of Mental Disorders, Fifth Edition*. Washington, DC: American Psychiatric Publishing, 2013.
Andrew, Donna T. 'The Secularisation of Suicide in England, 1660–1800'. *Past & Present* 119 (1988), 158–165.
Andrews, Jonathan. 'Bedlam Revisited: A History of Bethlem Hospital 1634–1770'. Unpublished PhD thesis, University of London, 1991.
'Napier, Richard (1559–1634), Astrological Physician and Church of England Clergyman'. *ODNB*, 21 May 2009, https://doi.org/10.1093/ref:odnb/19763.
Andrews, Jonathan, Asa Briggs, Roy Porter, Penny Tucker, and Keir Waddington. *The History of Bethlem*. London: Routledge, 1997.

Andrews, Jonathan, and Andrew Scull. *Customers and Patrons of the Mad-Trade: The Management of Lunacy in Eighteenth-Century London.* Berkeley: University of California Press, 2002.

[Anon.] 'Lunacy and Idiocy: The Old Law and Its Incubus'. *University of Chicago Law Review* 18(2) (1951), 361–368.

Arbesmann, Rudolph. 'The Concept of "Christus Medicus" in St. Augustine'. *Traditio* 10 (1954), 1–28.

Arrizabalaga, Jon. *The Articella in the Early Press, c. 1476–1534.* Cambridge: Wellcome Unit for the History of Medicine, 1998.

'Problematizing Retrospective Diagnosis in the History of Disease'. *Asclepio* 54(1) (2002), 51–70.

Ashworth, Jennifer. 'Aquinas on Analogy', in Jeffrey Hause (ed.), *Debates in Medieval Philosophy: Essential Readings and Contemporary Responses*, pp. 232–242. New York: Routledge, 2014.

Astbury, Leah. 'Being Well, Looking Ill: Childbirth and the Return to Health in Seventeenth-Century England'. *Social History of Medicine* 30(3) (2017), 500–519.

Aucante, Vincent. *La philosophie médicale de Descartes.* Paris: Presses Universitaires de France, 2006.

Babb, Lawrence. 'Melancholy and the Elizabethan Man of Letters'. *Huntingdon Library Quarterly* 4(3) (1941), 247–261.

The Elizabethan Malady: A Study of Melancholia in English Literature from 1580 to 1642. East Lansing: Michigan State College Press, 1951.

Bakker, Paul J. J. M., and Johannes M. M. H. Thijssen (eds.). *Mind, Cognition, and Representation: The Tradition of Commentaries on Aristotle's* De anima. London: Routledge, 2017.

Barraclough, Geoffrey. 'Psychohistory Is Bunk'. *The Guardian*, 3 March 1973.

Beck, Catherine. 'Patronage and Insanity: Tolerance, Reputation and Mental Disorder in the British Navy, 1740–1820'. *Historical Research* 94(263) (2021), 73–95.

Beier, Lucinda McCray. *Sufferers and Healers: The Experience of Illness in Seventeenth-Century England.* London: Routledge & Kegan Paul, 1987.

Berti, Enrico. 'Aristotle's Concept of Nature: Traditional Interpretation and Results of Recent Studies', in *Evolving Concepts of Nature: Proceedings of the Plenary Session of the Pontifical Academy of Sciences, 24–28 October 2014, Acta 23*. Vatican City: Pontifical Academy of Sciences, 2015.

Bertolacci, Amos. 'The Reception of Avicenna in Latin Medieval Culture', in Peter Adamson (ed.), *Interpreting Avicenna: Critical Essays*, pp. 242–269. Cambridge: Cambridge University Press, 2013.

Bigotti, Fabrizio. *Physiology of the Soul: Mind, Body and Matter in the Galenic Tradition of the Late Renaissance (1550–1630).* Turnhout: Brepols, 2019.

Birkwood, Katie. 'Thomas Willis: The Father of Neurology'. *Royal College of Physicians Online*, 20 May 2016, https://history.rcplondon.ac.uk/blog/thomas-willis-father-neurology.

Blum, Paul Richard. 'The Immortality of the Soul', in James Hankins (ed.), *The Cambridge Companion to Renaissance Philosophy*, pp. 211–233. Cambridge: Cambridge University Press, 2007.

Boer, S. W. de. *The Science of the Soul: The Commentary Tradition on Aristotle's De anima, c. 1260–c. 1360*. Leuven: Leuven University Press, 2013.

Braddick, Michael. *State Formation in Early Modern England, c.1550–1700*. Cambridge: Cambridge University Press, 2000.

Braddick, Michael, and John Walter (eds.). *Negotiating Power in Early Modern Society: Order, Hierarchy and Subordination in Britain and Ireland*. Cambridge: Cambridge University Press, 2001.

Branca, Vittore (ed.). *Umanesimo europeo e umanesimo veneziano*. Florence: Sansoni, 1964.

Brann, Noel. *The Debate Over the Origin of Genius during the Italian Renaissance: The Theories of Supernatural Frenzy and Natural Melancholy in Accord and Conflict on the Threshold of the Scientific Revolution*. Leiden: Brill, 2002.

Buchenau, Stefanie, and Roberto Lo Presti (eds.). *Human and Animal Cognition in Early Modern Philosophy and Medicine*. Pittsburgh, PA: University of Pittsburgh Press, 2017.

Bullough, Vern L. 'Medieval Concepts of Adultery'. *Arthuriana* 7(4) (1997), 5–15.

Burns, Norman T. *Christian Mortalism from Tyndale to Milton*. Cambridge, MA: Harvard University Press, 1972.

Bush, Sargent. 'Hooker, Thomas (1586?–1647), Minister in America'. *ODNB*, 3 January 2008, https://doi.org/10.1093/ref:odnb/13697 .

Butler, Sara M. 'Degrees of Culpability: Suicide Verdicts, Mercy, and the Jury in Medieval England'. *Journal of Medieval and Early Modern Studies* 36(2) (2006), 263–290.

Forensic Medicine and Death Investigation in Medieval England. London: Routledge, 2014.

Bynum, Caroline Walker. *The Resurrection of the Body in Western Christianity, 200–1336 CE*. New York: Columbia University Press, 1995.

'Why All the Fuss about the Body? A Medievalist's Perspective'. *Critical Enquiry* 22(1) (1995), 1–33.

Bynum, William F. 'The Anatomical Method, Natural Theology, and the Functions of the Brain'. *Isis* 64(4) (1973), 445–468.

'Phrenitis: What's in a Name?'. *Lancet* 356 (2000), 1936.

Bynum, William F., Roy Porter, and Michael Shepherd (eds.). *The Anatomy of Madness: Essays in the History of Psychiatry, Vol. 1: People and Ideas*. London: Tavistock, 1985.

The Anatomy of Madness: Essays in the History of Psychiatry, Vol. 2: Institutions and Society. London: Tavistock, 1985.

Cadden, Joan. *The Meanings of Sex Difference in the Middle Ages: Medicine, Science, and Culture*. Cambridge: Cambridge University Press, 1995.

Campbell, Gordon. 'Brownists', in *The Oxford Dictionary of the Renaissance*. Oxford: Oxford University Press, 2005.

Carley, James P. 'John Leland'. *ODNB*, 25 May 2006, https://doi.org/10.1093/ref:odnb/16416.

Caron, Louis. 'Thomas Willis, the Restoration, and the First Works of Neurology'. *Medical History* 59(4) (2015), 525–553.

Carpentieri, Nicola. 'On the Meaning of *Birsām* and *Sirsām*: A Survey of the Arabic Commentaries on the Hippocratic *Aphorisms*'. *MIDÉO* 32 (2017), 81–92.

Carpentieri, Nicola, and Taro Mimura. 'Arabic Commentaries on the Hippocratic *Aphorisms*, VI.11: A Medieval Medical Debate on Phrenitis'. *Oriens* 45(1–2) (2017), 176–202.

Carrera, Elena. 'The Emotions in Sixteenth-Century Spanish Spirituality'. *Journal of Religious History* 3 (2007), 235–252.

'Madness and Melancholy in Sixteenth- and Seventeenth-Century Spain: New Evidence, New Approaches'. *Bulletin of Spanish Studies* 87(8) (2010), 1–15.

'Understanding Mental Disturbance in Sixteenth- and Seventeenth-Century Spain: Medical Approaches'. *Bulletin of Spanish Studies* 87(8) (2010), 105–136.

Carrera, Elena. (ed.). *Emotions and Health 1200–1700*. Leiden: Brill, 2013.

Carter, Philippa. 'Childbirth, Madness, and Bodies in History'. *History Workshop Journal* 91(1) (2021), 29–50.

Cellamare, Davide. 'Anatomy and the Body in Renaissance Protestant Psychology'. *Early Science and Medicine* 19 (2014), 341–364.

'Confessional Science and Organisation of Disciplines: Anatomy, Psychology, and Anthropology between the Sixteenth and the Seventeenth Centuries'. *Quaestio* 17(4) (2017), 461–480.

'Review of *Controversies over the Soul and Its Origin*, by Leen Spruit'. *Early Science and Medicine* 25(2) (2020), 195–204.

Charalampous, Charis. 'William of Ockham's Mind/Body Dualism and Its Transmission to Early Modern Thinkers'. *Intellectual History Review* 23(4) (2013), 537–563.

Rethinking the Mind–Body Relationship in Early Modern Literature, Philosophy, and Medicine: The Renaissance of the Body. London: Routledge, 2016.

Chenu, M. D. 'Spiritus: le vocabulaire de l'âme au XIIe siècle'. *Revue des Sciences philosophiques et théologiques* 41(2) (1957), 209–232.

Clancy, Thomas H. *Papist Pamphleteers: The Allen-Persons Party and the Political Thought of the Counter-Reformation in England, 1572–1615*. Chicago: Loyola University Press, 1964.

Clark, Christopher. 'Professor Jonathan Steinberg 1934–2021, in memoriam'. Cambridge Faculty of History website, 8 March 2021, www.hist.cam.ac.uk/news/professor-jonathan-steinberg-1934-2021-memoriam.

Clark, Stuart. *Vanities of the Eye: Vision in Early Modern European Culture.* Oxford: Oxford University Press, 2007.

Clarke, Basil. *Mental Disorder in Earlier Britain: Exploratory Studies*. Cardiff: University of Wales, 1975.

Clarke, Desmond M., and Catherine Wilson (eds.). *The Oxford Handbook of Philosophy in Early Modern Europe*. Oxford: Oxford University Press, 2011.

Clarke, Edwin, and Kenneth Dewhurst (eds.). *An Illustrated History of Brain Function*. Oxford: Sandford, 1972.

Clarke, Edwin, and C. D. O'Malley. *The Human Brain and Spinal Cord: A Historical Study Illustrated by Writings from Antiquity to the Twentieth Century*. Berkeley: University of California Press, 1968.

Cook, Harold J. 'Sydenham, Thomas (bap. 1624, d. 1689), Physician'. *ODNB*, 19 May 2011, https://doi.org/10.1093/ref:odnb/26864.

Cooper, Thompson. 'Holland, Guy (1585/6–1660), Jesuit'. *ODNB*, 23 September 2004, https://doi.org/10.1093/ref:odnb/13520.

Cope, Esther S. *Handmaid of the Holy Spirit: Dame Eleanor Davies, Never Soe Mad a Ladie*. Ann Arbor: University of Michigan Press, 1992.

Corcilius, Klaus, and Dominik Perler (eds.). *Partitioning the Soul: Debates from Plato to Leibniz*. Berlin: De Gruyter, 2014.

Cottingham, John (ed.). *The Cambridge Companion to Descartes*. Cambridge: Cambridge University Press, 1992.

Cummings, Brian, and Freya Sierhuis (eds.). *Passions and Subjectivity in Early Modern Culture*. Farnham: Ashgate, 2013.

Cunningham, Andrew. *The Anatomical Renaissance: The Resurrection of the Anatomical Projects of the Ancients*. Aldershot: Scolar Press, 1997.

'Identifying Disease in the Past: Cutting the Gordian Knot'. *Asclepio* 54(1) (2002), 13–43.

Dales, R. C. *The Problem of the Rational Soul in the Thirteenth Century*. Leiden: Brill, 1995.

Davis, Natalie Zemon. *Fiction in the Archives: Pardon Tales and Their Tellers in Sixteenth-Century France*. Stanford, CA: Stanford University Press, 1987.

Demaitre, Luke. *Medieval Medicine: The Art of Healing from Head to Toe*. Santa Barbara, CA: Praeger, 2013.

Des Chene, Dennis. *Life's Form: Late Aristotelian Conceptions of the Soul*. Ithaca, NY: Cornell University Press, 2000.

Spirits and Clocks: Machine and Organism in Descartes. Ithaca, NY: Cornell University Press, 2001.

Distelzweig, Peter, Benjamin Goldberg, and Evan Ragland (eds.). *Early Modern Medicine and Natural Philosophy*. Dordrecht: Springer, 2015.

Dixon, Thomas. *From Passions to Emotions: The Creation of a Secular Psychological Category*. Cambridge: Cambridge University Press, 2003.

Dobson, Mary. *Contours of Death and Disease in Early Modern England*. Cambridge: Cambridge University Press, 1997.

Dols, Michael. *Majnūn: The Madman in Medieval Islamic Society*. Oxford: Clarendon Press, 1992.

Doob, Penelope. *Nebuchadnezzar's Children: Conventions of Madness in Middle English Literature*. New Haven, CT: Yale University Press, 1974.

Dos, Nandini (ed.). *Lives in Transit in Early Modern England: Identity and Belonging*. Amsterdam: Amsterdam University Press, 2022.

Duden, Barbara. *The Woman Beneath the Skin: A Doctor's Patients in Early Modern Germany*, trans. Thomas Dunlap. Cambridge, MA: Harvard University Press, 1991.

Edmond, Mary. 'Simon Forman's Vade-Mecum'. *The Book Collector* 26 (1977), 44–60.

Eigen, Joel P. 'Delusion in the Courtroom: The Role of Partial Insanity in Early Forensic Testimony'. *Medical History* 35 (1991), 25–49.

Essary, Kirk. 'Clear as Mud: Metaphor, Emotion and Meaning in Early Modern England'. *English Studies* 98(7) (2017), 689–703.

Farr, A. D. 'The First Human Blood Transfusion'. *Medical History* 24 (1980), 154–162.

Fessler, Alfred. 'The Management of Lunacy in Seventeenth-Century England: An Investigation of Quarter-Sessions Records'. *Proceedings of the Royal Society of Medicine* 49(11) (1956), 901–907.

Finger, Stanley. *Minds Behind the Brain: A History of the Pioneers and Their Discoveries*. Oxford: Oxford University Press, 2000.

Finucci, Valeria, and Kevin Brownlee (eds.). *Generation and Degeneration: Tropes of Reproduction in Literature and History from Antiquity to Early Modern Europe*. Durham, NC: Duke University Press, 2001.

Foucault, Michel. *Madness and Civilization: A History of Insanity in the Age of Reason*, trans. Richard Howard. London: Routledge, 2001.

Frank, Robert G. *Harvey and the Oxford Physiologists: A Study of Scientific Ideas and Social Interaction*. Los Angeles: University of California Press, 1978.

French, Roger. *Robert Whytt, The Soul, and Medicine*. London: Wellcome Institute for the History of Medicine, 1969.

Canonical Medicine: Gentile da Foligno and Scholasticism. Leiden: Brill, 2001.

French, Roger, and Andrew Cunningham. *Before Science: The Invention of the Friars' Natural Philosophy*. Abingdon: Ashgate, 1996.

French, Roger, and Andrew Wear (eds.). *The Medical Revolution of the Seventeenth Century*. Cambridge: Cambridge University Press, 1989.

Fudge, Erica. *Brutal Reasoning: Animals, Rationality, and Humanity in Early Modern England*. Ithaca, NY: Cornell University Press, 2006.

Furdell, Elizabeth Lane. 'Boorde, Andrew (c. 1490–1549), Physician and Author'. *ODNB*, 3 January 2008, https://doi.org/10.1093/ref:odnb/2870.

Garber, Daniel. *Descartes Embodied: Reading Cartesian Philosophy Through Cartesian Science*. Cambridge: Cambridge University Press, 2001.

Gaskill, Malcolm. 'Reporting Murder: Fiction in the Archives in Early Modern England'. *Social History* 23(1) (1998), 1–30.

Gaukroger, Stephen (ed.). *The Soft Underbelly of Reason: The Passions in the Seventeenth Century*. London: Routledge, 1998.

Gaukroger, Stephen, John Schuster, and John Sutton (eds.). *Descartes' Natural Philosophy*. London: Taylor & Francis, 2000.

Gibbons, B. J. 'Overton, Richard (fl. 1640–1663), Leveller and Pamphleteer'. *ODNB*, 27 May 2010, https://doi.org/10.1093/ref:odnb/20974.

Gillespie, Stuart, and Stuart Hardy (eds.). *The Cambridge Companion to Lucretius*. Cambridge: Cambridge University Press, 2007.

Gottfried, Robert S. *Doctors and Medicine in Medieval England, 1340–1530*. Princeton, NJ: Princeton University Press, 1986.

Gowing, Laura. *Gender Relations in Early Modern England*. London: Routledge, 2014.

Gowland, Angus. 'The Problem of Early Modern Melancholy'. *Past & Present* 191(1) (2006), 77–120.

The Worlds of Renaissance Melancholy: Robert Burton in Context. Cambridge: Cambridge University Press, 2006.

Green, Christopher D. 'Where Did the Ventricular Localization of Mental Faculties Come From?'. *Journal of History of the Behavioural Sciences* 39(2) (2003), 131–142.

Greengrass, Mark. *Christendom Destroyed: Europe 1518–1648*. London: Penguin, 2012.

Grell, Ole Peter, and Andrew Cunningham (eds.). *Medicine and the Reformation*. London: Routledge, 1993.

Religio Medici: Medicine and Religion in Seventeenth-Century England. Aldershot: Scolar Press, 1996.

Gunn, Steven. *Early Tudor Government, 1485–1558*. Basingstoke: Macmillan, 1995.

Gunn, Steven, and Tomasz Gromelski. 'For Whom the Bell Tolls: Accidental Deaths in Tudor England'. *Lancet* 380 (2012), 1222–1223.

Hackett, Helen. *The Elizabethan Mind: Searching for the Self in an Age of Uncertainty*. New Haven, CT: Yale University Press, 2022.

Hadass, Ofer. *Medicine, Religion, and Magic in Early Stuart England: Richard Napier's Medical Practice*. Philadelphia: Penn State University Press, 2018.

Hanawalt, Barbara. *Crime and Conflict in English Communities, 1300–1348*. Cambridge, MA: Harvard University Press, 1979.

Hankins, James (ed.). *The Cambridge Companion to Renaissance Philosophy*. Cambridge: Cambridge University Press, 2007.

Hankinson, R. J. (ed.). *The Cambridge Companion to Galen*. Cambridge: Cambridge University Press, 2008.

Hanson, Craig Ashley. *The English Virtuoso: Art, Medicine, and Antiquarianism in the Age of Empiricism*. Chicago: University of Chicago Press, 2009.

Harley, David. 'Medical Metaphors in English Moral Theology, 1550–1660'. *Journal of the History of Medicine and Allied Sciences* 48 (1993), 396–435.

'Political Post-Mortems and Morbid Anatomy in Seventeenth-Century England'. *Social History of Medicine* 7 (1994), 1–28.

'Explaining Salem: Calvinist Psychology and the Diagnosis of Possession'. *The American Historical Review* 101(2) (1996), 307–330.

'Rhetoric and the Social Construction of Sickness and Healing'. *Social History of Medicine* 12(3) (1999), 407–435.

Harvey, Elizabeth Ruth. *The Inward Wits: Psychological Theory in the Middle Ages and the Renaissance*. London: Warburg Institute, 1975.

Haskell, Yasmin (ed.). *Diseases of the Imagination and Imaginary Diseases in the Early Modern Period*. Turnhout: Brepols, 2011.

Healy, Margaret. 'Medicine, Metaphor, and "Crisis" in the Early Modern Social Body'. *Journal of Medieval and Early Modern Studies* 46(1) (2016), 117–139.

Healy, Róisín. 'Suicide in Early Modern and Modern Europe'. *The Historical Journal* 49(3) (2006), 903–919.

Hellworth, Jennifer Wynne. '"Be Unto Me as a Precious Ointment": Lady Grace Mildmay, Sixteenth-Century Female Practitioner'. *Dynamis: Acta Hispanica ad Medicinae Scientiarumque Historiam Illustrandam* 19 (1999), 95–117.

Henry, John. 'A Cambridge Platonist's Materialism: Henry More and the Concept of Soul'. *Journal of the Warburg and Courtauld Institutes* 49 (1986), 172–195.

'Medicine and Pneumatology: Henry More, Richard Baxter, and Francis Glisson's *Treatise on the Energetic Nature of Substance*'. *Medical History* 31 (1987), 15–40.

Heyd, Michael. *'Be Sober and Reasonable': The Critique of Enthusiasm in the Seventeenth and Early Eighteenth Centuries.* Leiden: Brill, 1995.

Hill, Boyd. 'The Grain and the Spirit in Mediaeval Anatomy'. *Speculum* 40(1) (1965), 63–73.

Hodgkin, Katharine. *Madness in Seventeenth-Century Autobiography*. Basingstoke: Palgrave Macmillan, 2007.

Women, Madness and Sin in Early Modern England: The Autobiographical Writings of Dionys Fitzherbert. London: Routledge, 2010.

'Scurvy Vapors and the Devil's Claw: Religion and the Body in Seventeenth-Century Women's Melancholy'. *Studies in the Literary Imagination* 44(2) (2011), 1–21.

Houston, Rab A. *Punishing the Dead? Suicide, Lordship, and Community in Britain, 1500–1830*. Oxford: Oxford University Press, 1998.

Humphries, Jane, and Jacob Weisdorf. 'The Wages of Women in England, 1260–1850'. *Journal of Economic History* 75(2) (2015), 405–447.

Hunnisett, Ralph F. *The Medieval Coroner*. Cambridge: Cambridge University Press, 1961.

Hunter, Elizabeth K. '"Between the Bridge and the Brook": Suicide and Salvation in England, c. 1500–1650'. *Reformation & Renaissance Review* 15(3) (2013), 237–257.

Hunter, Michael. *Science and Society in Restoration England.* Cambridge: Cambridge University Press, 1981.

Science and the Shape of Orthodoxy: Intellectual Change in Late Seventeenth-Century Britain. Woodbridge: Boydell, 1995.

Atheists and Atheism before the Enlightenment: The English and Scottish Experience. Cambridge: Cambridge University Press, 2023.

Hunter, Michael, and David Wootton (eds.). *Atheism from the Reformation to the Enlightenment*. Oxford: Oxford University Press, 1992.

Ingram, Martin. *Carnal Knowledge: Regulating Sex in England, 1470–1600*. Cambridge: Cambridge University Press, 2017.

Irwin, T. H. 'Who Discovered the Will?'. *Philosophical Perspectives* 6 (1992), 453–473.
Izenberg, Gerald. 'Psychohistory and Intellectual History'. *History and Theory* 14(2) (1975), 139–155.
Jackson, Mark. 'Fiction in the Archives? Sources for the Social History of Infanticide'. *Archives* 27 (2002), 173–185.
Jacquart, Danielle. 'Theory, Everyday Practice, and Three Fifteenth-Century Physicians'. *Osiris* 6 (1990), 140–160.
'Les Avatars de la phrénitis chez Avicenne et Rhazès', in Danielle Gourevitch (ed.), *Maladie et Maladies: Histoire et Conceptualisation. Mélanges en l'honneur de Mirko Grmek*, pp. 181–192. Geneva: Librairie Droz, 1992.
James, K. A. 'Barrow, Philip (d. 1600), Medical Writer'. *ODNB*, 3 January 2008, https://doi.org/10.1093/ref:odnb/1545.
James, Susan. *Passion and Action: The Emotions in Seventeenth-Century Philosophy.* Oxford: Oxford University Press, 1997.
Jarcho, Saul. 'Galen's Six Non-Naturals: A Bibliographic Note and Translation'. *Bulletin of the History of Medicine* 44(4) (1970), 372–377.
Jenner, Mark, and Patrick Wallis (eds.). *Medicine and the Market in England and Its Colonies, c.1450–1850*. London: Palgrave Macmillan, 2007.
Jones, Peter Murray. 'Medicine and Science', in Lotte Hellinga and J. B. Trapp (eds.), *The Cambridge History of the Book in Britain, vol. 3, 1400–1557*, pp. 433–448. Cambridge: Cambridge University Press, 2008.
The Medicine of the Friars in Medieval England. York: Boydell & Brewer, 2024.
Kassell, Lauren. 'How to Read Simon Forman's Casebooks: Medicine, Astrology, and Gender in Elizabethan London'. *Social History of Medicine* 12(1) (1999), 3–18.
Medicine and Magic in Elizabethan London: Simon Forman, Astrologer, Alchemist, and Physician. Oxford: Clarendon Press, 2005.
'Casebooks in Early Modern England: Medicine, Astrology, and Written Records'. *Bulletin of the History of Medicine* 88(4) (2014), 595–625.
'Forman, Simon (1552–1611), Astrologer and Medical Practitioner'. *ODNB*, 11 November 2021, https://doi.org/10.1093/ref:odnb/9884.
Kaufman, Sharon R., and Lynn M. Morgan. 'The Anthropology of the Beginnings and Ends of Life'. *Annual Review of Anthropology* 34 (2005), 317–341.
Keeble, Neil Howard. '"Self-Confidence and Self-Conceit Render Men Fools": Seventeenth-Century "Self-" Compounds, Puritan Discourse and Early Modern Subjectivity'. *Renaissance Studies* 37(3) (2023), 345–363.
Kermode, Jennifer, and Garthine Walker (eds.). *Women, Crime and the Courts in Early Modern England.* London: Routledge, 1994.
Kesselring, Krista. 'Bodies of Evidence: Sex and Murder (or Gender and Homicide) in Early Modern England'. *Gender & History* 27(2) (2015), 245–262.
Making Murder Public: Homicide in Early Modern England. Oxford: Oxford University Press, 2019.

'Law, Status, and the Lash: Judicial Whipping in Early Modern England'. *Journal of British Studies* 60(3) (2021), 511–533.
Kesselring, Krista, and Natalie Mears. *Star Chamber Matters: An Early Modern Court and Its Records.* London: University of London Press, 2021.
Kietzmann, Christian. 'Aristotle on the Definition of What It Is to Be Human', in Geert Keil and Nora Kreft (eds.), *Aristotle's Anthropology*, pp. 25–43. Cambridge: Cambridge University Press, 2019.
Kingdon, Robert M. 'Calvinism and Resistance Theory, 1550–1580', in J. H. Burns (ed.), *The Cambridge History of Political Thought, 1450–1700*, pp. 194–200. Cambridge: Cambridge University Press, 1991.
Kirkup, John. 'Wiseman, Richard (bap. 1620?, d. 1676), Surgeon'. *ODNB*, 3 January 2008, https://doi.org/10.1093/ref:odnb/29792.
Kishlansky, Mark. *A Monarchy Transformed: Britain, 1603–1714*. London: Penguin, 1996.
Klibansky, Raymond, Erwin Panofsky, and Fritz Saxl. *Saturn and Melancholy: Studies in the History of Natural Philosophy, Religion and Art*. London: Nelson, 1964.
Králová, Jana, and Tony Walter (eds.). *Social Death: Questioning the Life–Death Boundary*. London: Routledge, 2017.
Kroll, Jerome. 'A Reappraisal of Psychiatry in the Middle Ages'. *Archives of General Psychiatry* 19 (1973), 276–283.
Kroll, Jerome, and Bernard Bachrach. 'Sin and Mental Illness in the Middle Ages'. *Psychological Medicine* 14 (1984), 507–514.
Kuntz, Marion Leathers, and Paul Grimley Kuntz (eds.). *Jacob's Ladder and the Tree of Life: Concepts of Hierarchy and the Great Chain of Being*. New York: Peter Lang, 1987.
Kusukawa, Sachiko. *The Transformation of Natural Philosophy: The Case of Philip Melanchthon*. Cambridge: Cambridge University Press, 1995.
Picturing the Book of Nature: Image, Text and Argument in Sixteenth-Century Human Anatomy and Botany. Chicago: University of Chicago Press, 2012.
Andreas Vesalius: Anatomy and the World of Books. London: Reaktion Press, 2024.
Lakoff, George, and Mark Johnson. *Metaphors We Live By*. Chicago: University of Chicago Press, 1980.
Lamont, William. *Marginal Prynne, 1600–1669*. London: Routledge & Kegan Paul, 1962.
'Prynne, William (1600–1669), Pamphleteer and Lawyer'. *ODNB*, 19 May 2011, https://doi.org/10.1093/ref:odnb/22854.
Lane, Joan (ed.). *John Hall and His Patients: The Medical Practice of Shakespeare's Son-in-Law*. Stratford upon Avon: The Shakespeare Birthplace Trust, 1996.
'Hall, John (1574/5?–1635), Physician'. *ODNB*, 3 January 2008, https://doi.org/10.1093/ref:odnb/11968.
Lawlor, Clark. *From Melancholia to Prozac: A History of Depression*. Oxford: Oxford University Press, 2012.

Lawrence, Christopher, and Steven Shapin (eds.). *Science Incarnate: Historical Embodiments of Natural Knowledge*. Chicago: University of Chicago Press, 1998.

Leong, Elaine. *Recipes and Everyday Knowledge: Medicine, Science, and the Household in Early Modern England*. Chicago: University of Chicago Press, 2018.

Liu, Tai. 'Goodwin, John (c. 1594–1665), Independent Minister'. *ODNB*, 3 January 2008, https://doi.org/10.1093/ref:odnb/10994.

Looney, Jefferson. 'Undergraduate Education at Early Stuart Cambridge'. *History of Education* 10(1) (1981), 9–19.

Lovejoy, Arthur. *The Great Chain of Being: A Study of the History of an Idea*. Cambridge, MA: Harvard University Press, 1963.

Lund, Mary Ann. 'Robert Burton the Spiritual Physician: Religion and Medicine in *The Anatomy of Melancholy*'. *Review of English Studies* 57(232) (2006), 665–683.

Melancholy, Medicine and Religion in Early Modern England. Cambridge: Cambridge University Press, 2010.

MacDonald, Michael. 'Insanity and the Realities of History in Early Modern England'. *Psychological Medicine* 11(1) (1981), 11–25.

Mystical Bedlam: Madness, Anxiety and Healing in Seventeenth-Century England. Cambridge: Cambridge University Press, 1981.

'The Secularization of Suicide in England 1660–1800'. *Past and Present* 111(1) (1986), 50–100.

'*The Fearefull Estate of Francis Spira*: Narrative, Identity, and Emotion in Early Modern England'. *Journal of British Studies* 31(1) (1992), 32–61.

MacDonald, Michael, and Terence R. Murphy. *Sleepless Souls: Suicide in Early Modern England*. Oxford: Clarendon Press, 1990.

MacDonald, Scott, and Eleonore Stump (eds.). *Aquinas's Moral Theory: Essays in Honor of Norman Kretzmann*. Ithaca, NY: Cornell University Press, 1999.

Maclean, Ian. *The Renaissance Notion of Woman: A Study in the Fortunes of Scholasticism and Medical Science in European Intellectual Life*. Cambridge: Cambridge University Press, 1980.

Logic, Signs and Nature in the Renaissance: The Case of Learned Medicine. Cambridge: Cambridge University Press, 2002.

'The "Sceptical Crisis" Reconsidered: Galen, Rational Medicine and the *Libertas Philosophandi*'. *Early Science and Medicine* 11(3) (2006), 247–274.

MacLehose, William. 'The Pathological and the Normal: Mapping the Brain in Medieval Medicine'. *Progress in Brain Research* 243 (2018), 23–53.

Malament, Barbara C. (ed.). *After the Reformation: Essays in Honour of J. H. Hexter*. Philadelphia: University of Pennsylvania Press, 1980.

Manning, Gideon (ed.). *Matter and Form in Early Modern Science and Philosophy*. Leiden: Brill, 2012.

Manzoni, Tullio. 'The Cerebral Ventricles, the Animal Spirits, and the Dawn of Brain Localization of Function'. *Archives Italiennes de Biologie* 136 (1998), 103–152.

Marshall, Peter, and Alexandra Walsham (eds.). *Angels in the Early Modern World.* Cambridge: Cambridge University Press, 2006.

Martensen, Robert L. '"Habit of Reason": Anatomy and Anglicanism in Restoration England'. *Bulletin of the History of Medicine* 66(4) (1992), 511–535.

The Brain Takes Shape: An Early History. Oxford: Oxford University Press, 2004.

'Willis, Thomas (1621–1675), Physician and Natural Philosopher'. *ODNB,* 4 October 2007, https://doi.org/10.1093/ref:odnb/29587.

Martin, John. 'Inventing Sincerity, Refashioning Prudence: The Discovery of the Individual in Renaissance Europe'. *American Historical Review* 102(5) (1997), 1309–1342.

McDonald, Glenda C. 'Concepts and Treatments of Phrenitis in Ancient Medicine'. Unpublished PhD thesis, University of Newcastle, 2009.

'Galen on Mental Illness: A Physiological Approach to Phrenitis'. *Bulletin of the Institute of Classical Studies. Supplement* 114 (2014), 135–151.

McGee, J. Sears. 'Adams, Thomas (1583–1652), Church of England Clergyman'. *ODNB,* 24 May 2012, https://doi.org/10.1093/ref:odnb/131.

McGlynn, Margaret. 'Idiots, Lunatics, and the Royal Prerogative in Early Tudor England'. *Journal of Legal History* 26(1) (2005), 1–24.

Meconi, David, and Eleanore Stump (eds.). *The Cambridge Companion to Augustine,* 2nd ed. Cambridge: Cambridge University Press, 2014.

Mellyn, Elizabeth W. *Mad Tuscans and Their Families: A History of Mental Disorder in Early Modern Italy.* Philadelphia: University of Pennsylvania Press, 2014.

Mendelsohn, J. Andrew, and Annemarie Kinzelbach. 'Common Knowledge: Bodies, Evidence, and Expertise in Early Modern Germany'. *Isis* 108(2) (2017), 259–279.

Mengal, Paul. *La naissance de la psychologie.* Paris: L'Harmattan, 2005.

Midelfort, H. C. Erik. *Mad Princes of Renaissance Germany.* Charlottesville: University Press of Virginia, 1994.

A History of Madness in Sixteenth-Century Germany. Stanford, CA: Stanford University Press, 1999.

Miller, Jennifer, and Ken H. Rogers. 'The Strange Death of Edward Langford'. *Wiltshire Archaeological and Natural History Magazine* 62 (1967), 103–109.

Milward, Peter. *Religious Controversies of the Elizabethan Age: A Survey of Printed Sources.* London: Scolar Press, 1977.

Miner, Robert. *Thomas Aquinas on the Passions.* Cambridge: Cambridge University Press, 2009.

Mintz, Samuel. *The Hunting of Leviathan: Seventeenth-Century Reactions to the Materialism and Moral Philosophy of Thomas Hobbes.* Cambridge: Cambridge University Press, 1961.

Mólnar, Zoltán. 'Thomas Willis (1621–1675), The Founder of Clinical Neuroscience'. *Nature Reviews Neuroscience* 5 (2004), 329–335.

Muldrew, Craig. *The Economy of Obligation: The Culture of Credit and Social Relations in Early Modern England.* London: Palgrave Macmillan, 1998.

Muller, Richard A. *Christ and the Decree: Christology and Predestination in Reformed Theology from Calvin to Perkins.* Durham, NC: Labyrinth Press, 1986.
Grace and Freedom: William Perkins and the Early Modern Reformed Understanding of Free Choice and Divine Grace. Oxford: Oxford University Press, 2020.
Muratori, Cecilia (ed.). *The Animal Soul and the Human Mind: Renaissance Debates.* Pisa: Serra, 2013.
Murray, Alexander. *Suicide in the Middle Ages. Vol. 1, The Violent Against Themselves.* 3 vols. Oxford: Oxford University Press, 2008–2011.
Neely, Carol T. *Distracted Subjects: Madness and Gender in Shakespeare and Early Modern Culture.* Ithaca, NY: Cornell University Press, 2004.
Neugebauer, Richard. 'The Treatment of the Mentally Ill in Medieval and Early Modern England: A Reappraisal'. *Journal of the History of the Behavioural Sciences* 14 (1978), 158–169.
'Medieval and Early Modern Theories of Mental Illness'. *Archives of General Psychology* 36 (1979), 477–483.
Niebyl, Peter H. 'The Non-Naturals'. *Bulletin of the History of Medicine* 45(5) (1971), 486–492.
Nieuwenhove, Rik van. 'Contemplation, *Intellectus*, and *Simplex Intuitus* in Aquinas: Recovering a Neoplatonic Theme'. *American Catholic Philosophical Quarterly* 91(2) (2017), 199–225.
Norri, Juhani. *Dictionary of Medical Vocabulary in English, 1375–1500.* Abingdon: Ashgate, 2016.
Novak, Joseph A. 'Aquinas on the Incorruptibility of the Soul'. *History of Philosophy Quarterly* 4(4) (1987), 405–421.
Nutton, Vivian. *Galen: A Thinking Doctor in Imperial Rome.* New York: Routledge, 2020.
O'Brien, John. 'In Praise of the *Theologie Naturelle*'. *Review of English Studies,* 65(269) (2013), 236–251.
O'Daly, Gerard J. P. *Augustine's Philosophy of Mind.* Berkeley: University of California Press, 1987.
O'Neill, Ynez Violé. 'Meningeal Localization: A New Key to Some Medical Texts, Diagrams and Practices of the Middle Ages'. *Mediaevistik* 6 (1993), 211–238.
Osler, Margaret J. *Divine Will and the Mechanical Philosophy: Gassendi and Descartes on Contingency and Necessity in the Created World.* Cambridge: Cambridge University Press, 1994.
Osler, Margaret J., and Paul Lawrence Farber (eds.). *Religion, Science, and Worldview: Essays in Honor of Richard S. Westfall.* Cambridge: Cambridge University Press, 1985.
Overell, M. Anne. 'The Exploitation of Francesco Spiera'. *The Sixteenth Century Journal* 26(3) (1995), 619–637.
Pasnau, Robert. *Thomas Aquinas on Human Nature: A Philosophical Study of the Summa Theologiae 1a, 75–89.* Cambridge: Cambridge University Press, 2004.

Paster, Gail Kern. *Humoring the Body: Emotions and the Shakespearean Stage*. Chicago: University of Chicago Press, 2004.
Patrides, Constantinos A. *Premises and Motifs in Renaissance Thought and Literature*. Princeton, NJ: Princeton University Press, 1982.
Pearson, Giles. *Aristotle on Desire*. Cambridge: Cambridge University Press, 2012.
Peck, Linda Levy (ed.). *The Mental World of the Jacobean Court*. Cambridge: Cambridge University Press, 1991.
Peghaire, Julien. *Intellectus et Ratio selon S. Thomas d'Aquin*. Paris: J. Vrin, 1936.
Pender, Stephen, and Nancy S. Struever (eds.). *Rhetoric and Medicine in Early Modern Europe*. Farnham: Ashgate, 2012.
Plamper, Jan, et al. 'The History of Emotions: An Interview with William Reddy, Barbara Rosenwein and Peter Stearns'. *History & Theory* 49(2) (2010), 237–265.
Pollmann, Karla, and Willemien Otten (eds.). *The Oxford Guide to the Historical Reception of Augustine*. Oxford: Oxford University Press, 2013.
Pollock, Linda. *With Faith and Physic: The Life of a Tudor Gentlewoman Lady Grace Mildmay, 1552–1620*. London: Collins & Brown, 1993.
'Anger and the Negotiation of Relationships in Early Modern England'. *The Historical Journal* 47(3) (2004), 567–590.
'Mildmay [née Sharington], Grace, Lady Mildmay (c. 1552–1620), Memoirist and Medical Practitioner'. *ODNB*, 27 May 2010, https://doi.org/10.1093/ref:odnb/45817.
Pomata, Gianna. 'Sharing Cases: The *Observationes* in Early Modern Medicine'. *Early Science and Medicine* 15(3) (2010), 193–236.
'The Medical Case Narrative: Distant Reading of an Epistemic Genre'. *Literature and Medicine* 32(1) (2014), 1–23.
Pomper, Philip. 'Problems of a Naturalistic Psychohistory'. *History and Theory* 12(4) (1973), 367–388.
Popkin, Richard H. *The History of Scepticism: From Savonarola to Bayle*, 3rd ed. Oxford: Oxford University Press, 2003.
Pormann, Peter E. 'New Fragments from Rufus of Ephesus' *On Melancholy*'. *Classical Quarterly* 64(2) (2014), 649–656.
'Medicine on the Different Shores of the Mediterranean: Scientific Discourse Beyond Country and Creed'. Lecture given at the Alwaleed Centre, University of Edinburgh, 6 December 2017.
Pormann, Peter E. (ed.). *The Cambridge Companion to Hippocrates*. Cambridge: Cambridge University Press, 2018.
Porter, Roy. 'The Rage of Party: A Glorious Revolution in English Psychiatry?'. *Medical History* 27(1) (1983), 35–50.
'The Patient's View: Doing Medical History from Below'. *Theory and Society* 14 (1985), 175–198.
Mind-forg'd Manacles: A History of Madness in England from the Restoration to the Regency. London: Penguin, 1987.
A Social History of Madness: The World Through the Eyes of the Insane. New York: Weidenfeld & Nicolson, 1988.

'Margery Kempe and the Meaning of Madness'. *History Today* 38(2) (1998), 39–44.
Flesh in the Age of Reason: How the Enlightenment Changed the Way We See Our Bodies and Souls. London: Penguin, 2003.
Madmen: A Social History of Madhouses, Mad Doctors & Lunatics. Stroud: Tempus, 2004.
(ed.). *Patients and Practitioners: Lay Perceptions of Medicine in Pre-Industrial Society.* Cambridge: Cambridge University Press, 1985.
The Popularization of Medicine, 1650–1850. London: Routledge, 1992.
Disease, Medicine and Society in England, 1550 –1860, 2nd ed. Cambridge: Cambridge University Press, 1995.
Rewriting the Self: Histories from the Renaissance to the Present. London: Routledge, 1996.
Poynter, F. N. L. *The History and Philosophy of Knowledge of the Brain and Its Functions.* Oxford: Blackwell, 1958.
Rapple, Rory. 'Stanley, Sir William (1548–1630), Soldier'. *ODNB*, 4 October 2008, https://doi.org/10.1093/ref:odnb/26283.
Rather, L. J. 'The "Six Things Non-Natural": A Note on the Origins and Fate of a Doctrine and a Phrase'. *Clio Medica* 3(4) (1968), 337–347.
Reddy, William. *The Navigation of Feeling: A Framework for the History of Emotions.* Cambridge: Cambridge University Press, 2001.
Reed, Robert Rentoul. *Bedlam on the Jacobean Stage.* Cambridge, MA: Harvard University Press, 1952.
Ritchie, Carson I. A. 'Sir Richard Grenville and the Puritans'. *English Historical Review* 77(304) (1962), 518–523.
Rocca, Julius. *Galen on the Brain: Anatomical Knowledge and Physiological Speculation in the Second Century A. D.* Leiden: Brill, 2003.
Roffe, David, and Christine Roffe. 'Madness and Care in the Community: A Medieval Perspective'. *British Medical Journal* 311 (1995), 1708–1712.
Roper, Lyndal. 'Beyond Discourse Theory'. *Women's History Review* 19(2) (2010), 307–19.
Roper, Lyndal, et al. 'History of the Emotions'. *German History* 28(1) (2010), 67–80.
Rosen, George. 'The Mentally Ill and the Community in Western and Central Europe during the Late Middle Ages and the Renaissance'. *Journal of the History of Medicine* 19 (1964), 377–388.
Madness in Society. Chapters in the Historical Sociology of Mental Illness. Chicago: University of Chicago Press, 1968.
Rosenwein, Barbara. *Anger's Past: The Social Uses of an Emotion.* Ithaca, NY: Cornell University Press, 1998.
'Worrying about Emotions in History'. *American Historical Review* 107(3) (2002), 821–845.
Emotional Communities in the Early Middle Ages. Ithaca, NY: Cornell University Press, 2007.
Generations of Feeling: A History of Emotions, 600–1700. Cambridge: Cambridge University Press, 2015.

Rosenwein, Barbara, et al. '*AHR* Conversation: The Historical Study of the Emotions'. *American Historical Review* 117(5) (2012), 1487–1531.

Rousseau, G. S. (ed.). *The Languages of the Psyche: Mind and Body in Enlightenment Thought.* Berkeley: University of California Press, 1996.

Rublack, Ulinka. 'Fluxes: The Early Modern Body and the Emotions'. *History Workshop Journal* 53(1) (2002), 1–16.

Rublack, Ulinka. (ed.). *The Oxford Handbook of the Protestant Reformations.* Oxford: Oxford University Press, 2016.

Rushton, Peter. 'Lunatics and Idiots: Mental Disability, the Community, and the Poor Law in North-East England, 1600–1800'. *Medical History* 32(1) (1988), 34–50.

Russell, Donald, et al. (eds.). *On Prophecy, Dreams and Human Imagination: Synesius,* De insomniis. Tübingen: Mohr Siebeck, 2014.

Ryrie, Alec. *Being Protestant in Reformation Britain.* Oxford: Oxford University Press, 2013.

Saenz, Victor. 'Shame and Honor: Aristotle's *Thumos* as a Basic Desire'. *Apeiron* 51(1) (2018), 73–95.

Sahlins, Peter. *1668: The Year of the Animal in France*. New York: Zone Books, 2017.

Sakai, Akio. 'Phrenitis: Inflammation of the Mind and Body'. *History of Psychiatry* 2 (1991), 193–205.

Sawyer, Ronald C. 'Patients, Healers and Disease in the Southeast Midlands'. Unpublished PhD thesis, University of Wisconsin–Madison, 1986.

Scheer, Monique. 'Are Emotions a Kind of Practice (And Is That What Makes Them Have a History)?' *History and Theory* 51 (2012), 193–220.

Schleiner, Winfried. *Melancholy, Genius and Utopia in the Renaissance.* Wiesbaden: Harrassowitz, 1991.

Schmidt, Jeremy. *Melancholy and the Care of the Soul: Religion, Moral Philosophy and Madness in Early Modern England.* Aldershot: Ashgate, 2007.

Schmitt, Charles B., Quentin Skinner, Eckhard Kessler, and Jill Kraye (eds.). *The Cambridge History of Renaissance Philosophy.* Cambridge: Cambridge University Press, 1988.

Schoenfeldt, Michael. *Bodies and Selves in Early Modern England: Physiology and Inwardness in Spenser, Shakespeare, Herbert and Milton.* Cambridge: Cambridge University Press, 1999.

Schreiner, Susan. *Are You Alone Wise? The Search for Certainty in the Early Modern Period.* Oxford: Oxford University Press, 2012.

Scull, Andrew. *Madness in Civilization: The Cultural History of Insanity*. London: Thames & Hudson, 2015.

Seabourne, Gwen, and Alice Seabourne. 'The Law on Suicide in Medieval England'. *Journal of Legal History* 21(1) (2000), 21–48.

'Suicide or Accident? Self-Killing in Medieval England'. *British Journal of Psychiatry* 178 (2001), 42–47.

Seaver, P. S. 'Downham, John (1571–1652), Church of England Clergyman and Author'. *ODNB*, 3 January 2008, https://doi.org/10.1093/ref:odnb/7978.

Serjeantson, Richard. 'The Passions and Animal Language'. *Journal of the History of Ideas* 62(3) (2001), 425–444.

Shagan, Ethan. *The Rule of Moderation: Violence, Religion and the Politics of Restraint in Early Modern England.* Cambridge: Cambridge University Press, 2011.

Shapin, Steven. *Never Pure: Historical Studies of Science as if It Was Produced by People with Bodies, Situated in Time, Space, Culture, and Society, and Struggling for Credibility and Authority.* Baltimore, MD: Johns Hopkins University Press, 2010.

Shepard, Alexandra. *Meanings of Manhood in Early Modern England.* Oxford: Oxford University Press, 2003.

Shuger, Barbara. *Sacred Rhetoric: The Christian Grand Style in the English Renaissance.* Princeton, NJ: Princeton University Press, 1988.

Simpson, James. 'Unwritten Virtues, Selves, and Texts: Early Modern Self-Erasure'. *Journal of Medieval and Early Modern Studies* 52(3) (2022), 415–443.

Siraisi, Nancy. *Medieval and Early Renaissance Medicine: An Introduction to Knowledge and Practice.* Chicago: University of Chicago, 1990.

Skultans, Vieda. *English Madness: Ideas on Insanity, 1580–1890.* London: Routledge, 1979.

Sluhovsky, Moshe. *Believe Not Every Spirit: Possession, Mysticism and Discernment in Early Modern Catholicism.* Chicago: University of Chicago Press, 2007.

Smith, Helen. 'Metaphor, Cure, and Conversion in Early Modern England'. *Renaissance Quarterly* 67(2) (2014), 473–502.

Smith, C. U. M., and Harry Whitaker (eds.). *Brain, Mind and Consciousness in the History of Neuroscience.* Dordrecht: Springer, 2014.

Stachniewski, John. *The Persecutory Imagination: English Puritanism and the Literature of Religious Despair.* Oxford: Clarendon Press, 1991.

Stevenson, Lloyd G. '"New Diseases" in the Seventeenth Century'. *Bulletin of the History of Medicine* 39 (1965), 1–21.

Stevenson, S. J. 'The Rise of Suicide Verdicts in South East England, 1530–1590: The Legal Process'. *Continuity and Change* 2(1) (1987), 37–75.

Still, Arthur, and Irving Velody (eds.). *Rewriting the History of Madness: Studies in Foucault's* Histoire de la folie. London: Routledge, 1992.

Stretton, Tim. *Women Waging Law in Elizabethan England.* Cambridge: Cambridge University Press, 2005.

Sudhoff, Karl. 'Der "Micrologus" Text der "Anatomia" Richards des Englanders'. *Archiv für Geschichte der Medizin* 19 (1927), 209–239.

Sugg, Richard. *Smoke of the Soul: Medicine, Physiology and Religion in Early Modern England.* London: Springer, 2013.

Sullivan, Erin. *Beyond Melancholy, Sadness and Selfhood in Renaissance England.* Oxford: Oxford University Press, 2016.

Suzuki, Akihito. 'Lunacy in Seventeenth- and Eighteenth-Century England: Analysis of Quarter Sessions Records, Part I'. *History of Psychiatry* 2 (1991), 437–456.

'Lunacy in Seventeenth- and Eighteenth-Century England: Analysis of Quarter Sessions Records. Part II'. *History of Psychiatry* 3 (1991), 29–44.

Taavitsainen, Irma, and Paivi Pahta. 'Vernacularisation of Medical Writing in English: A Corpus-Based Study of Scholasticism'. *Early Science and Medicine* 3(2) (1998), 157–185.

Tellkamp, Jörg Alejandro. '*Vis aestimativa* and *vis cogitativa* in Thomas Aquinas's *Commentary on the Sentences*'. *The Thomist* 76 (2012), 611–640.

Thompson, Charles J. S. *The Quacks of Old London*. London: Brentano's, 1928.

Thomson, Ann. *Bodies of Thought: Science, Religion and the Soul in the Early Enlightenment.* Oxford: Oxford University Press, 2008.

Thumiger, Chiara. *A History of the Mind and Mental Health in Classical Greek Medical Thought.* Cambridge: Cambridge University Press, 2017.

Phrenitis and the Pathology of the Mind in Western Medical Thought, Fifth Century BCE to Twentieth Century CE. Cambridge: Cambridge University Press, 2023.

Thumiger, Chiara, and Peter N. Singer (eds.). *Mental Illness in Ancient Medicine: From Celsus to Paul of Aegina*. Leiden: Brill, 2018.

Tillyard, Eustace M. W. *The Elizabethan World Picture: A Study on the Idea of Order in the Age of Shakespeare, Donne, and Milton*. New York: Random House, 1961.

Turner, Wendy. *Care and Custody of the Mentally Ill, Incompetent, and Disabled in Medieval England.* Turnhout: Brepols, 2013.

Turner, Wendy (ed.). *Madness in Medieval Law and Custom*. Leiden: Brill, 2010.

Medicine and the Law in the Middle Ages. Leiden: Brill, 2014.

Tyacke, Nicholas (ed.). *The History of the University of Oxford. Vol 4: Seventeenth-Century Oxford.* Oxford: Oxford University Press, 1997.

Vaught, Jennifer C. (ed.). *Rhetorics of Bodily Disease and Health in Medieval and Early Modern England*. Farnham: Ashgate, 2010.

Vidal, Fernando. *Les sciences de l'âme: XVIe–XVIIIe siècle*. Paris: Honoré Champion Editeur, 2006.

The Sciences of the Soul: The Early Modern Origins of Psychology, trans. Saskia Brown. Chicago: Chicago University Press, 2011.

Vidal, Fernando, and Francisco Ortega. *Being Brains: Making the Cerebral Subject.* New York: Fordham University Press, 2017.

Walkden, Michael. 'The Gut–Mind Connection in Early Modern Medicine and Culture, c.1580–c.1740'. Unpublished PhD thesis, University of York, 2018.

Walker, Daniel P. 'The Astral Body in Renaissance Medicine'. *Journal of the Warburg and Courtauld Institutes* 21 (1958), 119–133.

'Medical Spirits and God and the Soul', in Marta Fattori and Massimo Bianchi (eds.), *Spiritus. IV° Colloquio internazionale del Lessico Intellectuale Europeo, Rome, 7–9 gennaio, 1983*, pp. 233–244. Rome: Edizioni dell'Ateneo, 1984.

'Medical Spirits in Philosophy and Theology from Ficino to Newton', in Jean Jacquot (ed.), *Arts du Spectacle et Histoire des Idées: Recueil Offert en Hommage à Jean Jacquot*, pp. 287–300. Tours: Centre d'Études Supérieures de la Renaissance, 1984.

Walker, Nigel. *Crime and Insanity in England, Vol. 1: The Historical Perspective.* Edinburgh: Edinburgh University Press, 1968.

'The Insanity Defence before 1800'. *Annals of the American Academy of Political and Social Science* 477 (1985), 25–30.

Wallis, Faith (ed.). *Medieval Medicine: A Reader.* Toronto: University of Toronto Press, 2010.

Walrath, Dana. *Aliceheimer's: Alzheimer's Through the Looking Glass.* University Park: Penn State University Press, 2016.

Walsham, Alexandra. '"Frantick Hacket": Prophecy, Sorcery, Insanity, and the Elizabethan Puritan Movement'. *The Historical Journal* 41(1) (1998), 27–66.

Providence in Early Modern England. Oxford: Oxford University Press, 1999.

'The Reformation and the "Disenchantment of the World" Reassessed'. *The Historical Journal* 51(2) (2008), 497–528.

Watt, Diane. 'Davies [née Touchet; other married name Douglas], Lady Eleanor (1590–1652), Prophetess'. *ODNB*, 3 January 2008, https://doi.org/10.1093/ref:odnb/7233.

Wear, Andrew. *Knowledge and Practice in English Medicine 1550–1680.* Cambridge: Cambridge University Press, 2000.

Wear, Andrew, R. K. French, and I. M. Lonie (eds.). *The Medical Renaissance of the Sixteenth Century.* Cambridge: Cambridge University Press, 1985.

Webster, Charles. *The Great Instauration: Science, Medicine and Reform, 1626–1660.* London: Duckworth, 1975.

Webster, Charles. (ed.). *Health, Medicine and Mortality in the Sixteenth Century.* Cambridge: Cambridge University Press, 1979.

Weisser, Olivia. 'Boils, Pushes and Wheals: Reading Bumps on the Body in Early Modern England'. *Social History of Medicine* 22(2) (2009), 321–339.

'Grieved and Disordered: Gender and Emotion in Early Modern Patient Narratives'. *Journal of Medieval and Early Modern Studies* 43 (2013), 247–273.

Ill Composed: Sickness, Gender and Belief in Early Modern England. New Haven, CT: Yale University Press, 2015.

Wells, Greg. *John Hall, Master of Physick: A Casebook from Shakespeare's Stratford.* Manchester: Manchester University Press, 2020.

Werrett, Simon. 'Wonders Never Cease: Descartes's *Météores* and the Rainbow Fountain'. *British Journal for the History of Science* 34(2) (2001), 129–147.

Williams, Owen. 'Exorcising Madness in Late Elizabethan England: *The Seduction of Arthington* and the Criminal Culpability of Demoniacs'. *Journal of British Studies* 47 (2008), 30–52.

Willis, Jonathan (ed.). *Sin and Salvation in Reformation England.* Farnham: Ashgate, 2015.

'"Strange Enthusiastical Exhortations": Distress, Religious Identity, and the English Reformation'. *Journal of Ecclesiastical History* 76(4) (2025), 760–789.

Wilson, Kenneth M. *Augustine's Conversion from Traditional Free Choice to 'Non-Free Free Will': A Comprehensive Methodology.* Tübingen: Mohr Siebeck, 2018.

Wilson, Philip K. 'Salmon, William (1644–1713), Medical Empiric and Author'. *ODNB*, 11 November 2021, https://doi.org/10.1093/ref:odnb/24559.
Wizeman, William. 'Somerville, John (1560–1583), Convicted Conspirator'. *ODNB*, 3 January 2008, https://doi.org/10.1093/ref:odnb/26022.
Wragge-Morley, Alexander. 'Imagining the Soul: Thomas Willis (1621–1675) on the Anatomy of the Brain and Nerves'. *Progress in Brain Research* 243 (2018), 55–56.
Wright, Edith A. 'Medieval Attitudes towards Mental Illness'. *Bulletin of the History of Medicine* 7 (1939), 352–356.
Wright, Jessica. 'Ventricular Localization in Late Antiquity: The Philosophical and Theological Roots of an Enduring Model of Brain Function'. *Progress in Brain Research* 243 (2018), 3–22.
The Care of the Brain in Early Christianity. Oakland: University of California Press, 2022.
Wright, John P., and Paul Potter (eds.). *Psyche and Soma: Physicians and Metaphysicians on the Mind-Body Problem from Antiquity to Enlightenment*. Oxford: Oxford University Press, 2000.
Yamamoto, Koji (ed.). *Stereotypes and Stereotyping in Early Modern England*. Manchester: Manchester University Press, 2022.
Yeoman, Louise. 'Archie's Invisible Worlds Discovered: Spirituality, Madness, and Johnston of Wariston's Family'. *Records of the Scottish Church History Society* 27 (1997), 156–186.
Yoshikawa, Naoë Kukita. 'Holy Medicine and Diseases of the Soul: Henry of Lancaster and *Le Livre de Seyntz Medicines*'. *Medical History* 53 (2009), 397–414.
Zalta, Edward N., and Uri Nodelman (eds.). *The Stanford Encyclopedia of Philosophy*. Stanford, CA: Stanford University Press, 2019.
Zimmer, Carl. *Soul Made Flesh: How the Secrets of the Brain Were Discovered in Seventeenth-Century England*. London: Penguin, 2005.

Index

For EU product safety concerns, contact us at Calle de José Abascal, 56–1°, 28003 Madrid, Spain or eugpsr@cambridge.org.

www.ingramcontent.com/pod-product-compliance
Ingram Content Group UK Ltd.
Pitfield, Milton Keynes, MK11 3LW, UK
UKHW020200290926
15471UKWH00005B/990
* 9 7 8 1 0 0 9 7 0 3 6 7 3 *